SMALL ANIMAL
WOUND MANAGEMENT

"For He wounds, but He also binds up,
He injures, but His hands also heal."
Job 5:18   NIV

SMALL ANIMAL WOUND MANAGEMENT

Steven F. Swaim, D.V.M., M.S.

Director of Scott-Ritchey Laboratories
Professor of Small Animal Surgery
Department of Small Animal Surgery and Medicine
College of Veterinary Medicine
Auburn University, Alabama

Ralph A. Henderson, Jr., D.V.M., M.S.

Chief of Small Animal Surgery
Professor of Small Animal Surgery
Department of Small Animal Surgery and Medicine
College of Veterinary Medicine
Auburn University, Alabama
Diplomate, American College of Veterinary Surgeons
    and American College of Veterinary Internal Medicine—
    Medical Oncology Specialty

Medical Illustrator:

Rhoda S. Pidgeon, B.F.A.

Medical Illustrator
1448 S.W. Oakley
Topeka, KS 66604

1990
LEA & FEBIGER
Philadelphia · London

Lea & Febiger
200 Chester Field Parkway
Malvern, PA 19355-9725
U.S.A.
(215) 251-2230

Lea & Febiger (UK) Ltd.
145a Croydon Road
Beckenham, Kent BR3 3RB
U.K.

Chapter and page reprints may be purchased from
Lea & Febiger in quantities of 100 or more.

Library of Congress Cataloging-in-Publication Data

Swaim, Steven F.
    Small animal wound management / Steven F. Swaim, Ralph A.
Henderson, Jr.; medical illustrator, Rhoda S. Pidgeon.
        p.   cm.
    Includes index.
    ISBN 0-8121-1239-3
    1. Dogs—Wounds and injuries—Treatment.   2. Cats—Wounds and
injuries—Treatment.   3. Veterinary traumatology.   4. Skin—Wounds
and injuries—Treatment.   I. Henderson, Ralph A.   II. Pidgeon,
Rhoda.   III. Title.
    [DNLM: 1. Veterinary Medicine.   2. Wounds and Injuries—therapy.
3. Wounds and Injuries—veterinary.   SF 914.3 S971s]
SF991.S92   1989
636.089'71—dc20
DNLM/DLC   89-12383
for Library of Congress   CIP

PRINTED IN THE UNITED STATES OF AMERICA

Print No.   3   2

Dedicated with love to our families:

Marj, Tom, and Matt

Diana, Sara, Amanda, and Lydia

Guy, David, and Elizabeth

PREFACE

Because the skin is a large and exposed organ of the body, it is susceptible to both major and minor trauma. Skin defects are caused not only by injury, but by surgical removal of pathologic growths involving this organ, such as tumors, cysts, and pyodermas. Regardless of the cause, the resulting skin defect requires open wound management and/or reconstruction. The purpose of this text is to provide veterinary practitioners, residents, interns, and students with information about the basic process of wound healing and several aspects of wound management and repair. Our intent is to present this information in a concise manner with the aid of photographs and clear, detailed, step-by-step drawings to assist in the performance of the various techniques. This book is not meant to provide an exhaustive coverage of pathophysiology, diagnostic alternatives, or perioperative care options. Rather, it gives the essentials of reasonable and necessary treatment and management.

Although other techniques and methods are available, those described in this text have been found practical and effective and, for the most part, are frequently used by the authors. The specifics of medication, bandages, sutures, and other supportive measures described are those we most commonly use, but these may vary according to individual patient needs. When the authors believed that suture size, pattern, or material was important to the procedure, this information was listed in the description.

When dealing with skin traumas and defects, the veterinary surgeon should consider the patient and its owner foremost and adhere to the philosophy that the simplest, least time-consuming, and most economical effective means of management and reconstruction should be considered first and more involved or complicated reconstructive procedures reserved for complicated lesions.

Surgery, like music, is learned initially by mimicking a teacher. The basic elements are mastered slowly, and repetitive tasks create patterns that are refined to become skills. Ultimately, the student uses these skills, combined with a thorough understanding of basic principles. When they are used against new obstacles, the student is often challenged to new composition, and a new operation is born. The authors, students themselves, offer these descriptions and drawings to be mimicked until they are no longer needed or are replaced by new procedures.

Auburn University
Alabama

Steven F. Swaim
Ralph A. Henderson
Rhoda S. Pidgeon

ACKNOWLEDGEMENTS

We are grateful to all who have assisted in making this book a reality. The technical advice and editorial assistance of Drs. Donna Angarano, James Milton, Paul Rumph, and Michael Peterson are most appreciated, as are the efforts and fine work of Gregg Greanoff and Brenda Kesler in their photographic support. The cooperation and help of Penny Pace in providing word processing support for this book are also appreciated. We thank Raymond Kersey and the staff of Lea & Febiger for their help in preparation of this book.

We are especially grateful for the loving encouragement and understanding of our families.

CONTENTS

WOUND HEALING

"I dressed the wound, and God healed it."—Ambroise Paré

The process of wound healing can be divided into four stages: (1) inflammatory, (2) debridement, (3) repair, and (4) maturation. The wound healing process is continuous, with overlapping of the various stages.

INFLAMMATORY STAGE

IMMEDIATE REACTIONS

After a full-thickness skin loss, the normal skin elasticity and the external tension produced by muscle pull in some areas enlarge the defect according to the amount and direction of force exerted on the skin. Immediately after injury, hemorrhage occurs, helping to cleanse the wound surface and provide it with cells that aid in the debridement process that follows. Small vessels constrict immediately after injury, helping to limit hemorrhage from the wound. Platelet aggregation and subsequent thrombus formation further attenuate hemorrhage. After 5 to 10 minutes vasodilation occurs, with leakage of fluid from venules, which provides fibrinogen and other clotting elements. Fibrin plugs form and occlude damaged lymphatics to stop lymphatic drainage from the area, localizing the inflammatory reaction to the immediate area of the wound.

If adequate coagulation factors are present, blood that has filled a wound forms a clot in which fibrinogen molecules crosslink to form fibrin. The undisturbed fibrin clot is hemostatic and provides a framework for the elements of repair. The clot dehydrates and contracts. As the clot's surface dehydrates, it forms a scab, which gives limited protection from external contamination, maintains internal homeostasis, and provides a surface beneath which epithelial cell migration and movement of the wound edges can occur (Figs. 1-1 and 1-2).

LATER REACTIONS

Capillary and venule permeability increases as gaps develop between endothelial cells. Plasma-like fluid containing enzymes, proteins, antibodies, and complement escapes from the vessels. In the tissues, these fluids dilute toxic substances and aid in the movement of cells into the injured area. Leukocytes, erythrocytes, and platelets become "sticky" within the vessels, and leukocytes escape into the tissues through endothelial gaps and concentrate at the injury site (Fig. 1-1).

DEBRIDEMENT STAGE

Several types of cells enter the wound during the inflammatory and debridement stages of healing (Fig. 1-1), and perform various functions. Neutrophils release various enzymes and prostaglandins of the E_2 series. The enzymes attack extracellular debris and facilitate the breakdown of necrotic material. Platelets that enter the wound in the early stages release potent locally acting growth factors for a short time. As monocytes enter the wound, they become macrophages, which play several

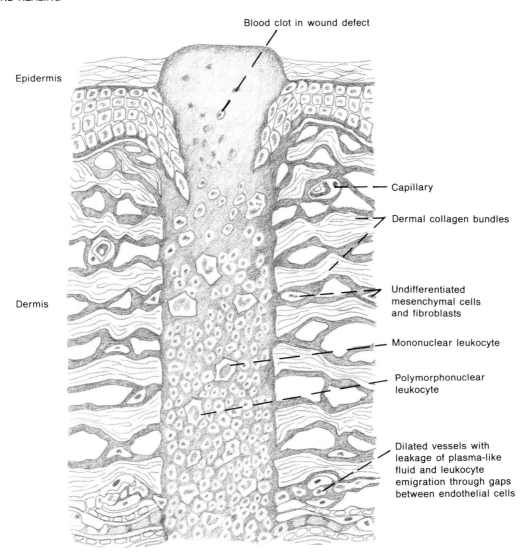

Blood clot in wound defect

Epidermis

Capillary

Dermal collagen bundles

Undifferentiated
mesenchymal cells
and fibroblasts

Mononuclear leukocyte

Polymorphonuclear
leukocyte

Dermis

Dilated vessels with
leakage of plasma-like
fluid and leukocyte
emigration through gaps
between endothelial cells

FIG. 1-1. Debridement stage of wound healing. Blood fills the wound gap, a clot unites wound edges, epithelial cells begin migrating across the defect, and polymorphonuclear cells and monocytes (macrophages) perform a debridement function.

roles. These cells take over the regulatory role of the platelets after 24 hours and continue to produce similar locally active growth factors until healing is complete. Macrophages release substances that stimulate fibroplasia, collagen synthesis, and angiogenesis. These cells also phagocytize necrotic tissue and debris; they attract fibroblasts into the wound and influence their maturation. Some monocytes coalesce into multinucleate giant cells.

The fluid that has escaped into the tissues, the migrating leukocytes, and dead tissue make up the inflammatory exudate, which becomes pus as the polymorphonuclear cells die and lyse. Open wounds appear septic, and their appearance worsens until the height of the debridement stage, when it begins to improve.

REPAIR STAGE

The repair stage of healing is composed of three processes: (1) fibroblast proliferation, (2) capillary infiltration, and (3) epithelial proliferation and migration. The first two processes manifest themselves in the form of granulation tissue in the wound. A major function of this tissue is wound contraction. Epithelial proliferation and migration provide the thin, hairless covering over the granulation tissue.

FIBROBLASTS AND CAPILLARY INGROWTH AND ORIENTATION

Fibroblasts originate from undifferentiated mesenchymal cells in nearby connective tissue (subcutaneous

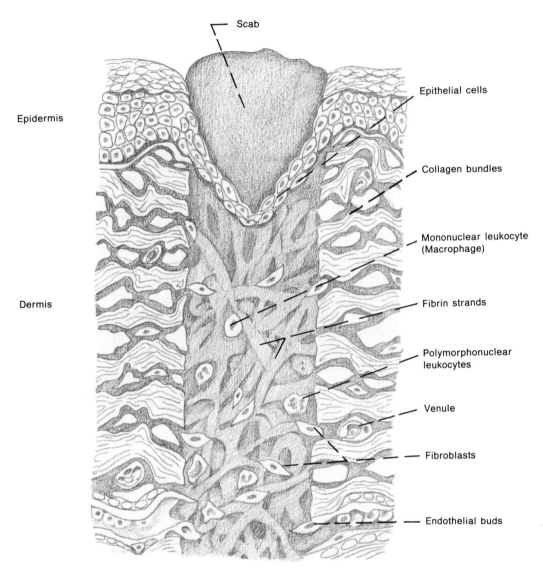

Scab

Epithelial cells

Collagen bundles

Mononuclear leukocyte
(Macrophage)

Fibrin strands

Polymorphonuclear
leukocytes

Venule

Fibroblasts

Endothelial buds

Epidermis

Dermis

FIG. 1-2. Early repair stage of wound healing. Epithelial migration and proliferation continue, macrophages function in stimulating the repair process, fibroblasts migrate into the wound along fibrin strands, and capillaries invade wound by budding.

tissue and fat). These resting cells and fibrocytes are primarily associated with adventitia of small blood vessels (Fig. 1-1). Fibroblasts advance along fibers within the fibrin clot that formed earlier and also move along capillaries growing into the wound (Fig. 1-2).

After wounding, a marked gradient of oxygen exists within the wound, with the center of the wound most deficient in oxygen. This gradient may be partially responsible for the branching and ingrowth of new blood vessels, in the form of capillaries, from the wound periphery into the wound (Fig. 1-2). The endothelial cells of the new capillaries growing into the wound contain a plasminogen activator that causes conversion of plasminogen to plasmin, the substance responsible for fibrinolysis and breakdown of the original fibrin network that was in the clot. The fibrin is replaced by collagen produced by the fibroblasts. Once the continuity of the connective tissue has been re-established, many of these new capillaries regress.

During the first 3 to 4 days after an incision-type wound, the fibrin strands of the clot in the wound are oriented vertically. Thus, ingrowing fibroblasts and the interweaving new collagen they produce have the same arrangement. The ingrowing new capillaries also have a vertical arrangement as a result of these structures being confined between the apposed edges of the wound. In

After 6 days

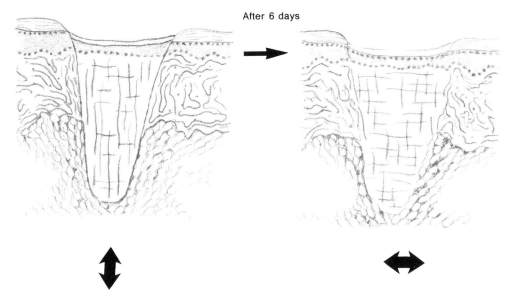

FIG. 1-3. Orientation of wound fibers. In early stages of wound repair, fibrin strands, fibroblasts, new collagen fibers, and new capillaries have a vertical orientation. As healing progresses, these structures become horizontally arranged.

addition, the upward and downward growth of the new fibroblasts entering the wound contribute to their vertical orientation. After about 6 days, the intraincisional fibroblasts, fibrils, and capillaries gradually change orientation until they lie parallel to the surface across the incision. Tension on the wound fibers seems to be the governing factor in reorientation of the fibers (Fig. 1-3).

When loss of tissue has occurred in a skin defect, the natural elasticity of the skin places tension on the fibrin clot adherent to the wound margins, thus orienting the fibrous components toward the wound margins. As ingrowing fibroblasts enter the wound, they are guided by these fibrous elements, the position and orientation of which bring cells toward the center of the defect.

PRODUCTS OF FIBROBLASTS AND WOUND STRENGTH

After fibroblasts have entered a wound, they begin to secrete the protein polysaccharides and various glycoproteins that constitute the wound's amorphous milieu of ground substance, which reaches its greatest point of development in about 3 to 5 days and is effective for collagen deposition. The mucopolysaccharides of this substance surround the fibroblasts and influence the aggregation and orientation of collagen.

The fibroblasts begin to synthesize collagen on the fourth or fifth day. In the early stages, tropocollagen molecules are extruded into the extracellular space and aggregate to form young collagen fibrils near the fibroblast. Continued bonding results in collagen fibers that become increasingly less soluble. Collagen bundles are small at first, but enlarge to gradually produce a dense collagenous scar that binds the edges of severed tissues together (Fig. 1-4).

As the collagen content of a wound increases, the wound glycoprotein and mucopolysaccharide contents decrease, as does the number of fibroblasts in the wound. The decrease in fibroblasts in the wound marks the end of the repair stage of healing and the beginning of the maturation stage. With the diminished number of synthesizing fibroblasts, the total collagen synthesis decreases and eventually balances the rate of collagen destruction. Collagen destruction may result from collagenase liberated by proliferating epithelial cells and fibroblasts that come into contact with new epithelium.

The early rise in wound tensile strength is caused by fibroblast production of collagen. The later slow gain in wound strength takes place over a long period and is caused by maturation and remodeling of the collagen present in the wound.

GRANULATION TISSUE

Bright red granular tissue begins to appear in a wound from 3 to 6 days after injury. This results from proliferation of capillary loops, which originate from cut capillaries in the wound. These loops grow into the wound immediately behind the fibroblasts, and each loop is capped by fibroblasts, macrophages, and other wandering cells, with fibroblasts predominating. These simple blood channels of the granulation tissue differentiate

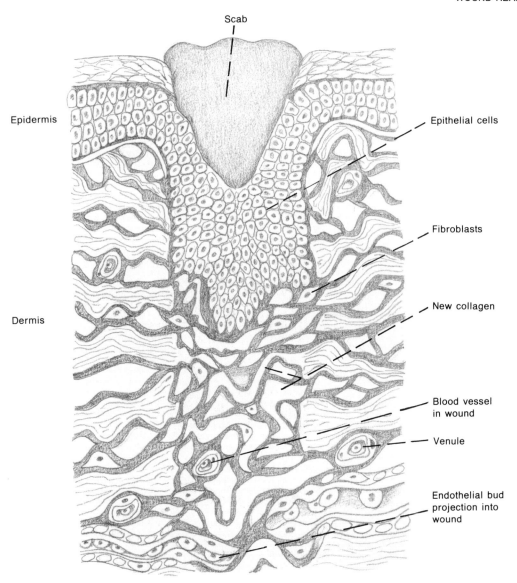

FIG. 1-4. Late repair stage of wound healing. Epithelium becomes thicker and develops irregular projections into dermis. New collagen formed by fibroblasts is randomly oriented.

progressively into arterioles, capillaries, and venules. In the same manner, although lagging behind blood vessel development, a system of lymphatic vessels is produced in the wound. The capillary loops, or "knuckles," cause a granular appearance in large open wounds. In small wounds, this tissue is beneath the scab (Fig. 1-2).

Granulation tissue is important in the healing of open wounds because it is extremely resistant to infection an serves as a barrier against systemic infection, provides a surface over which epithelium is able to migrate, plays a role in wound contraction, and contains the fibroblasts that produce the collagen for wound healing.

Wound Contraction

Wound contraction is the reduction in size of an open wound as the result of centripetal movement of the whole-thickness skin that surrounds the wound. Granulation tissue pulls the skin margins inward so that the area to be covered by epithelium is reduced. No new skin is formed in the process, but the surrounding skin is pulled toward the wound's center. In dogs, visible contraction of wounds usually begins about 5 to 9 days after wounding. In areas on animals where the skin is loosely attached to underlying structures, wound contraction can result in complete wound closure.

Within granulation tissue are fibroblasts that take on the characteristics of smooth muscle, including con-

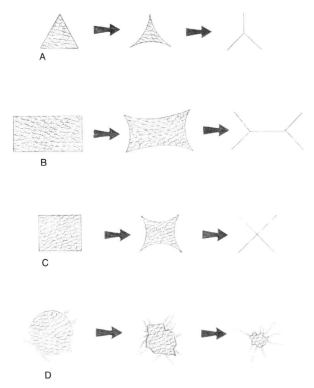

FIG. 1-5. Healing of various shaped wounds. A, Triangular wound. B, Rectangular wound. C, Square wound. D, Circular wound.

tractile ability. These cells attach to each other, the wound bed, the panniculus muscle, and the dermis at the wound edge. Contraction of these cells is responsible for wound contraction and stops when one side of a wound contacts the opposite side, myofibroblast tension equals tension of the surrounding skin, or the granulation tissue has a lack of healthy myofibroblasts.

Various-shaped wounds that heal by contraction result in various-shaped scars. Triangular, rectangular, and square wounds heal centripetally, with the corners remaining stationary and the sides moving centrally. The respective results are a three-pointed stellate scar, a double V-shaped scar with the points of the Vs pointing toward each other and connected by a thin line, and a four-pointed stellate scar. Circular wounds heal in a crumpled, unpredictable pattern, about 30% more slowly than rectangular, square, or triangular wounds (Fig. 1-5).

Complete healing of large wounds in loose skin is the primary advantage of contraction. The disadvantages of wound contraction are (1) formation of a web of tight skin over a flexor surface, limiting its movement; (2) stenosis of a body opening; (3) insufficient contraction resulting in epithelialization of the remaining wound; and (4) tightness of the skin after the wound has contracted closed, which limits body movement.

EPITHELIALIZATION

Epithelialization occurs independently of wound contraction and generally supplies a temporary covering while the wound contracts. Epithelialization begins with mobilization of the basal cells of the epidermis at the wound edge. These wound margin epithelial cells lose their firm attachment to the underlying dermis, enlarge, flatten, and extend downward and outward over the edge of the dermis. The activated cells then migrate out over the defect to replace the epithelial cell deficit (Fig. 1-6).

An incised wound can be covered by epithelial proliferation and migration at 48 hours. In open wounds, a

FIG. 1-6. Epithelialization of an open wound. A, Basal epidermal cells at wound edges lose their attachment to dermis. B, Epidermal cells at wound edges extend downward and outward over edge of dermis. C, Epithelial cell migration stops with contact inhibition. D, Epithelial cells proliferate and differentiate. (After Bryant, W.M.: Wound healing. Clin. Symposia *29*:2, 1977.)

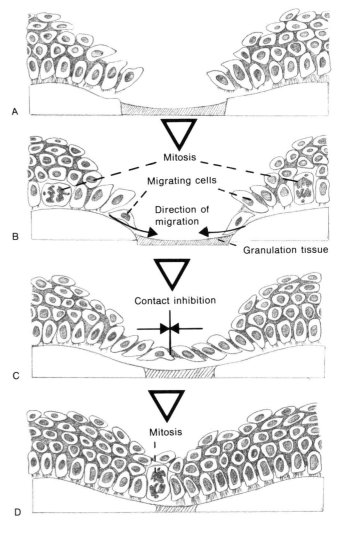

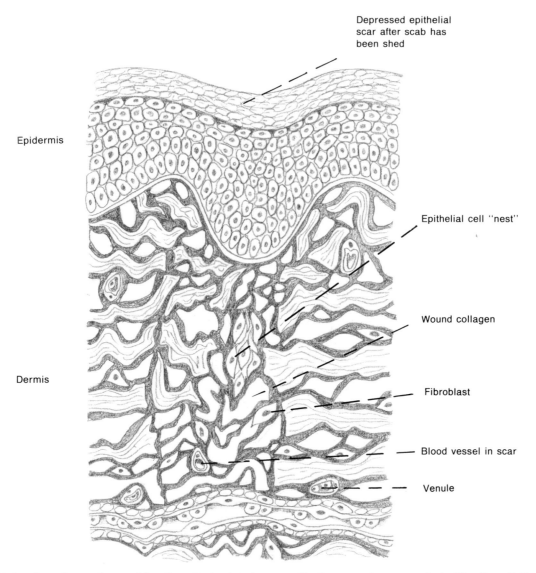

Depressed epithelial
scar after scab has
been shed

Epidermis

Epithelial cell "nest"

Wound collagen

Dermis

Fibroblast

Blood vessel in scar

Venule

FIG. 1-7. Maturation stage of wound healing. Scab sloughs as epithelium acquires normal stratification. Collagen fibers have increased bonding with purposefully oriented fibrils becoming thicker and more compact and forming bundles. Junction between wound and dermal collagen becomes more difficult to identify.

latent period of 4 to 5 days usually passes before epithelium starts to migrate from the wound margins across the developing granulation tissue bed. Adjacent to the wound edge, the epithelium is several cell layers thick, with cell differentiation, keratinization, and mitosis in the deep layers. Closer to the wound center, the epithelium is reduced to a single layer of flattened cells. Epithelialization is rapid at first, but as the line of cells from the wound margin extends, the epithelium dwindles to a monolayer as progress becomes slower. Days to weeks may pass before epithelialization becomes complete. In some large wounds, epithelialization may not give sufficient coverage, or the central epithelium may be so delicate that it is continually knocked off.

If a scab is present, the migrating epithelium moves under the scab until it contacts the underlying granulation tissue bed. The migrating epithelial cells produce collagenase, which dissolves the base of the scab so that it can be shed (Fig. 1-2).

Prominent downgrowths develop on the lower surface of the newly formed epithelium and invade the underlying connective tissue, giving rise to "pseudorete pegs" or epithelial spurs. These spurs may regress, leaving a relatively smooth undersurface on the epithelium, or separate from the epithelium, forming internally keratinizing epithelial "pearls," "nests," or "islands" that usually degenerate and disappear (Fig. 1-7). The smooth undersurface of the epithelium is responsible for its being easily knocked off the wound.

MATURATION STAGE

EARLY WOUND STRENGTH

A wound does not gain appreciably in strength during the first 4 to 6 days after it has been inflicted. Even within the first 24 hours, however, a properly coapted wound has some strength contributed by the fibrin of the clot. Within the first 5 days, epithelialization has occurred, and the adhesive forces of the epithelial cells add to wound strength, as does the ingrowth of capillaries into the ground substance (Fig. 1-2).

LATE WOUND STRENGTH

After the first 3 weeks of rapid collagen accumulation in a wound, its content stabilizes (Fig. 1-4). At this point, there seems to be a balance between deposition and dissolution of collagen. Various tissue collagenases participate in the dissolution of collagen by removing nonfunctional collagen fibers as functionally oriented fibers are preserved. Wound strength increases over time; however, its gain gradually decreases as time advances. The gain in strength is due to increased intermolecular and intramolecular cross-linkage of collagen fibers and the change in the physical weave of the fibers. The purposefully oriented collagen fibrils increase in thickness and compactness and tend to become grouped into bundles. The junction between collagen bundles of the dermis at the wound edge and newly formed collagen in the wound become progressively more difficult to define as fibers of the two intermingle (Fig. 1-7). Although its strength increases with time, a scar still remains 15 to 20% weaker than surrounding normal tissue.

REFERENCES AND SUGGESTED READING

1. Bryant, W.M.: Wound healing. Clin. Symp. 29:2, 1977.
2. Gabbiani, G, Hirschel, B.J., Ryan, G.B., Statkov, P.R., and Majno, G.: Granulation tissue as a contractile organ: A study of structures and function. J. Exp. Med. 135:719, 1972.
3. Johnston, D.E.: Wound healing and reconstructive surgery. Am. Anim. Hosp. Assoc. Sci. Proc. 2:383, 1975.
4. Johnston, D.E.: The process of wound healing. J. Am. Anim. Hosp. Assoc. 13:186, 1977.
5. Johnston, D.E.: Skin and subcutaneous tissue. In Pathophysiology in Small Animal Surgery. Edited by M.J. Bojrab. Philadelphia, W.B. Saunders, 1981.
6. Johnston D.E.: Wound healing. Arch. Am. Coll. Vet. Surg. 3:30, 1974.
7. Hunt, T.K., Knighton, D.R., Thakral, K.K., Goodson, W.H., and Andrews, W.S.: Studies on inflammation and wound healing: Angiogenesis and collagen synthesis stimulated in vivo by resident and activated wound macrophages. Surgery 96:48, 1984.
8. Lee, A.H., and Swaim, S.F.: Granulation tissue: How to take advantage of it in managment of open wounds. Compend. Contin. Educ. 10:163, 1988.
9. Madden, J.W.: Wound healing: Biologic and clinical features. In Davis-Christopher: Textbook of Surgery. 11th ed. Edited by D.C. Sabiston. Philadelphia, W.B. Saunders, 1977.
10. Ordman, L.J., and Gillman, T.: Studies in the healing of cutaneous wounds. Arch. Surg. 93:911, 1966.
11. Peacock, E.E.: Repair and regeneration. In Reconstructive Plastic Surgery: Principles and Procedures in Correction, Reconstruction, and Transplantation, 2nd ed., Vol I. Edited by J.M. Converse. Philadelphia, W.B. Saunders, 1977.
12. Peacock, E.E., Jr.: Wound Repair. 3rd ed. Philadelphia, W.B. Saunders, 1984.
13. Peyton, L.C.: Wound healing: The management of wounds and blemishes in the horse—Part I. Compend. Contin. Educ. 6:111, 1984.
14. Russell, P.S., and Billingham, R.E.: Some aspects of the repair process in mammals. Prog. Surg. 2:1, 1962.

WOUND MANAGEMENT

INITIAL MANAGEMENT

Initial management includes the preliminary procedures undertaken to prepare a wound and surrounding area for analgesia and debridement.

WOUND CLASSIFICATION

Wounds are classified according to contamination and increasing risk of infection, for example, clean, clean contaminated, contaminated, and dirty/infected. A clean wound is one created surgically under aseptic conditions when tissue trauma is minimal and exposure to microorganisms is strictly controlled. Considering the material covered in this book, an example of this type of wound is one created in removing skin neoplasms. Most of the wounds dealt with in this book, however, are associated with some form of trauma to the skin, and are therefore considered contaminated or infected wounds.

REFERENCE AND SUGGESTED READING

1. Committee on Control of Surgical Infections: Manual on Control of Infection in Surgical Patients. Edited by W.A. Altmeier, J.F. Burke, B.A. Pruitt, and W.R. Sandusky, Philadelphia, J.B. Lippincott Co., 1976.

CONTAMINATED/INFECTED WOUNDS

Preliminary Procedures

Definition and Indications. Contaminated and infected wounds are caused by various types of trauma.

Wounds are generally considered contaminated when the time lapse since infliction has been short. The tissues have been damaged and innoculated with microorganisms, but the microorganisms have not begun to grow in the devitalized tissue. An infected wound is one that has been present long enough for the microorganisms to begin growth in the devitalized tissues. Infected wounds are usually characterized by inflammation, pain, purulent exudate, and possibly fever, along with neutrophilia in late stages of infection.

The time at which a wound goes from contaminated to infected varies according to the blood supply remaining in the tissue, the amount and type of traumatized tissue, the number and pathogenicity of bacteria innoculated into the wound, the amount and type of foreign debris in the wound, and the patient's age and immunocompetence. For instance, a contaminated crushing-degloving injury to the limb of a dog in a barnyard becomes infected sooner than a clean laceration inflicted by a piece of glass on a paved street.

Technique. Preliminary procedures are those undertaken to (1) protect the wound during transport to veterinary facilities, (2) evaluate it for antimicrobial therapy, and (3) protect it during preparation of the surrounding area.

Wound management for transport. An occlusive dressing of dry gauze or an improvised bandage of clean linen held *firmly* in place will help to protect the wound, prevent further contamination, and stop all but the most severe hemorrhage. Care should be taken to ensure that all wound cavities are firmly packed to aid in hemostasis (Fig. 2-1A).

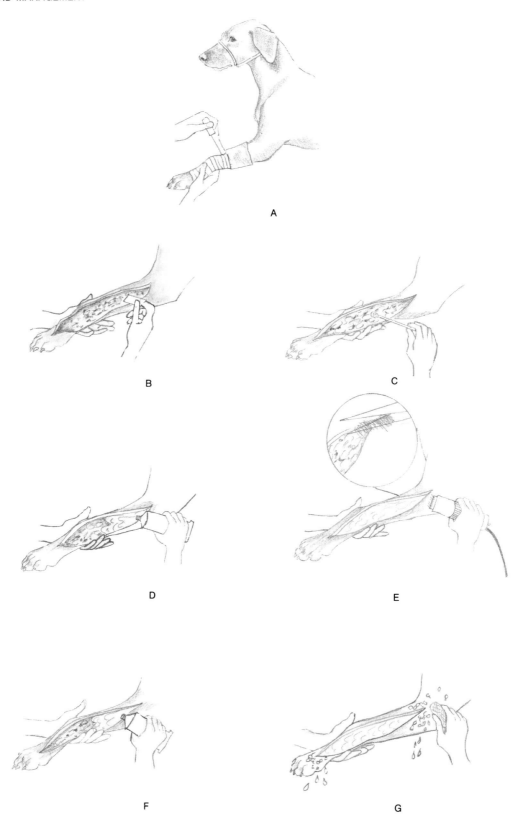

FIG. 2-1. Preliminary procedures for managing a contaminated/infected wound. A, Packing and wrapping a wound for transport. B, Direct smear of a severely infected wound for gram stain. C, Swabbing wound for culture and sensitivity. D, Water soluble lubricating gel placed in wound. E, Clipping hair around wound. Inset: Scissors dipped in mineral oil or water and clipping hair at wound edge. F, Replacing water-soluble lubricating gel. G, Scrubbing *around* the wound.

In the presence of an open fracture, the limb should be splinted without pulling exposed bone back into the wound. This is especially important in long bone fractures below the elbow and stifle joints to prevent additional soft tissue injury from movement of the bone fragments. In addition, exteriorized bone is contaminated and will contaminate deeper wound recesses if replacement into the wound is attempted.

Microbial Evaluation and Therapy. The systemic antibiotic selected for use should be effective against the bacteria that are expected in superficial wounds, namely staphylococci, streptococci, and *Escherichia coli.* The cephalosporins (for example, cephalothin* or cefazolin†) can be used for prophylaxis because of their good tissue penetration. In bite wounds, Pasteurella is a likely organism, and amoxicillin‡ or ampicillin can be considered for treatment. A gram-stained wound impression is helpful in evaluating the predominant bacterial population of infected wounds, and may be helpful in deciding on the initial systemic antibiotic therapy to be used (Fig. 2-1B). The authors use this technique on deep and potentially serious wounds. A swab of the wound is taken for bacterial culture and sensitivity (Fig. 2-1C). The culture and sensitivity results may later alter the treatment regimen. In many cases, culture and sensitivity tests support the initial antibiotic selection based on a gram-stained impression. The effectiveness of antibiotic therapy may be monitored by repeat cultures and sensitivity tests 3 to 4 days after the initial test. If these tests yield no growth, the initial therapy may be continued. A change in antibiotics should be considered, however, when (1) culture and sensitivity test results dictate another antibiotic, (2) little change occurs in the appearance of the wound after 2 to 3 days of initial therapy, or (3) the animal's general condition worsens and septicemia is possible.

Systemic antibiotics, when used, should be administered as soon as possible after wound infliction, preferably during the first 3 hours, to help ensure adequate levels within the wound fluids to contact bacteria before they become surrounded by coagulum. In heavily contaminated wounds, a combination of systemic and topical antibiotics is best.

Wound protection and preparation of the surrounding area. Protection of the wound is essential while preparing the surrounding area. Two commonly used protection techniques are packing the wound with moistened

sterile gauze sponges and filling the wound cavity with a water-soluble lubricating gel§ (Fig. 2-1D). Another technique is temporary closure with towel forceps or a continuous suture. Before preparing the area around head wounds, an eye ointment should be instilled to protect the cornea and conjunctiva.

If the animal is covered with dirt and debris, it should be bathed. A commercially available or improvised grill/tub arrangement may be used.

An ample area around the wound should be clipped with electric clippers and a No. 40 clipper blade, preferably in the presence of a vacuum suction system (Fig. 2-1E). Hair at the wound edges may be trimmed with scissors that have been dipped in mineral oil or water (Fig. 2-1E inset) so that the hair sticks to the blades instead of dropping into the wound. The ideal situation is to have a separate pair of clipper blades that have been disinfected for preparing the area around infected wounds to help prevent possible contamination of elective surgical sites.

After the area around the wound has been clipped, the original gauze sponges or gel should be replaced (Fig. 2-1F). Surgical scrub solution should be used to scrub the surrounding skin in the manner used for preparing the skin for aseptic surgery (Fig. 2-1G). Care must be taken to keep scrub solution out of the wound even though it is covered with a sponge or gel. The sponge or gel is removed just before wound debridement.

Skin antiseptics, when used, should be carefully applied so that they do not enter the wound. The area is draped, leaving adequate room to extend the incision as necessary.

Aftercare. After preparation of the surrounding area, the wound itself is prepared for analgesia and debridement.

Advantages and Disadvantages. Packing a wound with gauze or clean linen under pressure for transport of the animal may be safer than applying a tourniquet. If a tourniquet is not applied tightly enough, it may cause inadequate hemostasis; if it is applied too tightly, it may damage underlying neurovascular tissue. The application of towel forceps or a temporary continuous suture to close a wound while preparing the area around it may be painful if the tissues have not been rendered analgesic. Such closures also interfere with clipping the hair at the wound edge. Bathing an animal that is covered with dirt and debris helps protect the wound from secondary contamination from this source.

---

*Keflin, Eli Lilly and Co., Indianapolis, IN.

†Kefzol, Eli Lilly and Co., Indianapolis, IN.

‡Amoxicillin film-coated tablets or Amoxi-Drop suspension, Beecham Labs, Bristol, TN.

§K-Y Jelly, Johnson and Johnson, New Brunswick, NJ.

REFERENCES AND SUGGESTED READING

1. Aron, D.N.: Management of open musculoskeletal injuries. Semin. Vet. Med. Surg. *3*:290, 1988.

2. Bergamini, T.M., Lamont, P.M., Cheadle, W.G., and Polk, H.C.: Combined topical and systemic antibiotic prophylaxis in experimental wound infection. Am. J. Surg. *147*:753, 1984.
3. Bright R.M., and Probst, C.W.: Management of superficial skin wounds. *In* Textbook of Small Animal Surgery. Edited by D.H. Slatter. Philadelphia, W.B. Saunders, 1985.
4. Brown, T.R., Ehrlich, C.E., Stehman, F.B., Golichowski, A.M., and Madura, J.A.: A clinical evaluation of chlorhexidine gluconate spray as compared with iodophor scrub for preoperative skin preparation. Surg. Gynecol. Obstet. *158*:363, 1984.
5. Heath, M.M.: Surgical preparation: Part I. Preoperative preparation of the patient. Vet. Tech. *7*:253, 1985.
6. Hoover, N.W., and Ivins, J.C.: Wound debridement. Arch. Surg. *79*:701, 1959.
7. Jennings, P.B., and Heggers, J.P.: General principles in the care of open wounds. *In* Veterinary Trauma and Critical Care. Edited by I.M. Zaslow. Philadelphia, Lea & Febiger, 1984.
8. Kirk, R.W., and Bistner, S.I.: Handbook of Veterinary Procedures and Emergency Treatment. 4th ed. Philadelphia, W.B. Saunders, 1985.
9. Knowles, R.P.: Injuries to skin, muscles and tendon. *In* Some Techniques and Procedures in Small Animal Surgery. Bonner Springs, KS, Veterinary Medical Publishing Co., 1963.
10. Peacock, E.E., Jr: Wound Repair. 3rd ed. Philadelphia, W.B. Saunders, 1984.
11. Pope, E.R.: The important first steps: Initial management of feline wounds. Vet. Med. *81*:504, 1986.
12. Swaim, S.F., and Pope, E.R.: Limb degloving injuries: Pathophysiology and early management. Semin. Vet. Med. Surg. *3*:274, 1988.
13. Tobin, G.R.: Closure of contaminated wounds: Biological and technical considerations. Surg. Clin. North Am. *64*:639, 1984.

Anesthesia and Analgesia

Definition and Indications. General anesthesia or local or regional analgesia may be used for wound management. If the animal is in good physical condition and a good candidate for general anesthesia, this should be chosen; otherwise, local or regional analgesia should be used. The latter is generally used when the animal is a poor anesthetic candidate as a result of abnormalities induced by the trauma that caused the wound.

Techniques. It may be beneficial to lavage a wound initially with a 2% lidocaine solution, or to lay a surgical sponge soaked with 2% lidocaine on the wound for 1 to 2 minutes before irrigating and manipulating to remove foreign bodies (Fig. 2-2A). This appears to make these procedures more comfortable for the animal.

Local and regional analgesia are commonly used in combination with neuroleptanalgesia; in this case the tranquilizer calms the animal and the analgesic helps control the pain. Lidocaine, 1 or 2%, is injected through the intact skin at the wound periphery parallel to its edge with a 23 to 25 gauge needle. It should not be injected through wound tissues (Fig. 2-2B). Lidocaine without vasoconstrictors such as epinephrine is preferred for analgesia.

Ring block of a limb proximal to the area of injury is an effective and simple technique to induce analgesia in a limb for thorough debridement. With a 23 to 25 gauge needle, tissues proximal to the wound are infiltrated with the analgesic agent from the skin to the bone by encircling the limb (Fig. 2-2C).

Aftercare. After analgesia has been attained, debridement and lavage are undertaken.

Advantages and Disadvantages. Initial wound lavage with 2% lidocaine makes wound cleansing more comfortable for the animal; however, no surgical debridement can be performed. Although vasoconstrictors, such as epinephrine, may be added to help reduce hemorrhage and prolong the effect of the analgesic agent, they may also cause tissue necrosis along the wound edge, adversely affect tissue defenses, and potentiate infection. Therefore, lidocaine without epinephrine is preferred. With ring blocks, adequate analgesia distal to the injection site is common, but multiple injection sites are required to accomplish the procedure.

REFERENCES AND SUGGESTED READING

1. Edlich, R.F., Rodeheaver, G.T., Thacker, J.G. et al.: Management of soft tissue injury. Clin Plast Surg *4*:191, 1977.
2. Hoover, N.W., Ivins, J.C.: Wound debridement. Arch. Surg. *79*:701, 1959.
3. Skarda, R.T.: Local and regional analgesia. *In* Principles and Practice of Veterinary Anesthesia. Edited by C.E. Short. Baltimore, Williams and Wilkins, 1987.
4. Swaim, S.F., and Pope E.R.: Early management of limb degloving injuries. Semin. Vet. Med. Surg. *3*:274, 1988.
5. Tobin, G.R.: Closure of contaminated wounds: Biologic and technical considerations. Surg Clin North Am. *64*:639, 1984.
6. Zederfeldt, B., Jacobsson, S., and Ahonen, J.: Wounds and Wound Healing. London, Wolfe Medical Publishers, 1980.

Layer Debridement

Definition and Indications. Layer debridement involves removing devitalized tissues, beginning at the surface of the wound and progressing to the wound depths (Fig. 2-3). This technique should be used for lesions on the limbs and paws and other areas where tissue conservation for reconstruction is important.

Technique. Factors requiring attention during debridement are: (1) removal of devitalized, contaminated, and infected tissue, (2) removal of foreign debris, (3) obtaining adequate hemostasis, (4) delivering copious lavage solution to the wound, and (5) drainage of dead space. During debridement, the following should be avoided: (1) prolonged pressure and tearing by retractors, (2) massive ligatures with large necrotic portions of tissue distal to the ligature, (3) electrocoagulation causing plugs of necrotic tissue, and (4) extensive exploration that separates tissue planes and breaks down natural barriers to the spread of infection.

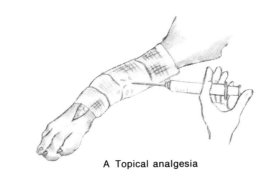

A Topical analgesia

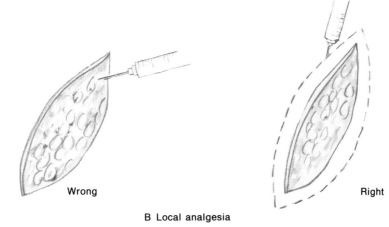

Wrong

Right

B Local analgesia

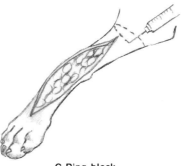

C Ring block

FIG. 2-2. Analgesia. A, Topical analgesia: Lidocaine applied to surgical sponges. B, Wrong: Analgesic injected through wound tissues. Right: Analgesic injected through intact skin. C, Ring block from skin to bone proximal to wound.

To help protect the wound from iatrogenic contamination, surgical gloves and a mask should be worn during debridement. Ideally, more than one set of instruments should be used to avoid reintroducing contaminated instruments back into the wound as it becomes progressively cleaner with debridement. In lieu of this, cold sterilization of instruments can be considered. The instruments are placed in antiseptic solution between uses and rinsed with saline to remove the germicide before each use.

Debridement should begin at the wound surface and progress to the depths, using toothed forceps and a sharp scissors or scalpel. Causing the tissue to bleed is not essential for adequate wound debridement. Capillary hemorrhage can be controlled with surface pressure and topical thombin. Fine-point electrocautery may be

Debridement of specific tissues is summarized in Table 2-1.

Table 2-1. Specific Tissue Debridement

Tissue	Appearance	Techniques and Comments

Skin	1. Turgid and dark flap
	  A. Sharp line of demarcation between normal and darker tissue (poor prognosis for darker tissue)
	  B. No sharp line of demarcation between normal and darker tissue (better prognosis for darker tissue)
	  C. Definite dark or pale flap
	2. Large, thick, flaps that are not contused and have a very tenuous pedicle of attachment
	3. Contused skin edges
		1. A. Observe for 24 to 48 hours. Trim definitely devitalized tissue.
		
		  B. Same as A.
		
		  C. Excise flap.
		2. Excise flap, remove all subcutaneous tissue, mesh it and place as a graft.
		3. Trim back until capillary oozing is seen (caution: reserve this technique for 12 to 24 hours after trauma to allow vessels to lose spasms of early trauma).

Fat	1. Contaminated with debris and blood stain	1. Excise to a healthy plane free of blood stains.
Fascia	1. Loose, ragged fragments	1. Excise with a thin border of normal fascia.
Blood vessels	1. Severed	1. Ligate if collateral circulation is intact.
Nerves	1. Exposed intact 2. Cleanly severed without trauma, identifiable ends 3. Severed with trauma and contamination, identifiable ends	1. Cleanse gently and cover. 2. Anastomose. 3. Defer definitive anastomosis until healthy wound tissue is present (21 days). Temporary anastomosis to prevent retraction.
Muscle	1. Friable, no bleeding, no contraction with stimulation, ground-in dirt, darker or paler than normal 2. Cat muscle normally appears pale	1. Excise muscle until remaining muscle bleeds and contracts normally (color may be deceptive unless obviously darker or lighter). 2. A. Debride cautiously. B. Use staged debridement, removing nonvital tissue as it becomes evident.
Tendons	1. Contaminated and denuded paratenon 2. Cleanly severed without trauma, identifiable ends 3. Severed with trauma and contamination, identifiable ends 4. Severed and frayed ends not identifiable with large gaps in tendon	1. Provide coverage. 2. Anastomose. 3. Defer anastomosis until healthy wound tissue is present (21 days). Temporary anastomosis to prevent retraction. 4. Trim frayed ends, no anastomosis.

Joints	1. Debris, clots, and cartilage fragments	1. A. Thorough lavage
		  B. Discard small pieces of bone and cartilage, replace large pieces and smooth sharp bone edges.
		  C. Suture joint capsule and ligaments partially or totally when possible.
		  D. Remove bullets or fragments from gunshot wounds.
		  E. Subcutaneous tissue and skin over joint are usually left open for delayed primary closure.
		  F. Immobilize joint.

Bone	1. Periosteal covering
	2. Dirt ground in
	3. Dirt in broken end
	4. Fragments
		1. Usually survives; needs protection.
		2. Remove with a brush, currette, or rongeur. Gentle massage during wound lavage.
		3. Remove with curette or cut off bone end.
		4. A. Remove small fragments with no muscle or periosteal attachment. Retain small fragments with tissue attachment.
		  B. Retain large fragments with or without attachments.
		  C. Use clinical judgment.
		  D. Better to remove too little than too much.
		  E. Immobilize fractures. Include a splint in the bandage or apply an external pin splint device in normal bone proximal and distal to wound. See Low-Velocity Gunshot Wounds, Chapter 4.

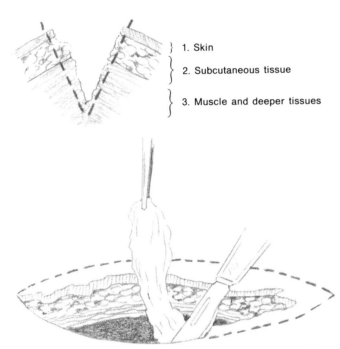

1. Skin

2. Subcutaneous tissue

3. Muscle and deeper tissues

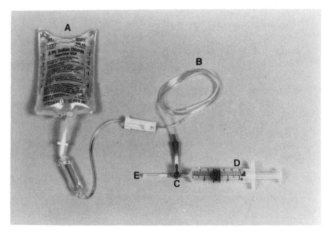

FIG. 2-4. Wound lavage apparatus. A, Container of lavage solution. B, Intravenous administration set. C, Three-way stopcock valve. D, 30 mL syringe. E, 18-gauge needle.

FIG. 2-3. Layer debridement. Skin is debrided first, followed by subcutaneous tissue, then muscle and deeper structures. (After Archibald, J. and Blakely C.L.: Basic procedures and preoperative considerations. *In* Canine Surgery, 2nd ed, Edited by J. Archibald. Santa Barbara, CA. American Veterinary Publishers, 1974, p. 30).

considered; however, care is necessary to prevent segments of charred tissue in the wound. If ligatures are necessary, 4-0 synthetic absorbable material is preferred.

During debridement, the wound should be lavaged with *copious* quantities of a lavage solution until all foreign material is removed from the wound (see Wound Lavage Solutions, Chapter 3). Lavage solution may be effectively delivered to a wound through a 30 ml syringe with an 18 gauge needle. A container of lavage solution can be connected to an intravenous administration set. A 3-way stopcock valve is attached to this set. The syringe and needle are attached to the three-way stopcock (Fig. 2-4). Turning the valve on the stopcock allows the syringe to be alternately filled and emptied to lavage the wound. Detergents are deleterious to tissues, and therefore should not be used in cleansing wounds.

Occasionally, staged debridement is performed. Obviously nonvital tissue is removed, leaving viable and questionable tissue. The wound is bandaged. When the bandage is changed, any tissue that has changed from questionable to obviously nonvital is removed.

When excision might jeopardize vital structures in the area or when the wound needs to be cleared of small amounts of necrotic tissue and debris following surgical

debridement, an enzymatic debriding agent on an adherent bandage may be used as an adjunct to layered debridement. Wet-to-dry or dry-to-dry bandages may also be considered to finish wound debridement (see Enzymes and Wound Dressing Materials, Contact Bandage Layer, Chapter 3).

Aftercare. Because some wounds are large, have extensive tissue damage, and are contaminated or infected, they are allowed to heal as open wounds. Some wounds are allowed to heal completely by contraction and epithelialization (see Wound Dressing Materials, Contact Bandage Layer—Open Wounds, and Topical Medications, Chapter 3). Other wounds are allowed to heal as open wounds until the tissues are healthy enough to allow closure (see Delayed Primary Closure, this chapter; and Secondary Closure, this chapter).

Advantages and Disadvantages. Layered debridement has the advantage of selectivity in debridement of tissue, thus conserving tissue that may eventually be used for closure. If the wound is to be treated as an open wound, each time the bandage is changed, the questionable tissue that was left on the wound at the previous bandage change can be re-evaluated and debrided if necessary (staged debridement). If initial debridement is done too aggressively, questionable tissue that may return to viability may be removed. This tissue could be used later for reconstruction.

Lavage of wounds with the syringe and needle is less damaging to tissues than jet lavage-type mechanisms.

REFERENCES AND SUGGESTED READING

1. Aron, D.N.: Management of open musculoskeletal injuries. Semin. Vet. Med. Surg. *3:*290, 1988.

2. Brinker, W.O., Piermattei, D.L., and Flo, G.L.: Handbook of Small Animal Orthopedics and Fracture Treatment. Philadelphia, W.B. Saunders, 1983.

3. Burke, J.F.: Infection. *In* Fundamentals of Wound Management. Edited by T.K. Hunt and T.E. Dunphy. New York, Appleton-Century-Crofts, 1979.

4. Committee on Trauma, American College of Surgeons: Early Care of the Critical Patient. 3rd ed. Philadelphia, W.B. Saunders, 1982.

5. Cummings, B.C.: Collateral circulation of the canine thoracic limb. *In* Some Techniques and Procedures in Small Animal Surgery. Bonner Springs, KS, Veterinary Medical Publishing Co. Inc., 1963.

6. Cummings, B.C.: Collateral circulation of the canine pelvic limb. *In* Some Techniques and Procedures in Small Animal Surgery. Bonner Springs, KS, Veterinary Medical Publishing Co. Inc., 1963.

7. Dudley, H.A.F.: Wounds and their treatment. *In* Hamilton Bailey's Emergency Surgery. 10th Ed. Edited by H.A.F. Dudley, Bristol, England, John A. Wright and Sons, 1977.

8. Edlich, R.F., Rodeheaver, G.T., Thacker, J.G., Winn, H.R., and Edgerton, M.T.: Manegement of soft tissue injury. Clin. Plast. Surg. *4*:191, 1977.

9. Edlich, R.F., Thacker, J.G., Buchanan, L., and Rodeheaver, G.T.: Modern concepts of treatment of traumatic wounds. Adv. Surg. *13*:169, 1979.

10. Hoover, N.W., and Ivins, J.C.: Wound debridement. Arch. Surg. *79*:701, 1959.

11. Jennings, P.B.: Surgical techniques utilized in the presence of infection. Arch. Offic. J. Am. Coll. Vet. Surg. *4*:43, 1975.

12. Jennings, P.B., and Heggers, J.P.: General principles in the care of open wounds. *In* Veterinary Trauma and Critical Care. Edited by I.M. Zaslow. Philadelphia, W.B. Saunders, 1984.

13. Johnston, D.E.: Wound healing and reconstructive surgery. Am. Anim. Hosp. Assoc. Sci. Proc. *2*:383, 1975.

14. Kirk, R.W., and Bistner, S.I.: Handbook of Veterinary Procedures and Emergency Treatment. 4th ed. Philadelphia, W.B. Saunders, 1985.

15. Knowles, R.P.: Injuries to skin, muscle, and tendon. *In* Some Techniques and Procedures in Small Animal Surgery. Bonner Springs, KS, Veterinary Medical Publishing Co. Inc., 1963.

16. Ndikuwera, J., Winstanley, E.W.: High pressure pulsatile lavage and high pressure syringe lavage in the treatment of contaminated wounds in dogs. J. Sm. Anim. Pract. *26*:3, 1985.

17. Peacock, E.E., Jr: Wound Repair. 3rd ed. Philadelphia, W.B. Saunders, 1984.

18. Reis, N.D., and Michaelson, M.: Crush injury of the lower limbs. J. Bone Joint Surg. *68A*:414, 1986.

19. Rudolph, R., Noe, J.M.: Initial treatment of the chronic wound. *In* Chronic Problem Wounds. Edited by R. Rudolph and J.M. Noe. Boston, Little, Brown and Co., 1983.

20. Swaim, S.F., Pope, E.R.: Early managemnt of limb degloving injuries. Semin. Vet. Med. Surg. *3*:274, 1988.

21. Tobin, G.R.: Closure of contaminated wounds: Biologic and technical consideration. Surg. Clin. North Am. *64*:639, 1984.

En Bloc Debridement

Definition and Indications. En bloc debridement is complete excision of the wound without entering the cavity of the wound itself. The technique is indicated for debriding wounds that are infected, and yet show no signs of systemic infection. The technique allows removal of infected tissue without breaking down barriers that have formed around the wound to prevent septicemia. The technique should be used only in areas where sufficient tissue is present to allow en bloc tissue removal. There should be no vital vessels, nerves, or tendons in an area of en bloc debridement.

Technique. The wound is packed with gauze, and several sutures are used to close the wound edges over the gauze (Fig. 2-5A and B). The entire wound is treated as a tumor (imagining the gauze and adjacent infected tissue as the tumor mass). The mass is excised with a

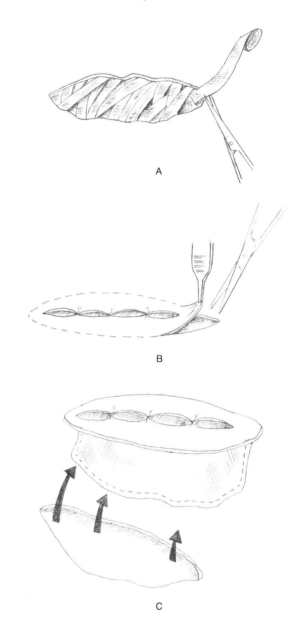

FIG. 2-5. En bloc debridement. A, Wound packed with gauze. B, Wound closed with a few sutures; beginning wound dissection. C, Wound removed with a margin of normal tissue.

margin of normal tissue so that the gauze is never exposed (Fig. 2-5C).

An alternative technique is to paint the tissues of the wound with sterile methylene blue. The wound is dissected out with a border of normal tissue so that no dye is exposed during dissection.

Aftercare. See Primary Closure, this chapter. After removal of the wound tissues, the remaining healthy tissues may be considered a clean wound and closed, provided that contaminated gloves and instruments have been changed.

Advantages and Disadvantages. En bloc debridement has the advantage of being a simple and certain way of eliminating all damaged and contaminated tissues. The technique, however, requires removal of a relatively large amount of tissue, leaving a large defect for closure. In addition, the areas on the body where it can be used are limited.

REFERENCES AND SUGGESTED READING

1. Committee on Trauma, American College of Surgeons: Early Care of the Critical Patient. 3rd ed. Philadelphia, W.B. Saunders, 1982.
2. Edlich, R.F., Rodeheaver, G., Thacker, J.G., and Edgerton, M.: Technical factors in wound management. *In* Fundamentals of Wound Management. Edited by T.K. Hunt, and T.E. Dunphy. New York, Appleton-Century-Crofts, 1979.
3. Edlich, R.F., Thacker, J.G., Buchanan, L., and Rodeheaver, G.T.: Modern concepts of treatment of traumatic wounds. Adv. Surg. *13*:169, 1979.
4. Hoover, N.W., and Ivins, J.C.: Wound debridement. Arch. Surg. *79*:701, 1959.
5. Peacock, E.E., Jr.: Wound Repair. 3rd ed. Philadelphia, W.B. Saunders, 1984.

SECONDARY MANAGEMENT

Secondary management includes procedures used in treatment of open wounds and in the closing of wounds that are suitable for closure.

OPEN WOUNDS

Definition and Indications. Because some wounds are large, have extensive tissue damage, and are contaminated or infected, they are allowed to heal completely by contraction and epithelialization (second-intention healing).

Techniques. To determine how much a wound will contract, the wound edges should be grasped with forceps, and gentle traction should be applied in an attempt to coapt the edges. Any deformity or defect produced by this maneuver (such as joint flexion or distortion of surrounding structures) will probably remain if the wound heals by contraction (see Wound Dressing Materials, Contact Bandage Layer—Open Wounds, and Topical Medication, Chapter 3).

Aftercare. Wounds on the body of a dog or cat where an abundance of skin overlies the panniculus carnosus muscle and there is a loose attachment to underlying structures usually heal completely by contraction and require no special aftercare. Even extremely large body wounds may heal completely or almost completely by contraction without interfering with the mechanical function of the underlying structures (Fig. 2-6A and B). The healing of some large wounds by contraction, however, may cause some abnormalities that require aftercare in the form of reconstructive surgery.

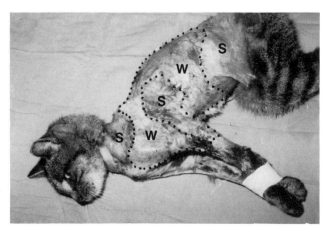

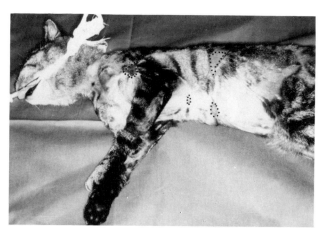

A   B

FIG. 2-6. Open wound healing. A, Large open wound on a cat. S = Intact skin, W = Wound. B, Nearly complete healing of the wound. Small wound areas left needing reconstruction (inside dotted lines).

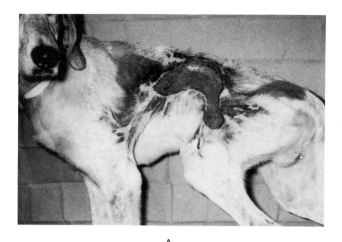 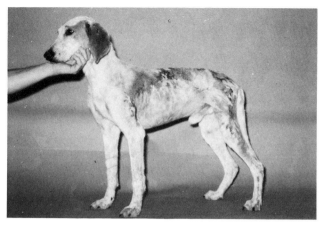

A

B

FIG. 2-7. Open wound healing—contracture. A, Web of skin and scar tissue across flexion surfaces of proximal joints of fore and hind limbs resulting from contraction. B, Contracture relieved by scar removal and reconstruction.

Advantages and Disadvantages. Healing by second intention has the advantage of allowing progressive debridement of tissues in the early stages of wound debridement, thus ensuring removal of only devitalized tissue. In addition, open wounds provide the optimum in wound drainage.

The time required for the healing of large wounds may be prolonged and the bandaging and medication may incur considerable expense. In addition, large open wounds may allow the loss of considerable fluids, electrolytes, and proteins as healing progresses.

Large wounds near the flexion surface of a proximal limb joint, when allowed to heal as an open wound, may result in a web of tight skin or scar tissue across the flexor surface that limits joint extension and requires reconstructive surgery to correct the abnormality (Fig. 2-7A and B). Similarly, large wounds on the distal limb may also result in contracture and deformity requiring reconstructive surgery (Fig. 2-8A–C). Second-intention healing of large wounds near a body orifice may result in stenosis of the orifice. Wounds on the limbs where mobility of surrounding tissue is insufficient to allow complete healing by contraction may heal by epithelialization. The epithelium is easily traumatized and abraded from the wound, however, and some areas may not epithelialize. Aftercare of such wounds may require placement of a graft to provide more durable tissue (Fig. 2-9A and B).

REFERENCES AND SUGGESTED READING

1. Billingham, R.E., and Medawar, P.B.: Contracture and intussusceptive growth in healing of extensive wounds in mammalian skin. J. Anat. *89*:114, 1955.

2. Dingwall, J.S.: Wound contraction. J. Am. Anim. Hosp. Assoc. *12*:668, 1976.
3. Johnston, D.E.: The process of wound healing. J. Am. Anim. Hosp. Assoc. *13*:186, 1977.
4. Peacock, E.E. Jr.: Wound Repair. 3rd ed. Philadelphia, W.B. Saunders, 1984.

CLOSED WOUNDS

Primary Closure

Definition and Indications. Primary wound closure entails closure of the wound relatively soon after it has been inflicted. Closure should be under good conditions and the surgeon should be convinced that healing will continue uneventfully. Ideally, primary closure should be performed when the animal is in good condition. Additional requirements are a short time lapse since injury and a minimal degree of contamination and tissue trauma or thorough debridement and lavage to provide tissue suitable for suturing. Closure should be possible in the presence of good hemostasis without creating tension or dead space. The clean wound created surgically under aseptic conditions is the best example of a wound for primary closure.

Technique. Layered closure should be used to eliminate dead space in primary wound closure. Depending on the size of the wound and/or the size of the animal, 3-0 to 4-0 suture material may be used to close the deeper tissues. Either absorbable or monofilament nonabsorbable simple interrupted sutures may be used in the deeper tissue. When placing sutures to close dead space, the surgeon should be careful not to include major vessels or nerves in the suture because they would essentially be ligated as the suture is tied, leading to impaired innervation, circulation,

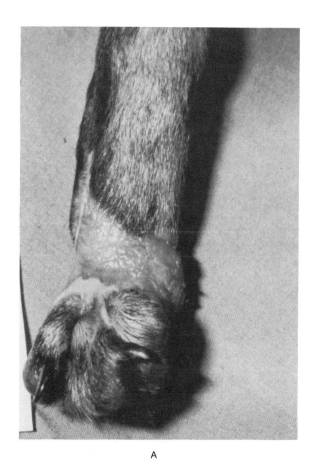

A

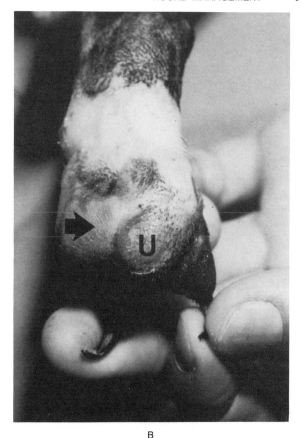

B

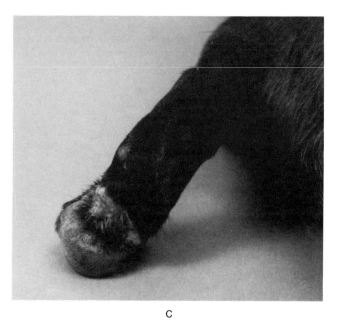

C

FIG. 2-8. Distal limb open wound healing—contracture. A, Distal limb contracture causing abnormal digit and metatarsal pad alignment. B, Metatarsal pad (arrow) pulled out of alignment. Ulcer adjacent to pad (U). C, Reconstructed foot after digit removal and metatarsal pad realignment. (B from Swaim, S.F.: Foot salvage techniques in dogs and cats: Options, "Do's" and "Don'ts". J. Am. Anim. Hosp. Assoc. *21*:511, 1985.)

and healing (Fig. 2-10). The smallest-diameter suture material and the fewest sutures that will effectively close the dead space without creating pockets should be used. Closure of subcutaneous tissue may be with similar suture materials in a simple continuous suture pattern.

When considerable trauma, foreign material, and contamination have been associated with the wound (as in a crushing injury), the surgeon should strongly consider placing a drain in the wound in addition to thorough lavage, debridement, and antimicrobial prophylaxis (see Drains, this chapter).

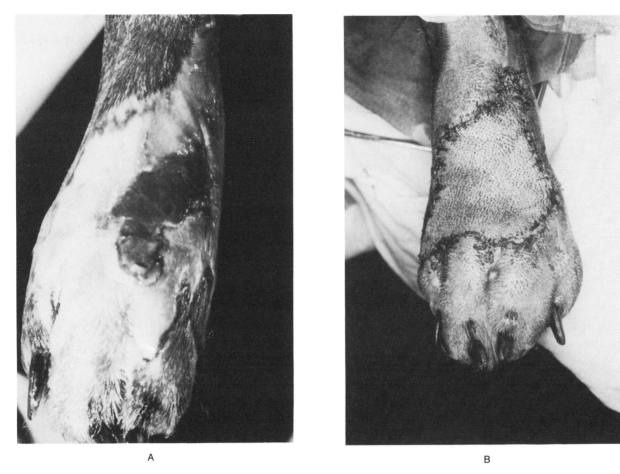

A   B

FIG. 2-9. Distal limb open wound healing—epithelialization. A, Epithelialization of a large wound on the dorsum of a paw. B, Correction of defect with a more durable skin graft. (B from Swaim, S.F.: Skin grafts. *In* textbook of Small Animal Surgery. Edited by D.H. Slatter. Philadelphia, W.B. Saunders Co. 1985, p. 492).

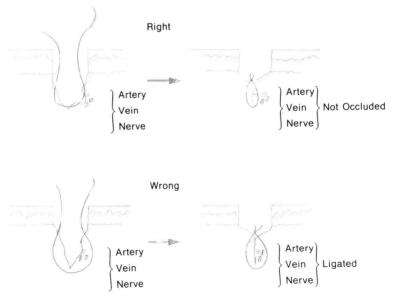

FIG. 2-10. Placing sutures to eliminate dead space. Right: Suture placed so that it does not include the artery, vein, or nerve. Wrong: Suture placed to include artery, vein, and nerve results in ligation.

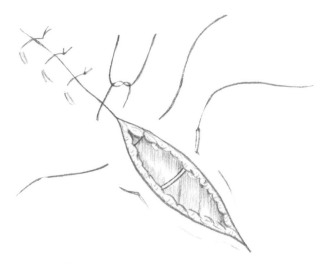

FIG. 2-11. Placing simple interrupted sutures.

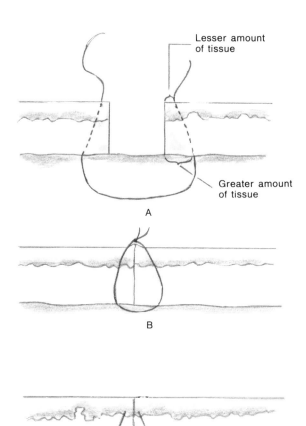

Lesser amount of tissue

Greater amount of tissue

A

B

C

FIG. 2-12. Ideal placement of simple interrupted suture. A, Suture is placed at an angle through the skin. B, When tied, suture tends to evert skin. C, After suture removal, scar flattens rather than widens.

Skin closure may be with 3-0 to 4-0 nonabsorbable suture material in one of several suture patterns or with staples.

Aftercare. Wounds that have been closed primarily should be observed over a 7- to 10- day period following closure to ensure that healing is progressing without complications. If a drain has been placed in a primarily closed wound, bandages should be applied to protect the wound and the drain, and the bandages should be changed periodically. If a drain has been placed, it should be removed when the amount of drainage noted in the bandage has decreased to a minimal amount (see Wound Dressing Materials, Contact Bandage Layer—Closed Wounds, Chapter 3, and Drains, this chapter).

Advantages and Disadvantages. If wounds are properly evaluated, managed, and closed they should heal in 7 to 10 days postoperatively. Improper evaluation, management, and closure, however, may result in a hematoma, seroma, and/or infection with the necessity for extended wound management.

REFERENCES AND SUGGESTED READING

1. Brown, P.W.: The prevention of infection in open wounds. Clin. Orthop. 96:42, 1973.
2. Dudley, H.A.F.: Wounds and their treatment. In Hamilton Bailey's Emergency Surgery. 10th ed. Edited by H.A.F. Dudley. Bristol, England, John A. Wright and Sons, 1977.
3. Edlich, R.F., Rodeheaver, G.T., Thacker, J.G., Winn, H.R., and Edgerton, M.T.: Management of soft tissue injury. Clin. Plast. Surg. 4:191, 1977.
4. Hoover, N.W., Ivins, J.C.: Wound debridement. Arch. Surg. 79:701, 1959.
5. Tobin, G.R.: Closure of contaminated wounds: Biologic and technical considerations. Surg. Clin. North Am. 64:639, 1984.

Skin Suture Patterns
Simple Interrupted Sutures

Definition and Indications. Each suture is a loop of suture material passed perpendicular to the plane of tissue, with its ends emerging on opposite sides of the wound an equal distance from the wound edge on each side (Fig. 2-11).

Technique. Ideally, simple interrupted sutures should be placed by passing the needle through the skin at a slight angle so that a slightly greater bite of the deeper part of the dermis is taken. When the needle is passed through the second side of the wound, it is again passed at a slight angle to include more dermis in the deeper aspect of the skin (Fig. 2-12A). This tends to evert the skin slightly so that the scars flatten rather than widen after suture removal (Fig. 2-12B and C). Enough sutures should be placed as close together as necessary to satisfactorily coapt the skin edges. Wounds in thick skin and those following tension lines require fewer sutures than wounds in thin skin and those cutting across tension lines.

Aftercare. Sutures should be removed 7 to 10 days after surgery.

Advantages and Disadvantages. The primary advantage of simple interrupted sutures is that if one suture fails, the others remain intact. In addition, the surgeon can adjust the tension of each suture at each wound segment according to the spreading forces that are present. The technique, however, uses a greater amount of suture material, and it takes relatively longer to place this suture pattern than continuous suture patterns. The pattern also has minimal holding power under stress.

REFERENCES AND SUGGESTED READINGS

1. Bellenger, C.R.: Sutures Part II. The use of sutures and alternative methods of closure. Compend. Contin. Educ. *4*:587, 1982.
2. Borges, A.F.: Elective Incisions and Scar Revision. Boston, Little, Brown and Co., 1973.
3. Braden, T.D.: Plastic and reconstructive surgery of the canine torso. Vet. Clin. North Am. *9*:285, 1979.
4. Epstein, E, and Epstein, E. Jr.: Skin Surgery. 5th ed. Springfield, IL, Charles C Thomas, 1982.
5. Grabb, W.C.: Basic techniques of plastic surgery. *In* Plastic Surgery. 3rd ed. Edited by W.C. Grabb and J.W. Smith. Boston, Little, Brown and Co., 1979.
6. Knecht, C.D., Allen, A.R., Williams, D.J., and Johnson, J.H.: Fundamental Techniques in Veterinary Surgery. 3rd ed. Philadelphia, W.B. Saunders, 1987.
7. McGregor, I.A.: Fundamental Techniques of Plastic Surgery. 7th ed. Edinburgh, Churchill Livingstone, 1980.
8. Stashak, T.S. Reconstructive surgery in the horse. J. Am. Vet. Med. Assoc. *170*:143, 1977.

Simple Continuous Sutures

Definition and Indications. This pattern consists of a progressive series of sutures inserted without interruption perpendicular to the plane of the tissue, with only the beginning and end of the suture being tied. These sutures are indicated in tissues that require minimal holding but maximal tissue apposition. They are also effectively used to suture subcutaneous tissue and fascia in nontension planes.

Technique. The pattern is started at one commissure of the wound with a simple interrupted suture. The remainder of the suture can be placed so that it advances above or beneath the skin. A modification of this is the "running suture," in which the deep and superficial portions of the suture are advanced (Fig. 2-13A–C). To end the suture when a swaged-on needle has been used, the needled end may be tied to the last available suture

loop (Fig. 2-13D). Another technique involves placing an additional suture close to and in reverse direction from the normally placed last suture. The needled end is tied to the resulting narrow loop (Fig. 2-13E). If an eyed needle has been used, the needle is advanced through the tissues, and the short end of the suture is held on the proximal end of the needle passage. A loop is pulled through with the needle and tied to the single end on the contralateral side (Fig. 2-13F).

Aftercare. Sutures should be removed 7 to 10 days after surgery.

Advantages and Disadvantages. These sutures can be placed more rapidly than interrupted sutures. They have an advantage over the continuous lock suture pattern in that they allow tension adjustment after placement. Also, they create an air- and liquid-tight seal. These sutures are weaker than simple interrupted sutures; they tend to pucker the skin, and if placed too tightly, may strangulate the wound edge. Also, if a break occurs anywhere along the suture, the entire suture line may disrupt.

REFERENCES AND SUGGESTED READING

1. Bellenger, C.R.: Sutures: Part II. The use of sutures and alternative methods of closure. Compend. Contin. Educ. *4*:587, 1982.
2. Borges, A.F.: Elective Incisions and Scar Revision. Boston, Little, Brown and Co., 1973.
3. Forrester, J.C.: Suture materials and their uses. Nurs. Mirror *140*:48, 1975.
4. Knecht, C.D., Allen, A.R., Williams, D.J., and Johnson, J.H.: Fundamental Techniques in Veterinary Surgery. 3rd ed. Philadelphia, W.B. Saunders Co. 1987.
5. McGregor, I. A.: Fundamental Techniques of Plastic Surgery. 7th ed. Edinburgh, Churchill Livingstone, 1980.

Continuous-Lock Sutures

Definition and Indications. This is a continuous-lock pattern, also called a "blanket stitch" or Ford interlocking suture. It is a progressive series of sutures inserted uninterruptedly in the skin like a simple continuous suture; however, each passage through the tissue is partially locked. It is indicated when speed as well as some suture security are needed for closure.

Technique. Following the placement of each suture, the needle passes above the unused suture material to lock the suture in place as it is tightened (Fig. 2-14A). To end a lock stitch when an eyed needle has been used, the needle is introduced in the opposite direction from that previously used, with the suture end being held on the side of insertion (Fig. 2-14B). A loop of suture formed on the side opposite that of introduction is tied to the single end (Fig. 2-14C). When a swaged-on needle is used, the final tie is similar to that used for a simple continuous suture.

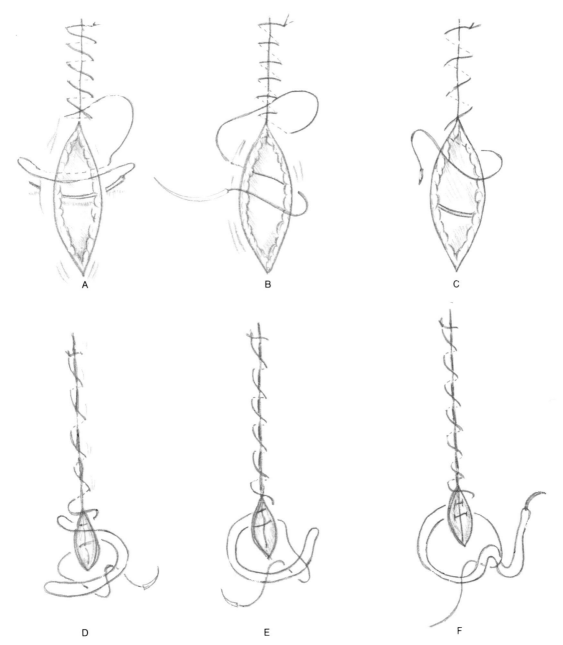

FIG. 2-13. Simple continuous suture: A, Advancing above skin. B, Advancing below skin. C, Advancing above and below skin ("running suture"). Ending of a simple continuous suture: D, Swadged-on needle—needled end of suture is tied to last available suture loop. E, Swadged-on needle—additional suture placed close to and in reverse direction from normally placed last suture, needled end of suture is tied to resulting loop. F, Eyed needle—needle advanced through tissues; short end of suture is held on proximal end of needle passage; a loop is pulled through with needle and tied to single end on contralateral side. (A and B after Archibald, J., and Blakely, C.L.: Sutures. *In* Canine Surgery. 2nd ed. Edited by J. Archibald. Santa Barbara, CA, American Veterinary Publishers, 1974. p 44. C through F after Knecht, C.D., Allen A.R., Williams, D.J., and Johnson, J.H.: Fundamental Techniques in Veterinary Surgery. 3rd ed. Philadelphia, W.B. Saunders, 1987, p. 58.)

Aftercare.   Sutures should be removed 7 to 10 days after surgery.

Advantages and Disadvantages.   Suture placement is more rapid than that for an interrupted suture pattern, and the pattern has greater stability than other continuous patterns in the event of a partial break along the suture line. This pattern, however, requires an increased amount of suture material, and does not readily allow tension adjustment after placement. It may pucker the skin and, if placed too tightly, may

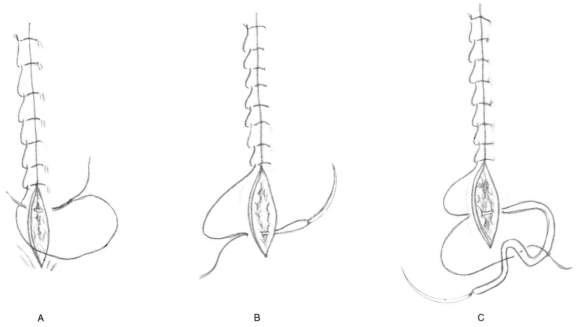

A   B   C

FIG. 2-14. Continuous-lock sutures. A, Needle is passed above unused portion of suture material with each suture. B and C, Ending of a continuous-lock suture: B, With eyed needle—needle introduced in opposite direction from that previously used, with suture end held on side of insertion. C, A loop of suture formed on side opposite that of introduction is tied to single end.

strangulate the skin edges. It is more difficult to remove than a simple continuous suture.

REFERENCE AND SUGGESTED READING

1. Knecht, C.D., Allen, A.R., Williams, D.J., and Johnson, J.H.: Fundamental Techniques of Veterinary Surgery. 3rd ed. Philadelphia, W.B. Saunders, 1987.

Continuous Horizontal Mattress Sutures
Definition and Indications. This pattern is a progressive series of sutures placed uninterruptedly in the same plane as the tissue. It is indicated when speed is necessary in wound closure, when some eversion is not objectionable, and when some tension is desired. A similar pattern may be used as a subcutaneous suture pattern to close deep tissues and as a continuous intradermal suture.

Technique. A simple interrupted suture is placed to start the suture pattern. The suture material is advanced 7 to 8 mm above the skin and parallel to the incision line between each passage of the suture under the skin, which is made perpendicular to the incision line (Fig. 2-15).

Aftercare. Sutures should be removed 7 to 10 days after surgery.

Advantages and Disadvantages. Wound closure is more rapid than when an interrupted suture pattern is used, and the pattern permits accurate approximation of the wound edges with reduced tension. This pattern does not have good security, and a break anywhere along the suture may cause the entire line to disrupt.

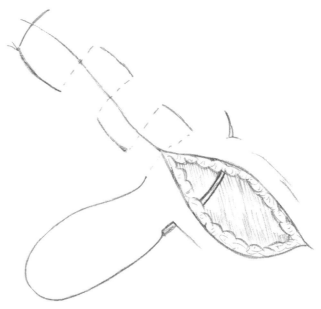

FIG. 2-15. Continuous horizontal mattress suture.

REFERENCE AND SUGGESTED READING

1. Knecht, C.D., Allen, A.R., Williams, D.J., and Johnson, J.H.: Fundamental Techniques of Veterinary Surgery. 3rd ed. Philadelphia, W.B. Saunders, 1987.

Cross Sutures

Definition and Indications. The cross-stitch or "baseball stitch" is a double simple continuous suture pattern. It is indicated for suturing thick skin when haste is required.

Technique. A simple continuous line is placed, followed by placement of a second line from the opposite direction (Fig. 2-16). The first row of sutures is placed deep, wide, and loose to approximate the full thickness of the skin edges. The second row is used for fine approximation of the superficial wound edges. If the wound appears almost completely closed after the first row of sutures has been placed, the returning second row of sutures may skip over a number of loops until the starting knot is reached. It is better to have the loops too loose than too tight. If they are loose, a few simple interrupted sutures can be added to complete skin apposition where indicated.

Aftercare. Sutures should be removed 7 to 10 days after surgery.

Advantages and Disadvantages. This suture pattern can be placed with relative rapidity and the double

row gives much greater security to the suture line. The suture pattern requires increased suture material for placement.

REFERENCE AND SUGGESTED READING

1. Borges, A.F.: Elective Incisions and Scar Revision. Boston, Little, Brown, and Co., 1973.

X-Mattress (Cruciate) Sutures

Definition and Indications. These sutures are similar to cross sutures, but are placed in an interrupted pattern. This pattern is particularly useful for suturing the skin of stumps as found in tail and digit amputations.

Technique. The needle is inserted 3 to 4 mm from the wound edge on one side and passed to the opposite

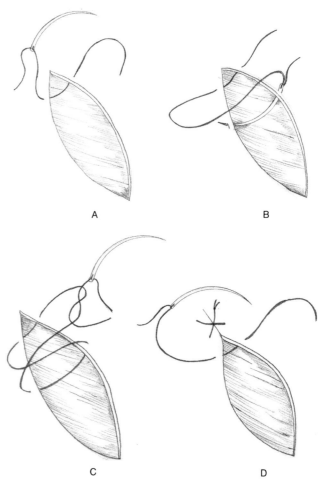

FIG. 2-17. X-Mattress sutures. A, First passage of suture, like simple interrupted suture. B, Advancement of needle across wound with second passage parallel to first. C, Tying suture. D, First suture tied, second being placed.

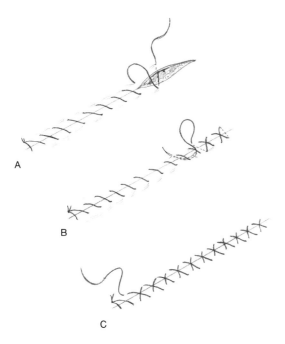

FIG. 2-16. Cross sutures. A, First row of simple continuous sutures. B, Second row of simple continuous sutures. C, Completed suture.

side of the wound as in placement of a simple inter-rupted suture (Fig. 2-17A). The needle is then advanced 5 mm and crosses the wound without penetrating the tissue. The needle is passed a second time through the skin parallel to the first passage (Fig. 2-17B). The suture ends, which are on opposite sides of the wound, are tied together, forming an "X" on the skin surface (Fig. 2-17C and D).

Aftercare.   Sutures should be removed 7 to 10 days after surgery.

Advantages and Disadvantages.   These serve as tension sutures to provide strength and prevent eversion of the wound edges. Their interrupted pattern gives security to the suture line. Increased suture material and time, however, are required for placement of sutures.

REFERENCE AND SUGGESTED READING

1. Knecht, C.D., Allen, A.R., Williams, D.J., and Johnson, J.H.: Fundamental Techniques of Veterinary Surgery. 3rd ed. Philadelphia, W.B. Saunders, 1987.

Staples

Definition and Indications.   Staples are metallic devices that appose and hold together the skin edges when dispensed by an applicator. Numerous manufacturers make staple-dispensing devices. They are indicated when speed is necessary for wound closure.

Technique.   The staple applicator is held over the skin edges with the indicator arrow of the dispensing port situated over the nearly apposed wound edges (Fig. 2-18A). Compressing the handle of the staple applicator inserts and bends a staple into the skin with one half of the staple on each side of the incision line (Fig. 2-18B and C). The staple thus holds the wound edges in apposition for healing.

Aftercare.   The incision line is usually covered with a bandage to prevent the animal from disturbing the staples. Staples are removed 7 to 10 days after surgery with a special staple-removing instrument.

Advantages and Disadvantages.   The main advantage of staple closure is the speed with which it is accomplished. Long incisions can be closed in a matter of seconds. The simple and rapid application of staples and their inert composition are favorable factors, causing little inflammation, resisting infection, and resulting in minimal iatrogenic trauma when inserted. Their expense may be considered a disadvantage, but if reduction of surgical time is an important factor, they may be well worth the expense. Occassionally, staples may rotate in the skin and must be manipulated into the proper position for application of the removal instrument when the staples are removed (Fig. 2-18D through G).

REFERENCES AND SUGGESTED READING

1. Adams, S.B.: The practical use of skin stapling units in horses. Eq. Pract. *3*:45, 1981.
2. Bellenger, C.R.: Sutures: Part II. The use of sutures and alternative methods of closure. Compend. Contin. Educ. *4*:587, 1982.
3. Hess, J.L., DeYoung, D.W., Riley, M.G.I., and McCurnin, D.M.: Comparison of stainless steel staple and synthetic suture material on skin wound healing. J. Am. Anim. Hosp. Assoc. *15*:569, 1979.
4. Johnson, A., Rodeheaver, G.T., Durand, L.S., Edgerton, M.T., and Edlich, R.F.: Automatic disposable stapling devices for wound closure. Ann. Emerg. Med. *10*:631, 1981.
5. Porter, D.B.: A clinical evaluation of the Proximate(R) stapling system for closing skin incisions. Vet. Med. Sm. Anim. Clin. *76*:320, 1981.
6. Stillman, R.M., Marino, C.A., and Seligman, S.J.: Skin staples in potentially contaminated wounds. Arch. Surg. *119*:821, 1984.

Delayed Primary Closure

Definition and Indications.   Delayed primary closure is wound closure after local infection has been adequately controlled, usually 3 to 5 days from the time of infliction. It is indicated for wounds that show evidence of heavy contamination, purulent exudate, residual necrotic or questionable tissue, edema, erythema at the margins, lymphangitis, and skin tension.

Technique.   During the 3- to 5-day period before closure, the wound should be managed as an open wound (see Contaminated and Infected Wounds, this chapter; Wound Dressing Materials, Contact Bandage Layer—Open Wounds and Topical Medications, Chapter 3). At the time of daily bandage change, staged debridement should be performed whereby obviously nonvital tissue is removed each day. At the time of delayed closure, the techniques are the same as those used for primary closure (see Primary Closure, this chapter). If there is any doubt about the status of the wound tissue at the time of closure, a drain should be placed in the wound (see Drains, this chapter).

Aftercare.   See Primary Closure, this chapter.

Advantages and Disadvantages.   Delayed primary closure is beneficial because it allows the surgeon to observe the progression of the early healing process. It allows staged debridement of the wound, adherent bandage wound debridement, and maximal wound drainage. Delayed primary closure of wounds provides better mechanical strength than primary closure. If closure is properly performed, healing should be complete in 7 to 10 days. If the procedures are performed improperly, wound infection may result, with a need for extended wound management.

REFERENCES AND SUGGESTED READING

1. Brown, P.W.: The prevention of infection in open wounds. Clin. Orthop. *96*:42, 1973.

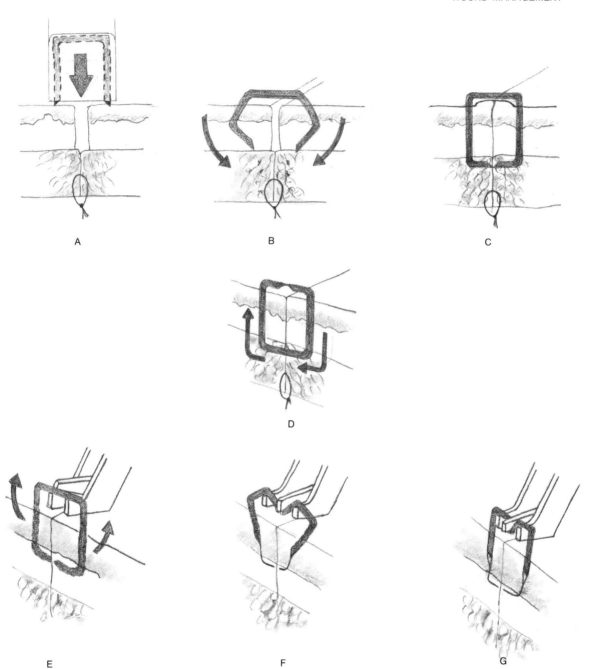

FIG. 2-18. Skin staples. A, Dispensing port of staple applicator centered over almost-apposed wound edges. B, Dynamics of staple insertion. C, Staple applied with half on each side of wound. D, Rotation of staple during healing. E, Insertion of staple remover. F, Bending staple for removal. G, Staple bent for removal.

2. Danielsen, C.C., and Fogdestam, I.: Delayed primary closure: Collagen synthesis and content in healing rat skin incisions. J. Surg. Res. *31*:210, 1981.

3. Dudley, H.A.F.: Wounds and their treatment. *In* Hamilton Bailey's Emergency Surgery. 10th ed. Edited by H.A.F. Dudley, Bristol, England, John A. Wright and Sons, 1977.

4. Edlich, R.F., Rodeheaver, G.T., Thacker, J.G., Winn, H.R., and Edgerton, M.T.: Management of soft tissue injury. Clin. Plast. Surg. *4*:191, 1977.

5. Fogdestam, I.: A biomechanical study of healing rat skin incisions after delayed primary closure. Surg. Gynecol. Obstet. *153*:191, 1981.

6. Furneaux, R.W.: Management of contaminated wounds. Canine Pract. *2*:22, 1975.

7. Hoover, N.W., Ivins, J.C.: Wound debridement. Arch. Surg. *79*:701, 1959.

8. Shepard, G.H.: The healing of wounds after delayed primary closure: An experimental study. Plast. Reconstr. Surg. *48*:358, 1971.

Secondary Closure

Definition and Indications. Secondary closure of a wound is closure 5 days after the time of injury, when the wound has formed a bed of healthy granulation tissue. Such closure is indicated when it has been necessary to leave the wound open longer than 5 days to provide adequate management of infection. Secondary closure is also performed when a wound is presented to the surgeon when it is already in the reparative stage of healing and has a well-developed bed of healthy granulation tissue. Another indication is for closure of a wound that has disrupted and in which granulation tissue has formed.

Technique. Before secondary closure, a wound should be managed as an open wound (see Wound Dressing Materials, Contact Bandage Layer—Open Wounds and Topical Medications, Chapter 3). At the time of daily bandage change, staged debridement should be performed, so that obviously nonvital tissue is removed each day. Beyond the fourth or fifth day after injury, the proliferative phase of wound healing progresses. Granulation tissue continues to form; the skin edges become increasingly adherent to underlying tissue with the wound tissue becoming less pliable; and the epithelium begins to advance over the granulation tissue.

With small wounds that have not progressed too far into the proliferative stages of healing, it may be possible to appose and suture the wound edges in the presence of granulation tissue (Fig. 2-19). Such closure should be done after cleansing the wound surface with an antiseptic solution. Secondary closure should be done before epithelial tissue has begun to migrate over the granulation tissue.

Wounds in the later proliferative stages of healing require some dissection to achieve secondary closure. The surface of the wound should be cleansed with a surgical sponge soaked in an antiseptic solution (Fig. 2-20A). A surgical sponge soaked in the same solution should be placed over the granulation tissue for 2 to 3 minutes. An incision is made around the wound at the junction of the epithelial tissue with haired skin. Any epithelial tissue covering the edge of the granulation tissue should also be removed (Fig. 2-20B). The skin around the wound is undermined, and the skin edges are advanced across the granulation tissue and sutured together (Fig. 2-20C and D). On large wounds, "walking" sutures of 3-0 absorbable suture material (see "Walking" Sutures, Chapter 5) are used to advance the skin over the granulation tissue on the defect until the wound edges are apposed. "Biting" deeply into the granulation tissue with the "walking" sutures provides good security. The wound edges are sutured together once they are apposed. If there is any doubt about the condition of the tissues at the time of surgery, a drain may be placed in the area.

When a wound has been disrupted and has already formed granulation tissue, it should be resutured without disrupting the granulation tissue that is present. The underlying causes for disruption, however, should be corrected before resuturing. These causes include undue tension on the skin edges, use of improper suture material, improper knot tying, poor suturing technique, necrosis and ischemia of tissues, hematomas, infection, poor nutritional status of the patient, and retention of foreign material in the wound.

Aftercare. See Primary Closure, this chapter.

Advantages and Disadvantages. Delaying wound closure helps ensure that all infection and necrotic tissue have been removed and the wound is in the reparative stage. Thus, healing can progress without complication. Because the wound is already in the reparative stage of healing, it will gain tensile strength faster than a primarily closed wound.

Closure of wounds in the presence of granulation tissue may be more difficult because of the lack of pliability of the tissue. Suturing granulating skin edges of a disrupted wound does not provide the cosmetic appearance of a primarily closed wound. Tensile strength of the wound is attained sooner, however and with time and maturation, the appearance of the scar improves.

REFERENCES AND SUGGESTED READING

1. Brown, P.W.: The prevention of infection in open wounds. Clin. Orthop. *96*:42, 1973.
2. Dudley, H.A.F.: Wounds and their treatment. *In* Hamilton Bailey's Emergency Surgery. 10th ed. Edited by H.A.F. Dudley. Bristol, England, John A. Wright & Sons, 1977.
3. Hackett, R.P.: Delayed wound closure: A review and report of use of the technique on three equine limb wounds. Vet. Surg. *12*:48, 1983.
4. Kirk, R.W., and Bistner, S.I.: Handbook of Veterinary Procedures and Emergency Treatment. 4th ed. Philadelphia, W.B. Saunders, 1985.
5. Lee, A.H.: The tensile strength of primary and secondary skin closures. M.S. Thesis, Auburn University, AL 36849, June, 1985.
6. Lee, A.H., and Swaim, S.F.: Granulation tissue: How to take advantage of it in management of open wounds. Compend. Contin. Educ. *10*:163, 1987.

DRAINS

Passive Drains

Definition and Indications. Passive drains are those that drain a wound by means of pressure differentials, overflow and gravity. Tubular drains are composed of rubber or plastic tubes or catheters with thicker walls that are not easily collapsed. They have a single lumen

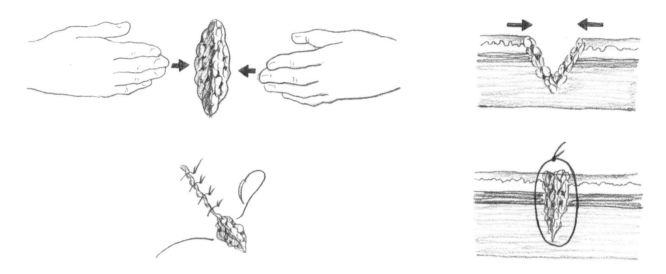

FIG. 2-19. Secondary closure of a small wound. A, Manipulating wound edges to ascertain if they can be apposed. B, Suturing wound edges together in presence of granulation tissue. (From Lee, A.H., and Swaim, S.F.: Granulation tissue: How to take advantage of it in management of open wounds. Compend. Contin. Educ. *10*:163, 1988.)

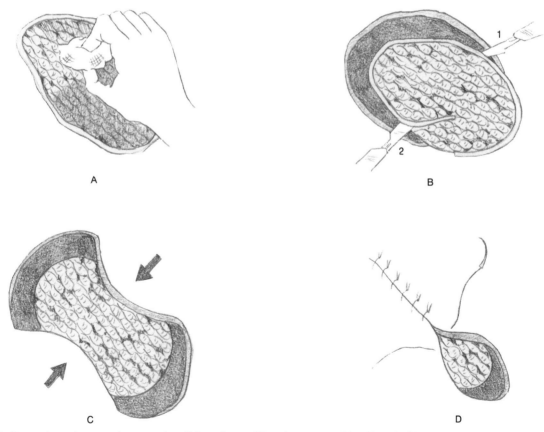

FIG. 2-20. Secondary closure of a wound well into the proliferative stage of healing. A, Cleansing wound surface. B, Incision at junction of epithelium and haired skin (1), removal of epithelium covering the edge of granulation tissue (2). C, After surrounding skin is undermined, it is advanced over granulation tissue. D, Skin is sutured over granulation tissue. (From Lee, A.H., and Swaim, S.F.: Granulation tissue: How to take advantage of it in management of open wounds. Compend. Contin. Educ. *10*:163, 1988.)

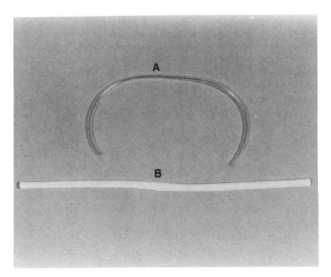

FIG. 2-21. Two types of passive drains. A, Fenestrated tube drain. B, Penrose drain.

with or without side holes (Fig. 2-21A). These drains may also be made of soft, thin latex rubber that is basically cylindrical in shape; however, because of their thin walls, they are easily collapsed (Penrose drains, Fig. 2-21B). Wound drainage is indicated: (1) when there is an abscess cavity, (2) in the presence of foreign material or tissue of questionable viability that cannot be excised, (3) when massive contamination is inevitable (such as in wounds near the anal area), and (4) when it is necessary to obliterate dead space to prevent blood, exudate, or serum accumulation.

Technique. *Single-exit drain.* Generally, fenestrations are not cut in flat (Penrose) drains. If fenestrations are cut in tube drains, however, they should be cut in an oval shape and should be no more than 1/3 the diameter of the drain to prevent kinking of the tube.

The proximal end of the drain is placed in the most proximal aspect of the wound and anchored to the tissue in the area by a buried simple interrupted absorbable suture. The suture is placed through the edge of the drain and the tissue (Fig. 2-22A and B). The suture should incorporate a very small amount of the drain so that it can hold the drain in place and yet allow it to be removed easily in a few days by merely pulling on its distal portion, tearing the suture from the drain (Fig. 2-22C). An alternative for fixing the drain in the proximal portion of the wound is to pass a nonabsorbable suture through the skin and drain and tie it outside the skin (Fig. 2-23A and B). The suture is removed before the drain (Fig. 2-23C).

A pair of hemostatic forceps is used to make a tunnel between the ventral aspect of the wound and a point just under the skin ventral to the ventral aspect of the wound (Fig. 2-24A). An incision is made in the skin at this point for the emergence of the distal end of the drain. The incision should be large enough to allow the drain to exit, with some space around the drain. The distal end of the drain is pulled through this incision and tacked to the edge of the incision with a simple interrupted nonabsorbable suture (Fig. 2-24B). The wound is then closed (Fig. 2-24C; see Primary Closure, this chapter).

If a wound that is already closed requires drainage (for example, an unruptured abscess), an instrument with long blades, such as Doyen intestinal forceps, may be used to place the proximal end of the drain in the wound depths by means of a stab incision near the ventral aspect of the wound. Using the tip of the forceps as a palpable landmark, a simple interrupted suture is placed through the skin into the drain to anchor the proximal end of the drain in the wound (Fig. 2-25A). The drain is anchored to the edge of this incision with a tacking suture (Fig. 2-25B).

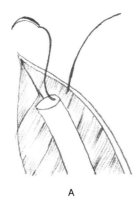
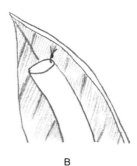
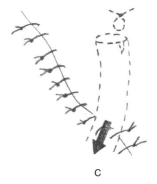

A   B   C

FIG. 2-22. Internal anchoring of proximal end of a drain in a wound. A, Simple interrupted absorbable suture placed through wound tissue and drain edge. B, Suture tied. C, Tension on distal end of drain breaks it free from suture at time of removal. (From Swaim, S.F., and Lee, A.H.: Wound drainage techniques. *In* Current Techniques in Small Animal Surgery. 3rd ed. Edited by M.J. Bojrab. Philadelphia, Lea and Febiger, 1990, p. 30.)

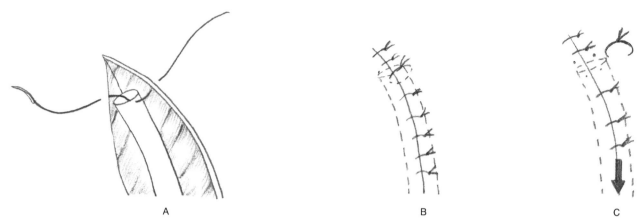

FIG. 2-23. External anchoring of proximal end of a drain in a wound. A, A simple interrupted nonabsorbable suture placed through skin and drain. B, Suture tied outside of skin. C, Suture cut and removed; allows drain removal. (From Swaim, S.F., and Lee, A.H.: Wound drainage techniques. *In* Current Techniques in Small Animal Surgery. 3rd ed. Edited by M.J. Bojrab. Philadelphia, Lea and Febiger, 1990, p. 30.)

Double-exit drain. In addition to making a port of exit for the drain ventral to the most ventral aspect of the wound, a similar exit port is made near the dorsal edge of the wound to allow exit of the proximal end of the drain (Fig. 2-26).

Aftercare. Several layers of wide-mesh absorbent gauze should be placed over the end of the drain. This procedure is followed by application of an absorbent intermediate bandage layer and a porous adhesive tape tertiary layer. The bandage protects the wound and drain from molestation by the animal and yields information about the wound drainage. The bandage should be changed frequently to remove drainage from the wound area and for inspection of the nature and amount of drainage, which determines how long the drain should remain in place. With infection, the discharge should

progress from exudative to transudative and should decrease in amount as healing progresses. When drainage has decreased to a small amount and remains about the same in nature and amount from one bandage change to the next, the drain should be removed.

With a double-exit drain, antibiotics or antiseptics may be used to lavage the wound from the proximal tube emergence site.

Advantages and Disadvantages. Penrose drains are easily sterilized and readily available. Because they are soft and malleable, they do not exert undue pressure on adjacent blood vessels or other structures; however, they may cause some tissue inflammation. The disadvantage of the proximal buried tacking suture is that the drain may tear at the time of removal, leaving a piece of drain attached to the suture in the wound.

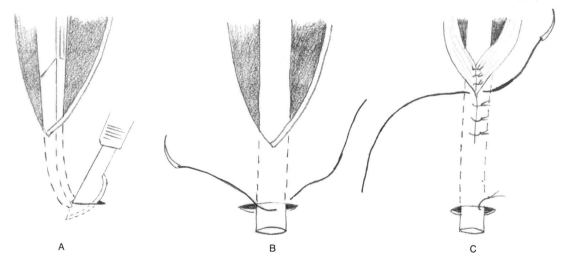

FIG. 2-24. Placing distal end of a drain. A, Incision over tip of hemostats tunneled subcutaneously near distal aspect of wound. B, Distal end of drain pulled through incision and anchored with simple interrupted suture. C, Wound being closed.

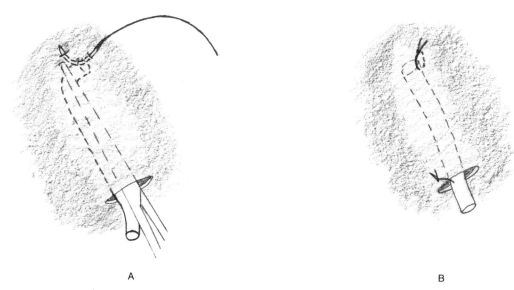

A   B

FIG. 2-25. Drainage of a closed wound (unruptured abscess). A, Long-bladed instrument places drain in wound depths through a distal stab incision. Drain anchored to skin with a simple interrupted suture using tips of instrument as a landmark for suture placement. B, Drain anchored at edge of stab incision.

Tube drains are inexpensive and readily available, and plastic tubes seem to cause less tissue reaction than rubber tube drains. The stiffness of the tubes may cause postoperative discomfort, however. If the tube is fenestrated, drainage can occur both from within and outside the lumen.

With double-exit drains, lavaging the wound from the proximal tube emergence site exposes the length of the wound tract to the solution. The solution, however, may only follow the path of least resistance, the drain tract, and not reach the crevices of the wound. If pressure is

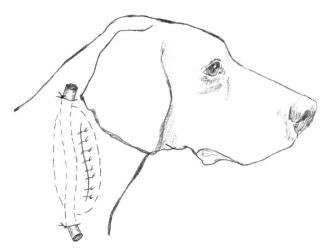

FIG. 2-26. Double-exit drain, exiting proximal and distal to wound. (After Swaim, S.F., and Lee A.H.: Wound drainage techniques. *In* Current Techniques in Small Animal Surgery. 3rd ed. Edited by M.J. Bojrab. Philadelphia, Lea & Febiger, 1990, p. 31.)

applied to the lavage solution or if the distal drain port is occluded, the solution may spread wound debris into normal tissue.

REFERENCES AND SUGGESTED READING

1. Hampel, N.L., and Johnson, R.G.: Principles of surgical drains and drainage. J. Am. Anim. Hosp. Assoc. *21:*21, 1985.
2. Lee, A.H., Swaim, S.F., and Henderson, R.A.: Surgical drainage. Compend. Contin. Educ. *8:*94, 1986.
3. Swaim, S.F., and Lee, A.H.: Wound drainage techniques. *In* Current Techniques in Small Animal Surgery. 3rd ed. Edited by M.J. Bojrab. Philadelphia, Lea & Febiger, 1990, p. 30.

Active Drains

Definition and Indications. Active closed-suction drainage occurs when a vacuum is applied to a drainage tube with no external air vent. The indications for such drainage are the same as for passive drains; however, the wound should be free of foreign material and necrotic tissue, which could plug the drain tube.

Technique. The necessary items for a closed suction drain are a butterfly scalp needle apparatus and a standard 5 to 10 mL evacuated blood collection tube. The syringe adapter of a butterfly scalp needle apparatus is cut off the tubing and holes are cut into the sides of the tubing (Fig. 2-27). After thorough wound lavage and debridement, the fenestrated portion of the tube is inserted through a small puncture wound near the site to be drained, with the puncture wound no larger than the diameter of the tube. The tube is secured to the skin at the puncture hole with a nonabsorbable suture (Fig. 2-28A). After wound closure, the needle on the free end

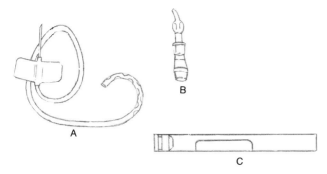

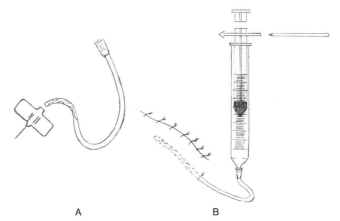

FIG. 2-27. Closed-suction drain. A, Butterfly scalp needle apparatus with fenestrated tube. B, Syringe adapter removed from butterfly scalp needle apparatus. C, Evacuated blood collection tube. (From Swaim, S.F., and Lee, A.H.: Wound drainage techniques. *In* Current Techniques in Small Animal Surgery. 3rd ed. Edited by M.J. Bojrab. Philadelphia, Lea & Febiger, 1990, p. 32.)

FIG. 2-29. Placement of modified closed suction drain. A, Butterfly needle removed from catheter and tube fenestrated. B, Fenestrated tube placed in wound through *small* stab incision and anchored with a suture at incision. Wound closed. Plastic syringe attached to Luer-Lok and plunger withdrawn for desired amount of negative pressure. A metal pin inserted across plunger to hold it at desired level. (From Swaim S.F., and Lee A.H.: Wound drainage techniques. *In* Current Techniques in Small Animal Surgery. 3rd ed. Edited by M.J. Bojrab. Philadelphia, Lea & Febiger, 1990, p. 32.)

of the tube is inserted into a standard 5 to 10 mL evacuated blood collection tube (Fig. 2-28B). A bandage is placed over the wound and the tube incorporated in the bandage. For large wounds, two drain apparatuses may be necessary.

A modification of the closed-suction apparatus can be made with various sized syringes. The butterfly needle is removed from the catheter and the tube is fenestrated. The Luer-Lok is left on the catheter (Fig. 2-29A). The catheter is placed in the wound as previously described, the wound is closed, and a plastic syringe is attached to

the Luer-Lok of the tube. The syringe plunger is withdrawn enough to create the desired negative pressure, then a metal pin is used to hold the plunger at the desired level within the syringe barrel (Fig. 2-29B). A bandage is applied as previously described.

Aftercare. The bandages over the wounds are changed periodically and new vacuum tubes or syringes are placed on the drain tube. When fluid is no longer being drained from the wound, the tacking suture is removed and the tube is taken from the wound.

Advantages and Disadvantages. Closed-suction drains allow wounds and dressings to be kept dry, prevent bacterial ascension through and around the drain, provide continuous drainage to decrease drainage time, and eliminate the need for irrigation. Few complications are encountered with such drains. The volume and nature of the drainage fluid can be accurately assessed. When used under skin grafts, these drains help hold the graft in contact with the wound bed to enhance revascularization and graft "take."

A disadvantage of closed-suction drainage is that high negative pressure may cause injury to the tissues. In a highly productive wound, 10 mL evacuated blood tubes may require several changes daily.

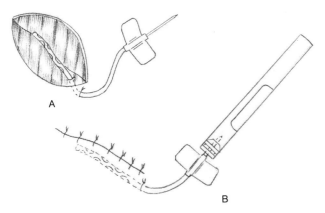

FIG. 2-28. Placement of closed-suction drain. A, Fenestrated end of tube is placed into wound through *small* stab incision. Tube is anchored with a simple interrupted suture at incision. B, Wound is closed and needle of butterfly scalp needle apparatus is inserted into evacuated blood collection tube. (From Swaim, S.F., and Lee, A.H.: Wound drainage techniques. *In* Current Techniques in Small Animal Surgery. 3rd ed. Edited by M.J. Bojrab. Philadelphia, Lea and Febiger, 1990, p. 32.)

REFERENCES AND SUGGESTED READING

See Passive Drains, this chapter.

3

WOUND DRESSING MATERIALS AND TOPICAL MEDICATIONS

WOUND DRESSING MATERIALS

Bandages are generally composed of three layers, each with its own properties and functions. The contact (primary) layer rests on the wound and may be adherent or nonadherent. Adherent bandages are preferred if the wound is in the inflammatory stage of healing, but nonadherent are preferred if it is in the repair stage. The intermediate (secondary) layer is bulky for absorbency and padding. The outer (tertiary) layer holds the other layers in place (Fig. 3-1).

CONTACT BANDAGE LAYER— OPEN WOUNDS

Adherent Materials

Definition and Indications. Adherent bandage material used as the contact bandage layer has wide mesh openings without cotton filler (Fig. 3-2A). The wide mesh entraps loose necrotic tissue and foreign bodies, which are then removed when the dressing is changed. In addition, exudate penetrates the dressing and dries by evaporation, attaching the dressing to the crust or scab that forms.

Adherent bandages are indicated after incomplete surgical debridement. Adherence of the bandage material to the wound helps complete the debridement of the wound each time the dressing is removed. The most common adherent dressings are dry-to-dry and wet-to-

dry dressings. Dry-to-dry dressings are indicated when a wound has copious quantities of a low-viscosity exudate that does not tend to aggregate, but wet-to-dry dressings are used when a viscous exudate is present on the wound surface (Fig. 3-2B).

Technique. *Dry-to-Dry Dressing.* Dry-to-dry dressings are applied to the wound in a dry state and covered with an absorbent intermediate bandage layer and a porous outer bandage layer. Because of the good absorptive capacity of the dry dressing, necrotic tissue and foreign material adhere to it well. The bandage should remain in place until both the contact and intermediate layers have absorbed fluid and debris from the wound, and the fluid has evaporated from the bandage, resulting in a dry contact layer. At this time, the bandage is removed, and with it the entrapped necrotic tissue and foreign debris (Fig. 3-2C).

Wet-to-Dry Dressing. Wide-mesh gauze is applied to the wound from a container of wetting solution such as sterile saline or 1:40 dilution (0.05%) of chlorhexidine diacetate* solution. Alternately, sterile dry gauze may be placed on the wound and then saturated with the wetting solution from a sterilized spray or pour bottle. The wetting solution dilutes the viscous exudate so that it is readily absorbed. The gauze is covered by an absorbent intermediate bandage layer and a porous outer bandage. As the bandage dries by evaporation, necrotic tissue and foreign debris adhere to the bandage and are removed with it (Fig. 3-2C).

Aftercare. All dry-to-dry and wet-to-dry bandages should be changed at least daily. To help make bandage

---

*Nolvasan solution, Fort Dodge Laboratories, Fort Dodge, IA.

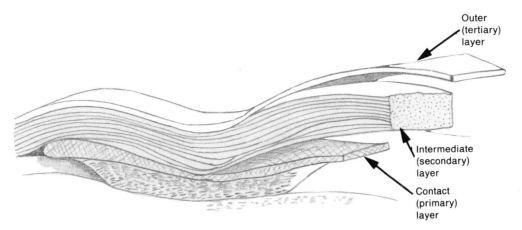

FIG. 3-1. Component layers of a bandage. (From Swaim, S.F., and Wilhalf, D.: The physics, physiology and chemistry of bandaging open wounds. Compend. Contin. Educ. 7:146, 1985).

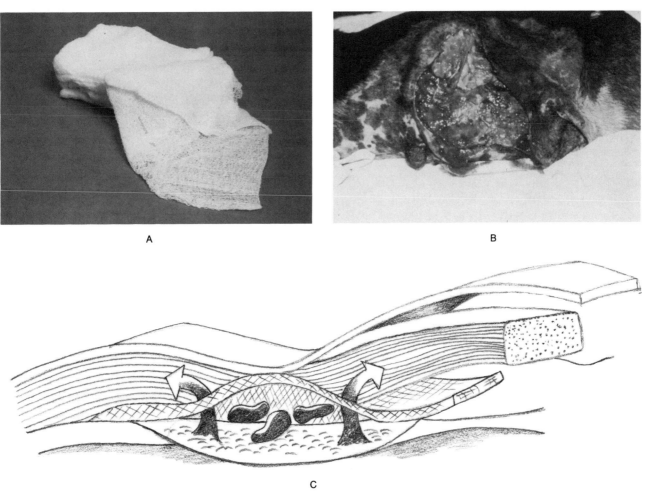

FIG. 3-2. Adherent contact bandage layer. A, Wide mesh gauze. B, Wound on which a wet-to-dry adherent contact layer is indicated because of necrotic tissue, foreign matter, and viscous exudate. C, Principle of dry-to-dry and wet-to-dry adherent contact bandages: Fluid absorbed into intermediate layer and evaporates (arrows). Necrotic tissue and debris adhere to gauze contact layer for removal with bandage change. (B and C, from Swaim, S.F., and Wilhalf, D.: The physics, physiology and chemistry of bandaging open wounds. Compend. Contin. Educ. 7:146, 1985).

changing more comfortable for the animal, the contact layer may be moistened with 2% lidocaine a minute or two before removing it from the wound.

Advantages and Disadvantages. The advantage of adherent dressings is that they provide a means of completing debridement of a contaminated or infected wound. The main disadvantage to adherent bandages is that they are painful to remove and may injure viable cells during dressing changes. In addition, the tissues may become desiccated if they are subjected too long to a dry environment. At the other extreme, if bandages are too wet, tissues may macerate, and if fluid reaches the outer bandage layer, bacteria may move centrally toward the wound. If a 0.05% chlorhexidine solution is used in a wet-to-dry bandage, it may not be sufficient to control a heavy pseudomonas wound infection. Although a 0.1% or 0.5% solution in a bandage may control infection better, these dilutions tend to slow the development of granulation tissue.

REFERENCES AND SUGGESTED READING

1. Bojrab, M.J.: Wound Management. Mod. Vet. Pract. *63*:867, 1982.
2. Lawrence, J.C.: What materials for dressings? Injury *13*:500, 1982.
3. Lee, A.H., Swaim, S.F., McGuire, J.A., and Hughes, K.S.: Effects of chlorhexidine diacetate, povidone iodine, and polyhydroxydine on wound healing in dogs. J. Am. Anim. Hosp. Assoc. *24*:77, 1988.
4. Noe, J.M., and Kalish, S.: The problem of adherence in dressed wounds. Surg. Gynecol. Obstet. *147*:185, 1978.
5. Noe, J.M., and Kalish, S.: Dressing materials and their selection. In Chronic Problem Wounds. Edited by R. Rudolph and J.M. Noe. Boston, Little, Brown and Co., 1983.
6. Rudolph, R., and Noe, J.M.: Initial treatment of the chronic wound. In Chronic Problem Wounds. Edited by R. Rudolph and J.M. Noe, Boston, Little, Brown and Co., 1983.
7. Swaim, S.F., and Wilhalf, D.: The physics, physiology, and chemistry of bandaging open wounds. Compend. Contin. Educ. *7*:146, 1985.

Nonadherent Semiocclusive Materials

Definition and Indications. Nonadherent bandages used as the contact layer are usually classified as semiocclusive because they retain enough moisture to prevent tissue dehydration and promote epithelialization while allowing excess fluid to be absorbed from the wound, thus preventing maceration (Fig. 3-3A). Some of the commercial nonadherent bandages[*,†] have a degree of absorbency also. Autoclaving gauzes with petrolatum or impregnating them with polyethylene glycol or a nitrofurazone/polyethylene glycol combination[‡,§] renders the gauzes nonadherent. Placing a petrolatum-base antibiotic ointment[‖] on gauze also provides a nonadherent bandage (see Antibiotics and Antibacterials, this chapter).

Nonadherent bandages are indicated when a wound is in the reparative stage of healing with a bed of granulation tissue, production of a serosanguineous exudate, and epithelialization occurring from the wound edges (Fig. 3-3B). The nonadherency of the bandage prevents damage to the newly formed tissue when the bandages are changed.

Technique. These dressings are applied to the wound, followed by an absorbent intermediate bandage layer and a porous outer bandage layer. The bandage is left in place for 1 or 2 days depending on the amount of drainage from the wound.

If petrolatum-impregnated gauzes are to be used, they may be prepared by placing a stack of gauzes in a container and spooning petrolatum on them (Fig. 3-3C). The container is covered and autoclaved. The petrolatum melts and wicks through the gauzes by gravity. At each bandage change, the cover is removed from the container, and a gauze is removed from the top of the stack and placed on the wound. If this type of petrolatum gauze or a commercial petrolatum gauze[#] is used, its use should be discontinued in favor of a nonadherent dressing that does not contain petrolatum when epithelium begins to grow over the granulation tissue.

Semiocclusive nonadherent nitrofurazone/polyethylene glycol gauze is prepared by applying a thin layer of the medication on the gauze with a tongue depressor just before placing it on the wound. Semiocclusive nonadherent petrolatum-base antibiotic ointment gauze is prepared in a similar manner.

Aftercare. Bandages are left in place for 1 to 2 days, depending on the amount of drainage from the wound.

Advantages and Disadvantages. Nonadherent bandages provide a suitable environment for healing, and bandage removal does not interfere with wound healing. Nitrofurazone/polyethylene glycol gauzes have the advantage of being antibacterial and hydrophilic. The hydrophilic property draws homeostatic fluid through the tissues to bathe the wound and dilute wound coagulum so that it can be absorbed. Gauzes with petrolatum-base antibiotic ointment provide antibacterial activity along with nonadherence. Wounds covered with nonadherent bandages impregnated with

---

*Release-nonadhering dressing, Johnson & Johnson, New Brunswick, NJ.

†Telfa Adhesive Pads, The Kendall Co., Hospital Products, Boston, MA.

‡Furacin dressing, Norden Laboratories, Inc., Lincoln, NE.

§Nitrofurazone solution 0.2%, Tech America Vet. Prod., Kansas City, MO.

‖Neosporin ointment, Burroughs Wellcome, Research, Triangle Park, NC.

#Adaptic-nonadhering dressing, Johnson & Johnson, New Brunswick, NJ.

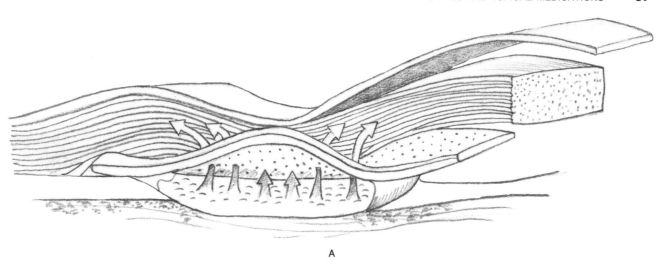

A

FIG. 3-3. Nonadherent contact bandage layer. A, Principle of nonadherent contact bandages: Excess fluid absorbed into intermediate layer and evaporates (long arrows). Some fluid retained (short arrows).

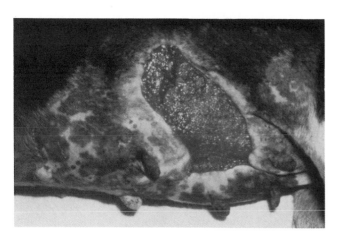

B

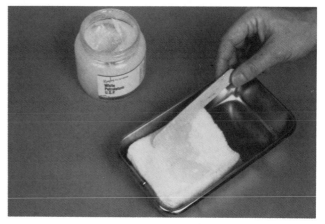

C

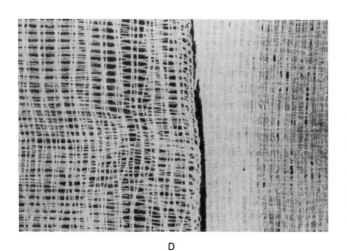

D

B, Wound on which a nonadherent contact layer is indicated because of granulation tissue, serosanguineous exudate, and epithelialization beginning. C, Making petrolatum non-adherent gauzes: Placing petrolatum on gauzes before autoclaving them. D, Problem of inconsistency with nonadherent sponges prepared by autoclaving petrolatum and gauze: Left, top gauze of stack has light coating; Right, bottom gauze of stack has occlusive coating. (A, from Swaim, S.F., and Wilhalf, D.: The physics, physiology and chemistry of bandaging open wounds. Compend. Contin. Educ. *7*:146, 1985; B from Swaim, S.F.: Etiology, pathophysiology and management of soft tissue wounds. Amer. Anim. Hosp. Assoc. Sci. Proc. 457, 1982; D, from Lee, A.H., Swaim, S.F., McGuire, J.A., and Hughes, K.S.: Effects of nonadherent dressing materials on the healing of open wounds in dogs. J. Amer. Vet. Med. Assoc. *190*:416, 1987).

petrolatum tend to epithelialize more slowly than wounds covered with other types of nonadherent bandages. Petrolatum-impregnated gauzes prepared by autoclaving result in an inconsistent deposition of petrolatum. Gauzes at the top of the stack are impregnated lightly, but the bottom of the stack may become so heavily impregnated that the interstices are occluded, creating an occlusive bandage (Fig. 3-3D). Because little or no fluid can drain from beneath these bandages, they may lead to tissue maceration.

REFERENCES AND SUGGESTED READING

1. Bojrab, M.J.: Wound management. Mod. Vet. Pract. *63*:867, 1982.
2. Eaglstein, W.H., and Mertz, P.M.: "Inert" vehicles do affect wound healing. J. Invest. Dermatol. *74*:90, 1980.
3. Eaglstein, W.H., and Mertz, P.M.: Effect of topical medicaments on the rate of repair of superficial wounds. *In* The Surgical Wound. Edited by P. Dineen and G. Hildick-Smith. Philadelphia, Lea & Febiger, 1981.
4. Lee, A.H., Swaim, S.F., Yang, S.T., Wilken, L.O., Miller, D.P., Wilt, G.R., and Hughes, K.S.: The effects of petrolatum, polyethylene glycol, nitrofurazone, and a hydroactive dressing on open wound healing. J. Am. Anim. Hosp. Assoc. *22*:443, 1986.
5. Lee, A.H., Swaim, S.F., McGuire, J.A., and Hughes, K.S.: Effects of nonadherent dressing materials on the healing of open wounds in dogs. J. Am. Vet. Med. Assoc. *190*:416, 1987.
6. Linsky, C.B., Rovee, D.T., and Low, T.: Effects of dressings on wound inflammation and scar tissue. *In* The Surgical Wound. Edited by P. Dineen and G. Hildick-Smith. Philadelphia, Lea & Febiger, 1981.
7. Noe, J.M., and Kalish, S.: The mechanism of capillarity in surgical dressings. Surg. Gynecol. Obstet. *143*:454, 1976.
8. Noe, J.M., and Kalish, S.: The problem of adherence in dressed wounds. Surg. Gynecol. Obstet. *147*:185, 1978.
9. Noe, J.M., and Kalish, S.: Dressing materials and their selection. *In* Chronic Problem Wounds. Edited by R. Rudolph and J.M. Noe. Boston, Little, Brown and Co., 1983.
10. Swaim, S.F., and Wilhalf, D.: The physics, physiology and chemistry of bandaging open wounds. Compend. Contin. Educ. *7*:146, 1985.

Nonadherent Occlusive Material

Definition and Indications. An occlusive nonadherent bandage material is commercially available. It is composed of a hydrocolloid material on one surface* (Fig. 3-4A). The hydrocolloid over the skin around the wound adheres to this skin, but the hydrocolloid over the wound absorbs wound fluids to create a nonadherent occlusive hydrocolloid gel.

Hydrocolloid bandages are indicated for covering wounds in the repair stage of healing, that is, wounds with an established granulation tissue bed, advanced contraction, decreased fluid production, and the beginning of epithelialization.

Technique. The skin around the wound should be cleaned and dried and the surface of the granulation tissue gently wiped with an antiseptic solution. The package containing the hydrocolloid dressing is warmed between the surgeon's hands to soften the hydrocolloid material and make it moldable to the body contours. The material is cut to the proper shape and size before the covering is peeled off (Fig. 3-4B). After the covering is removed from the hydrocolloid surface of the dressing, it is centered over the wound (Fig. 3-4C). Light pressure is applied around the edges of the bandage until it adheres to the skin (Fig. 3-4D).

Aftercare. The dressing is left in place for 2 to 3 days or until the outer surface of the dressing over the wound feels like a fluid-filled blister. At this time, the dressing is removed, the gel is wiped from the wound surface and surrounding skin, and a second dressing may be applied. If the wound produces more fluid than anticipated and the gel begins to leak from under its edge, the dressing should be changed. When epithelium covers the wound, these dressings are discontinued.

Advantages and Disadvantages. Wounds dressed with hydrocolloid material epithelialize more rapidly than those dressed with semiocclusive material. Wound contraction, however, is reduced because adherence of the hydrocolloid material to the skin around the wound splints the wound edges against wound contractile elements. The hydrocolloid gel is tenacious and may be difficult to clean from the skin surrounding the wound.

REFERENCES AND SUGGESTED READING

1. Alvarez, O.M., Mertz, P.M, and Eaglstein, W.H.: The effect of occlusive dressings on collagen synthesis and reepithelialization in superficial wounds. J. Surg. Res. *35*:142, 1983.
2. Lee, A.H., Swaim, S.F., Yang, S.L., Wilken, L.O., Miller, D.P., Wilt, G.R., Hughes, K.S.: The effects of petrolatum, polyethylene glycol, nitrofurazone, and a hydroactive dressing on open wounds. J. Am. Anim. Hosp. Assoc. *22*:443, 1986.
3. Leipziger, L.S., Glushkov, DiBernado, B., Shafaie, F., Noble, J., Nichols, J., and Alvarez, O.M.: Dermal wound repair: Role of collagen matrix implants and synthetic polymer dressings. J. Amer. Acad. Dermatol. *12*:2, 1985.

CONTACT BANDAGE LAYER— CLOSED WOUNDS

Definition and Indications. As with open wounds, this is the layer that contacts the wound. It serves to absorb fluid that drains from the wound.

---

*Dermaheal, Solvay Veterinary, Inc., Princeton, NJ.

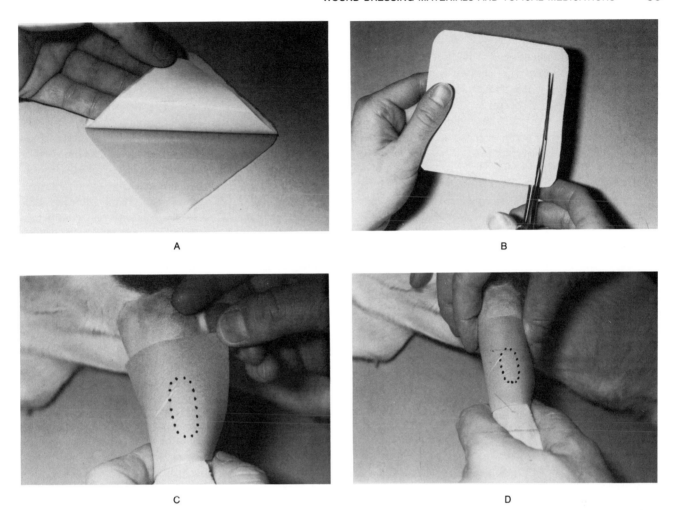

FIG. 3-4. Nonadherent occlusive material. A, Commercially available nonadherent bandage material. Covering being removed from hydrocolloid bandage surface. B, Trimming bandage material before removing covering. C, Hydrocolloid dressing surface centered over wound (dotted line) as bandage is applied. D, Light pressure around bandage edges adheres it to skin but not wound. Dotted line = underlying wound.

Technique.   On a closed wound that will have minimal to no drainage, a nonadherent dressing pad*,† with some absorptive properties is indicated. On a closed wound that will have a drain, several layers of wide-mesh absorbent gauzes should be placed over the end of the drain.

Aftercare.   The frequency of bandage change depends on the amount of wound drainage. With little or no drainage, the bandage may be removed after 7 days. With heavy drainage, it should be changed daily.

Advantages and Disadvantages.   The nonadherent bandage over a wound with slight or no drainage allows

absorption of that drainage and is comfortable because it does not adhere to the wound. With a heavily draining wound, observation of the gauzes placed over the drain informs the surgeon of the amount and nature of wound drainage so that drain removal can be performed when drainage becomes minimal and of serosanguineous nature.

REFERENCES AND SUGGESTED READING

1. Bojrab, M.J.: A Handbook of Veterinary Wound Management. Boston, Kendall Co., 1981.
2. Lee, A.H., Swaim, S.F., and Henderson, R.A.: Surgical Drainage. Compend. Contin. Educ. *8*:94, 1986.
3. Swaim, S.F., and Lee, A.H.: Wound drainage techniques. *In* Current Techniques in Small Animal Surgery. 3rd ed. Edited by M.J., Bojrab. Philadelphia, Lea & Febiger, 1990, p. 30.

*Release-nonadhering dressing, Johnson & Johnson, New Brunswick, NJ.

†Telfa Adhesive Pads, The Kendall Co., Hospital Products, Boston, MA.

INTERMEDIATE BANDAGE LAYER

Definition and Indications. The intermediate bandage layer that overlies the contact bandage layer is primarily absorptive, so it should have good capillary action[*,†] (Fig. 3-5A). Absorption of exudate removes bacteria from the wound. The intermediate bandage layer also serves as a protective pad from trauma and as a splint to retard movement.

Technique. When a bandage is applied to a wound, the contact layer should remain in close contact with the wound, and the intermediate layer in close contact with the contact layer to promote maximum absorption. Excessive pressure should not be applied to attain this contact, however. Pressure over the intermediate layer governs the amount of fluid absorbed from the wound, and excessive pressure limits the absorptive capacity of the bandage (Fig. 3-5B) and may induce pressure sores or restrict vascular flow.

Aftercare. The bandage should be changed frequently (at least daily) on heavily draining wounds to remove exudate that has been absorbed into the bandage. It is changed less often when wounds reach the reparative stage of healing. When the bandage is changed, unwrapping the intermediate bandage layer is less painful than trying to manipulate scissors through it.

Advantages and Disadvantages. The main advantage of the intermediate bandage layer is its ability to absorb and store exudate away from the wound. If the bandage allows evaporation of fluid from absorbed exudate, the partially dry atmosphere of concentrated exudate retards bacterial growth. If a wound is highly productive, however, evaporation cannot keep up with absorption, and if the bandage is not changed frequently enough, the wound fluids serve as a culture media for bacteria in the bandage.

REFERENCES AND SUGGESTED READING

1. Bojrab, M.J.: Wound management. Mod. Vet. Pract. *63*:867, 1982.
2. Noe, J.M., and Kalish, S.: The mechanism of capillarity in surgical dressings. Surg. Gynecol. Obstet. *143*:454, 1976.
3. Noe, J.M., and Kalish, S.: Dressing materials and their selection. *In* Chronic Problem Wounds. Edited by R. Rudolph, J.M. Noe. Boston, Little, Brown and Co., 1983.
4. Swaim, S.F., and Wilhalf, D.: The physics, physiology and chemistry of bandaging open wounds. Compend. Contin. Educ. *7*:146, 1985.

*Sof-Band bulky bandage, Johnson and Johnson, New Brunswick, NJ.
†Kerlix roll, The Kendall Co., Hospital Products, Boston, MA.

OUTER BANDAGE LAYER

Porous Adhesive Tape

Definition and Indications. The outer bandage layer serves to hold the other bandage layers in place. Porous adhesive tape provides one type of outer bandage layer (Fig. 3-6A). This material is indicated for wounds producing exudate or transudate because the evaporation of the fluid through the tape creates a partially dry atmosphere.

Technique. Tape may be applied over the underlying bandage materials by rolling it *carefully* off the roll. Pulling a length of tape off the bandage roll while securing the tape near the bandage with one hand is best because tension can be adjusted (Fig. 3-6B). An alternative is pre-tearing strips of tape and applying them to the bandage (Fig. 3-6C). Each wrap of tape should overlap the previous wrap. At the ends of the bandage, the tape should overlap, with half the tape width on the bandage and the other half on the skin. Additional wraps as needed may incorporate hair or be wrapped around the trunk to prevent slippage.

Aftercare. On heavily draining wounds, the bandage should be changed at least daily to remove exudate that has been absorbed. Bandage changes may be less frequent on wounds in the reparative stage of healing. Wound fluid that reaches the outer bandage layer predisposes to exogenous bacterial contamination, so the bandage should be changed immediately if wound fluid is noticed or the outer layer of the bandage becomes wet.

Advantages and Disadvantages. Evaporation of fluid from the bandage and wound is the primary advantage of porous adhesive tape. The adhesive nature of the tape helps affix the ends of the bandage to the skin to prevent slippage and loss.

The pores of the tape, which allow evaporation of fluid from the bandage, also allow the ingress of exogenous fluid into the bandage, which could result in secondary contamination of the wound. The adherence of the tape to the skin can cause pain and irritation when a bandage is removed.

REFERENCES AND SUGGESTED READING

1. Bojrab: M.J.: Wound Management. Mod. Vet. Pract. *63*:867, 1982.
2. Swaim, S.F., and Wilhalf, D.: The physics, physiology, and chemistry of bandaging open wounds. Compend. Contin. Educ. *7*:146, 1985.

Elastic Adhesive Tape—Pressure Bandage

Definition and Indications. Elastic adhesive tape is compliant (Fig. 3-7A) and applies continuous, dynamic pressure to the wound as the patient moves. Pressure

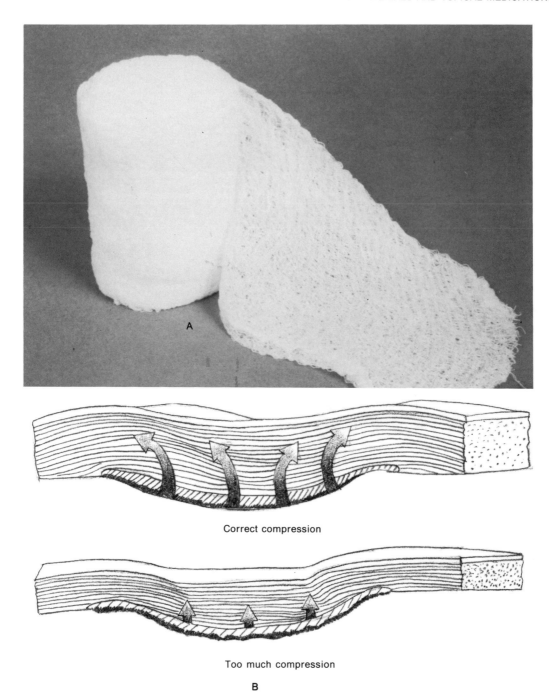

FIG. 3-5. Intermediate bandage layer. A, Material with strong capillarity for absorption. B, Application of intermediate bandage layer: Correct compression = proper absorption (longer arrows). Too much compression = poor absorption (shorter arrows). (B after Swaim, S.F., and Wilhalf, D.: The physics, physiology and chemistry of bandaging open wounds. Compend. Contin. Educ. *7*:146, 1985).

application is indicated to help control minor hemorrhage; however, a pressure pack should not be used for more than 24 to 48 hours. Pressure bandages may also be used to help control edema around a wound; pressure controls transudative passive edema more effectively than exudative inflammatory edema. Pressure bandages are also helpful in containing exuberant granulation tissue below the level of the skin.

Technique. The elastic adhesive tape should be wrapped over the underlying bandage materials carefully so that even but not excessive pressure is applied. Pulling a length of tape off the bandage roll while

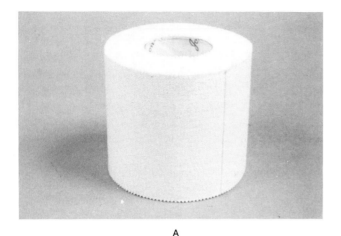

A

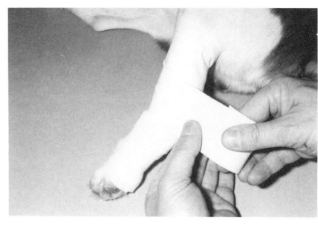

B

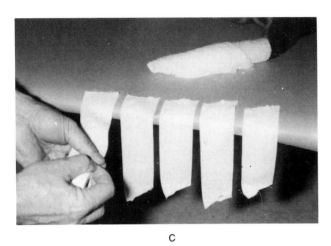

C

FIG. 3-6. Outer bandage layer. A, Porous adhesive tape. B, Applying tape from roll: Pulling a length of tape off roll while holding tape near bandage with one hand. C, Pretearing tape strips before application.

securing the tape near the bandage with one hand helps ensure application of that length of tape under the proper tension (Fig. 3-7B). Each wrap of the tape should overlap the previous wrap by 1/3 to 1/2 (Fig. 3-7C).

When pressure bandages are applied to a limb, the third and fourth digits should be left exposed just enough that they can be used for monitoring sensation and circulation.

When elastic tape is applied over a very convex surface (such as the point of the hock or elbow), efforts should be made to reduce the amount of pressure over these areas. The more convex the surface, the greater is the pressure exerted by the bandage on the surface. With this phenomenon, the added compression of an elastic tape over such an area could cause pressure problems. Additional padding over such surfaces tends to increase rather than decrease pressure (Fig. 3-7D and E).

Aftercare. The exposed digits on a limb should be observed for hypothermia, swelling, and loss of sensation, signs that the bandage may be too tight. In addition, the animal may lick or chew the bandage,

indicating that it is too tight. When any of these signs are observed, the bandages should be removed and the limb examined.

Advantages and Disadvantages. The advantages of pressure bandages are related to their indications. In addition, elastic tapes tend to adhere to themselves; therefore, minimal external taping is needed to affix the bandage in place. There is no discomfort with bandage removal because the tape does not adhere to the skin. The primary disadvantages of pressure bandages are circulatory impairment and ischemic necrosis, as well as neuropathies if they are applied too tightly.

REFERENCES AND SUGGESTED READING

1. Bojrab, M.J.: Wound Management. Mod. Vet. Pract. 63:867, 1982.
2. Knecht, C.D., Allen, A.R., Williams, D.J., and Johnson, J.H.: Fundamental Techniques in Veterinary Surgery. 3rd ed. Philadelphia, WB Saunders, 1987.

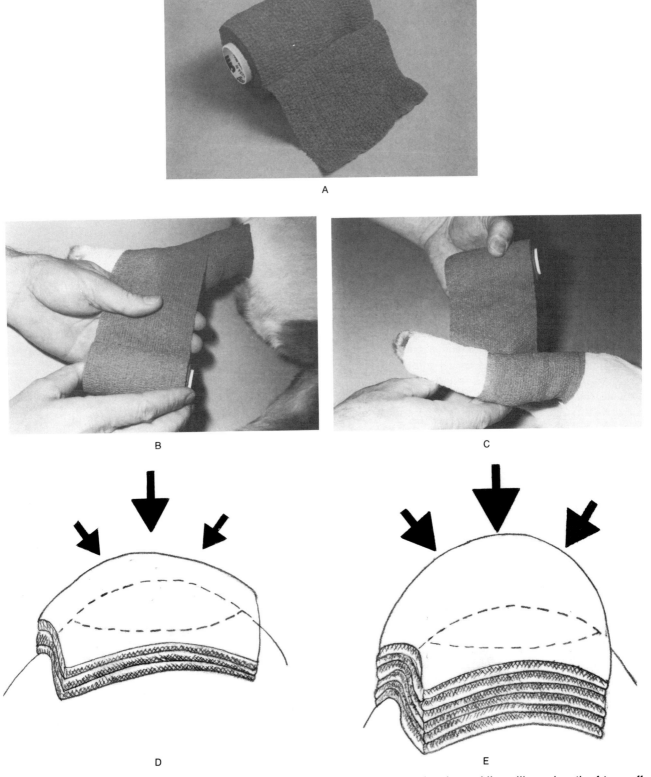

FIG. 3-7. Outer bandage layer. A, Elastic adhesive tape. B, Securing tape near bandage while pulling a length of tape off roll. C, Each tape wrap overlaps previous wrap. D, Bandage padding over a convex surface increases pressure over surface. E, Additional padding on a convex surface further increases pressure. (D and E from Swaim, S.F., and Wilhalf, D.: The physics, physiology and chemistry of bandaging open wounds. Compend. Contin. Educ. *7*:146, 1985).

3. Noe, J.M., and Kalish, S.: Dressing materials and their selection. *In* Chronic Problem Wounds. Edited by R. Rudolph and J.M. Noe. Boston, Little, Brown and Co., 1983.
4. Swaim, S.F., and Wilhalf, D.: The physics, physiology and chemistry of bandaging open wounds. Compend. Contin. Educ. *7*:146, 1985.

Waterproof Adhesive Tape

Definition and Indications. Waterproof adhesive tape is nonporous and creates an occlusive bandage (Fig. 3-8A) that protects the wound from exogenous fluid and bacteria. Waterproof tape is indicated as the outer bandage layer for relatively dry wounds and those that need to be protected from exogenous contamination because its slick surface makes it more difficult for the animal to remove the tape or contaminate it with saliva (Fig. 3-8B).

Technique. See Porous Adhesive Tape, this chapter.

Aftercare. If retention of large amounts of fluid (endogenous or exogenous) in the bandage is suspected, the bandage should be changed.

Advantages and Disadvantages. The advantages of waterproof tape are related to its indications. It may help to waterproof a bandage and aid in preventing wound molestation. If fluid does get into the bandage, however, or if the wound is producing considerable exudate, the tissues may become macerated as a result of fluid retention. In addition, the moist environment favors bacterial growth.

REFERENCE

1. Swaim, S.F., and Wilhalf, D.: The physics, physiology, and chemistry of bandaging open wounds. Compend. Contin. Educ. *7*:146, 1985.

TOPICAL MEDICATIONS

The medications discussed in this chapter do not constitute an exhaustive list of the topical agents used to treat wounds, but information on some of the substances used by the authors in wound management is presented.

WOUND LAVAGE SOLUTIONS

Isotonic Saline, Lactated Ringer's, or Ringer's Solutions

Definition and Indications. Isotonic saline, lactated Ringer's or Ringer's solution may be used for lavaging contaminated or infected wounds to reduce the bacterial numbers in the wound by means of their washing action.

Technique. See Layer Debridement, Chapter 2.

Aftercare. Wound lavage with isotonic saline, lactated Ringer's, or Ringer's solution requires no special aftercare.

Advantages and Disadvantages. These solutions are isotonic, isosmotic, and sterile and therefore are physiologic, causing no damage to the tissues. When such solutions are used in large quantities to lavage a

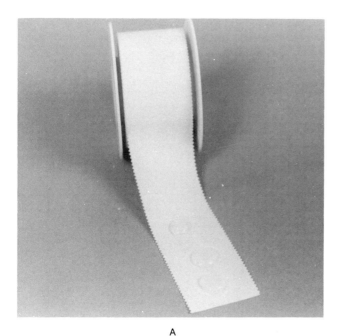

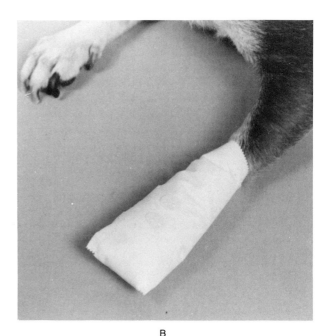

A

B

FIG. 3-8. Outer bandage layer. A, Nonporous waterproof adhesive tape. B, Nonporous waterproof adhesive tape as outer bandage layer. Note beads of water on tape surface.

wound, there may be some tissue retention, appearing as edema. These solutions do not have antibacterial properties and depend on the mechanical process of lavage to rid the wound of bacteria and debris.

REFERENCES AND SUGGESTED READING

1. Aron, D.N.: Management of musculoskeletal injuries. Semin. Vet. Med. Surg. 3:290, 1988.
2. Daly, W.R.: Wound infections. In Textbook of Small Animal Surgery. Edited by D.H. Slatter. Philadelphia, W.B. Saunders, 1985.

Chlorhexidine

Definition and Indications. Although available in several forms, chlorhexidine used for wound lavage should be in diacetate form*, prepared as a 0.05% solution by diluting 1 part of 2% stock solution with 40 parts of water. The solution is indicated for lavaging contaminated or infected wounds to reduce bacterial numbers and expose any remaining bacteria to its antimicrobial activity.

Technique. See Layer Debridement, Chapter 2.

Aftercare. Wound lavage with chlorhexidine requires no special aftercare.

Advantages and Disadvantages. Chlorhexidine has a wide spectrum of antimicrobial activity and a sustained residual activity. Systemic absorption, toxicosis, and inactivation by organic matter do not seem to be disadvantages of chlorhexidine. When diluted with physiologic saline, chlorhexidine diacetate forms a precipitate. Some gram-negative bacteria appear to be highly resistant to chlorhexidine.

REFERENCES AND SUGGESTED READING

1. Amber E.I., Henderson, R.A., Swaim, S.F., and Gray, B.W.: A comparison of antimicrobial efficacy and tissue reaction of four antiseptics on canine wounds. Vet. Surg. 12:63, 1983.
2. Amber E.I., and Swaim, S.F.: An update on common wound antiseptics. Aust. Vet. Pract. 14:29, 1984.
3. Lee, A.H., Swaim, S.F., McGuire, J.A., and Hughes, K.S.: The effects of chlorhexidine diacetate, povidone iodine, and polyhydroxydine on wound healing in dogs. J. Amer. Anim. Hosp. Assoc. 24:77, 1988.
4. Platt, J., and Bucknall, R.A.: An experimental evaluation of antiseptic wound irrigation. J. Hosp. Infect. 5:181, 1984.
5. Russell, A.D.: Chlorhexidine: Antibacterial action and bacterial resistance. Infection 14:212, 1986.
6. Sebben, J.E.: Surgical antiseptics. J. Amer. Acad. Dermatol. 9:759, 1983.

*Nolvasan solution Fort Dodge Laboratories, Fort Dodge, IA.
†Betadine solution, The Purdue Frederick Co., Norwalk, CT.

7. Swaim, S.F., and Lee, A.H.: Topical wound medications: A review. J. Am. Vet. Med. Assoc. 190:1588, 1987.

Povidone Iodine

Definition and Indications. Povidone iodine is a complex of iodine with polyvinylpyrrolidone.† It slowly releases iodine from the complex as "free iodine," which provides the antimicrobial efficacy. Dilute solutions have been found more bactericidal in vitro than full-strength solutions, because more available "free iodine" is present in the weaker solutions. Povidone iodine is indicated as an antiseptic for lavaging contaminated and infected wounds to reduce bacterial numbers and expose any remaining bacteria to its antimicrobial activity.

Technique. See Layer Debridement, Chapter 2. Wounds should be thoroughly cleansed of blood, exudate, and organic soil before application of povidone iodine. A 1% dilution of stock solution can be prepared by diluting 1 part of solution (10% povidone iodine) with 9 parts of sterile water or electrolyte solution. If povidone iodine lavage is the only topical medication applied to the wound, it should be applied often during the day because it has only a 4 to 6 hour bactericidal activity.

Aftercare. Wound lavage with povidone iodine requires no special aftercare.

Advantages and Disadvantages. Povidone iodine provides a broad spectrum of antimicrobial activity. Complexing iodine with polyvinylpyrrolidone eliminates the staining, instability, and irritation of free iodine; however, it also decreases the bactericidal activity of the iodine.

The inactivation of povidone iodine by blood, exudate, and organic soil is a disadvantage because it results in a short residual action of povidone iodine.

Povidone iodine is systemically absorbed, and excess systemic iodine concentration can result from absorption through the skin, mucous membranes, severe burns, large wounds, and body cavities. Newborn infants have been reported to be particularly sensitive to iodine exposure, with resulting transient hypothyroidism. If the thyroid glands and kidneys are normal, transient nonclinical hypothyroidism may result. Clinical hypothyroidism, however, has been reported in human burn patients treated with povidone iodine. Clinical hyperthyroidism and thyroid hyperplasia have also been reported with povidone iodine use. The low pH of povidone iodine can cause or exacerbate metabolic acidosis when it is absorbed; therefore it should be used with discretion, especially in large wounds or exposed body cavities.

The detergent form of povidone iodine has been found deleterious to wound tissues. Such detergents are irritating and can potentiate wound infection.

REFERENCES AND SUGGESTED READING

1. Amber, E.I., Henderson, R.A., Swaim, S.F., and Gray, B.W.: A comparison of antimicrobial efficacy and tissue reaction of four antiseptics on canine wounds. Vet. Surg. 12:63, 1983.
2. Amber, E.I., and Swaim, S.F.: An update on common wound antiseptics. Aust. Vet. Pract. 14:29, 1984.
3. Balogh, D., Bauer, M., and Riccabona, G.: The influence of povidone-iodine treatment on thyroid hormones in severe burns. J. Hosp. Infect. 6:(Suppl):147, 1985.
4. Berkelman, R.L., Holland, B.W., and Anderson R.L.: Increased bactericidal activity of dilute preparations of povidone-iodine solution. J. Clin. Microbiol. 15:635, 1982.
5. Georgiade, N.G., and Harris, W.A.: Open and closed treatment of wounds with povidone-iodine. Plast. Reconst. Surg. 52:640, 1973.
6. L'Allemand, D., Gruters, A., Heidemann, P., and Schurnbrand, P.: Iodine-induced alterations of thyroid function in newborn infants after prenatal and perinatal exposure to povidone-iodine. J. Pediatr. 102:935, 1983.
7. Mertz, P.M., Alvarez, O.M., Smerbeck, R.V., and Eaglstein, W.H.: A new in vivo model for evaluation of topical antiseptics on superficial wounds. Arch. Dermatol. 120:58, 1984.
8. Pietsch, J., Meakins, J.L.: Complications of povidone-iodine absorption in topically treated burn patients. Lancet 1:280, 1976.
9. Rodeheaver, G., Bellamy, W., Kody, E.M., Spatafora, G., Fitton, L., Leyden, K., and Edlich, R.: Bactericidal activity and toxicity of iodine-containing solutions in wounds. Arch. Surg. 117:181, 1982.
10. Schneider, W., Ahuja, S., Klebe, I.: Clinical and bacteriological studies of the polyvinylpyrrolidone-iodine complex. In World Congress on Antisepsis. New York, PH Publishing Co., 1976.
11. Silva, J.E.: Effects of iodine and iodine containing compounds on thyroid function. Med. Clin. North Am. 69:881, 1985.
12. Swaim, S.F., and Lee, A.H: Topical wound medications: A review. J. Am. Vet. Assoc. 190:1588, 1987.
13. Viljanto, J: Disinfection of surgical wounds without inhibition of normal wound healing. Arch. Surg. 115:253, 1980.
14. Zamora, J.L.: Povidone-iodine and wound infection. Surgery 95:121, 1984.

Hydrogen Peroxide
Definition and Indications. Hydrogen peroxide is a commonly used wound irrigant that is converted into a foam of water and oxygen when it contacts wound tissue. When used, hydrogen peroxide should be reserved for one-time initial irrigation of dirty wounds that may contain anaerobic organisms.

Technique. Hydrogen peroxide may be used to irrigate wounds but should not be delivered to wounds under pressure, as are other lavage solutions. Because of its foaming expansion, pressure delivery or restricted drainage forces the agent and debris between tissue planes, enlarging the wound and creating emphysema of the tissues.

Aftercare. Wound lavage with hydrogen peroxide requires no special aftercare.

*Clorox, The Clorox Co., Oakland, CA.

Advantages and Disadvantages. The foaming action of hydrogen peroxide may be beneficial in removing dirt and debris from deep wounds when used in initial wound management. It may also be beneficial for removing clots from wounds and in obtaining hemostasis. Hydrogen peroxide has little value as an antiseptic because of its minimal bactericidal potency. It is more effective as a sporicide. It injures cells in the commercially available 3% solution and even at lower concentrations.

REFERENCES AND SUGGESTED READING

1. Baldry, M.G.C.: The bactericidal, fungicidal and sporicidal properties of hydrogen peroxide and peracetic acid. J. Appl. Bacteriol. 54:417, 1983.
2. Lineweaver, W., McMorris, S., Soucy, D., and Howard, R.: Cellular and bacterial toxicities of topical antimicrobials. Plast. Reconst. Surg. 75:394, 1985.
3. Lineweaver, W., Howard, R., Soucy, D., McMorris, S., Freeman, J., Crain, C., Robertson, J., and Rumley, T.: Topical antimicrobial toxicity. Arch. Surg. 120:267, 1985.
4. Lineweaver, W., McMorris., S., and Howard, R.: Effects of topical disinfectants and antibiotics on human fibroblasts. Surg. Forum 33:37, 1982.
5. Reybrouck, G.: The bactericidal activity of aqueous disinfectants applied on living tissues. Pharm. Weekbl. (Sci.) 7:100, 1985.
6. Stringer, M.D., Lawrence, J.C., and Lilly, H.A.: Antiseptics and the casualty wound. J. Hosp. Infect. 4:410, 1983.
7. Swaim, S.F., and Lee, A.H.: Topical wound medications: A review. J. Am. Vet. Med. Assoc. 190:1588, 1987.

Dakin's Solution
Definition and Indications. Dakin's solution is a 0.5% solution of sodium hypochlorite*, which can be prepared at one-tenth the strength of commercial laundry bleaches. It was first used as an effective irrigant of human wounds in World War I. Free chlorine and oxygen are released into the tissues to kill bacteria and liquify tissue debris.

Technique. See Layer Debridement, Chapter 2. Half-strength (0.25%) Dakin's solution is used on most human wounds. This may be prepared using the following formula:

1 liter Dakin's solution:
Sodium hypochlorite 5%	50 ml
Sodium bicarbonate	30 ml
Sterile distilled water Q.S.A.D.	1000 ml

If half-strength Dakin's solution causes discomfort, quarter-strength (0.125%) solution has been advocated, and this is the authors' preferred dilution for use in animal wounds. Once the solution is prepared, it will deteriorate within a few days, and therefore it should be used promptly. The solution should be protected from light.

Aftercare. Lavaging a wound with Dakin's solution requires no special aftercare.

Advantages and Disadvantages. Dakin's solution has been found more effective than either chlorhexidine or povidone-iodine against *Staphylococcus aureus*, a common wound contaminant. Full-strength solution, however, retards wound epithelialization in rats.

REFERENCES AND SUGGESTED READING

1. Lineweaver, W., Howard, R., Soucy, D., McMorris, S. Freeman, J., Crain, C., Robertson, J., Rumley, T.: Topical antimicrobial toxicity. Arch. Surg. *120*:267, 1985.
2. Reybrouck, G.: The bactericidal activity of aqueous disinfectants applied on living tissues. Pharm. Weekbl. (Sci.) *7*:100, 1985.
3. Rudolph, R., Fisher, J.C., and Ninneman, J.L.: Skin Grafting. Boston Little, Brown and Co., 1979.
4. Rudolph, R., Noe, J.M.: Initial treatment of the chronic wound. *In* Chronic Problem Wounds. Edited by R. Rudolph and J.M. Noe. Boston, Little, Brown and Co., 1983.
5. Swaim, S.F., and Lee A.H.: Topical wound medications: A review. J. Am. Vet. Med. Assoc. *190*:1588, 1987.

ANTIBIOTICS AND ANTIBACTERIALS

Bacitracin–Neomycin–Polymixin

Definition and Indications. Bacitracin, neomycin, and polymixin are three bactericidal antibiotics that are commonly combined in a petrolatum base* for topical application, generally to smaller wounds.

Technique. These three antibiotics are usually in the form of an ointment and may be placed on a piece of gauze to make a nonadherent semiocclusive contact bandage or on a commerical nonadherent dressing (see Nonadherent Semiocclusive Materials, this chapter). Because of poor absorption by the wound tissues, these agents should be placed on the wound in an early stage, before the organisms invade the tissues. The wound should be covered by a bandage.

Aftercare. When bacitracin, neomycin, and polymixin ointment are used, the skin around the wound should be observed for evidence of possible allergic reaction to the drugs, especially neomycin. Bandages should be changed as necessary according to the amount of wound drainage and clinical judgment. Bandages are changed more frequently in the early stages of wound healing.

Advantages and Disadvantages. The primary advantage of bacitracin-neomycin-polymixin is its wide spectrum of bactericidal activity. Neomycin is particularly effective against *Staphylococcus aureus* and bacitracin against *Streptococcus pyogenes*. Neomycin and polymyxin provide coverage against some gram-negative organisms. These antibiotics stimulate re-epithelialization of wounds, and it has been determined that the zinc bacitracin component is responsible for this enhanced healing. When they are used in ointment form on a fine mesh gauze, the contact layer of a bandage may be rendered nonadherent. Its poor absorption by the tissues can be both advantageous and disadvantageous. It is advantageous from the standpoint that high concentrations of the antibiotics can be applied to the wound without fear of systemic absorption and toxicity. The disadvantage is that these antibiotics are not as effective on infected wounds. With massive topical application on large wounds, systemic absorption is possible, and systemic side effects such as nephrotoxicity, ototoxicity, and neurotoxicity may occur. A disadvantage of the triple antibiotics is their ineffectiveness against *Pseudomonas* species.

REFERENCES AND SUGGESTED READING

1. Eaglstein, W.H., Mertz, P., and Alvarez, O.M.: Effects of topically applied agents on healing wounds. Clin. in Dermatol. *2*:112, 1984.
2. Glotzer, D.J., Goodman, W.S., and Geronimus, L.H.: Topical antibiotic prophylaxis in contaminated wounds. Arch. Surg. *100*:589, 1970.
3. Leyden, J.J., and Sulzberger, M.B.: Topical antibiotics and minor skin trauma. Am. Fam. Physician *23*:121, 1982.
4. Noyes, H.E., Chi, N.H., Linh, L.T., Mo, D.H., Punyashthiti, K., and Puch, C.: Delayed topical antimicrobials as adjuncts to systemic antibiotic therapy of war wounds: Bacteriologic studies. Milit. Med. *132*:461, 1967.
5. Rudolph, R.: Nonsurgical maintenance of the chronic problem wound. *In* Chronic Problem Wounds. Edited by R. Rudolph, and J.M. Noe. Boston, Little, Brown and Co., 1983.
6. Swaim, S.F., and Lee, A.H.: Topical wound medications: A review. J. Am. Vet. Med. Assoc. *190*:1588, 1987.

Silver Sulfadiazine

Definition and Indications. Silver sulfadiazine, 1%, is a water-miscible cream† with a broad spectrum of antimicrobial activity. It is indicated for treatment of burns and other skin wounds with necrotic tissue.

Technique. Silver sulfadiazine may be applied to a wound by placing it on the contact layer of a bandage. When used to treat burns, it is applied as a 1/16-inch-thick layer on the wound.

Aftercare. Topical application of silver sulfadiazine requires no special aftercare. Bandages should be changed as necessary according to the amount of wound drainage and clinical judgement, with bandage changes more frequent in the early stages of healing.

---

*Neosporin ointment, Burroughs Wellcome Co., Research Triangle Park, NC.
†Silvidene Creme, Marion Laboratories, Inc., Kansas City, MO.

Advantages and Disadvantages. Advantages of silver sulfadiazine include its lack of toxicity and its wide antimicrobial activity against most gram-negative and gram-positive bacteria as well as most fungi. It is also painless and nonstaining. It enhances re-epithelialization of wounds. A major advantage is the ability of its antimicrobial activity to penetrate eschar and necrotic tissue. It may, however, delay the separation of eschar from burn wounds.

REFERENCES AND SUGGESTED READING

1. Eaglstein, W.H., and Mertz, P.M.: Effect of topical medicaments on the rate of repair of superficial wounds. In The Surgical Wound. Edited by P. Dineen and G. Hildick-Smith. Philadelphia, Lea & Febiger, 1981.
2. Eaglstein, W.H., Mertz, P.M., Alvarez, O.M.: Effect of topically applied agents on healing wounds. Clin. in Dermatol. 2:112, 1984.
3. Muller, G.H., Kirk, R.W., and Scott, D.W.: Small Animal Dermatology. 3rd ed. Philadelphia, W.B. Saunders Co., 1983.
4. Stefanides, M.M., Copeland, C.E., Kominos, S.D., and Yee, R.B.: In vitro penetration of topical antiseptics through eschar of burn patients. Ann. Surg. 183:358, 1976.
5. Swaim, S.F., and Lee, A.H.: Topical wound medications: A review. J. Am. Vet. Med. Assoc. 190:1588, 1987.

Nitrofurazone

Definition and Indications. Nitrofurazone is a widely used broad spectrum topical antimicrobial medication. It is available in water-soluble base (dressing), solution, and powder forms. It is used in the topical treatment of wounds.

Techniques. The authors prefer the water-soluble dressing formulation* of nitrofurazone for treating open wounds. The medication may be spread on a fine-mesh gauze sponge as the contact layer of a bandage. Gauze may also be soaked in the nitrofurazone solution† before placement on the wound. (see Nonadherent Semiocclusive Material, this chapter).

Aftercare. Wound treatment with nitrofurazone ointment requires no special aftercare. Bandages should be changed as necessary according to the amount of wound drainage and clinical judgment, with bandage changes more frequent in the early stages of healing.

Advantages and Disadvantages. The polyethylene glycol vehicle of the nitrofurazone is bland, nontoxic, nonirritating, and water-soluble, and renders the bandage nonadherent. This is beneficial for wounds in the repair stage. The hydrophilic nature of polyethylene glycol brings homeostatic body fluid up through the

wounded tissues to help dilute tenacious exudates for better absorption. It increases the capillarity of the contact bandage layer so that wound fluid is more effectively transported up through the contact layer to the absorbent intermediate layer. The fact that polyethylene glycol is water-soluble can be disadvantageous because it may be leeched out of the contact bandage layer on a highly productive wound. Although it has been reported to slow wound epithelialization, this has not been the authors' experience.

REFERENCES AND SUGGESTED READING

1. Eaglstein, W.H., and Mertz, P.M.: Effect of topical medicaments on the repair of superficial wounds. In The Surgical Wound. Edited by P. Dineen and G. Hildick-Smith. Philadelphia, Lea & Febiger, 1981.
2. Eaglstein, W.H., Mertz, P.M., and Alvarez, O.M.: Effect of topically applied agents on healing wounds. Clin. in Dermatol. 2:112, 1984.
3. Lee, A.H., Swaim, S.F., Yang, S.L., Wilken, L.O., Miller, D.P., Wilt, G.R., and Hughes, K.S.: The effects of petrolatum, polyethylene glycol, nitrofurazone, and a hydroactive dressing on open wound healing. J. Am. Anim. Hosp. Assoc. 22:443, 1986.
4. Muller, G.H., Kirk, R.W., and Scott, D.W.: Small Animal Dermatology. 3rd ed. Philadelphia, W.B. Saunders Co., 1983.
5. Noe, J.M., and Kalish, S.: The mechanism of capillarity in surgical dressings. Surg. Gynecol. Obstet. 143:454, 1976.
6. Noe, J.M., and Kalish, S.: The problem of adherence in dressed wounds. Surg. Gynecol. Obstet. 147:185, 1978.
7. Noe, J.M., and Kalish, S.: Dressing materials and their selection. In Chronic Problem Wounds. Edited by R. Rudolph and J.M. Noe. Boston, Little, Brown and Co., 1983.
8. Swaim, S.F., and Wilhalf, D.: The physics, physiology, and chemistry of bandaging open wounds. Compend. Contin. Educ. 7:146, 1985.
9. Swaim, S.F. and Lee, A.H.: Topical wound medications: A review. J. Am. Vet. Med. Assoc. 190:1588, 1987.

Gentamicin Sulfate

Definition and Indications. Gentamicin sulfate is a wide spectrum antibiotic available in a 0.1% ointment‡ for topical therapy of bacterial infections in wounds. It is especially effective against some of the gram-negative organisms that infect wounds, such as Pseudomonas aeruginosa, Escherichia coli, and Proteus vulgaris. It has been found especially effective in preparing granulating wounds for application of a skin graft and for postoperative control of bacteria following graft application.

Technique. A thin coating of ointment on a fine-mesh gauze sponge or an absorbent nonadherent dressing pad should be placed over the wound.

Aftercare. Topical application of gentamicin sulfate ointment requires no special aftercare. Bandages should be changed as necessary, however, according to the amount of wound drainage and clinical judgment, with bandage changes being more frequent in the early stages of healing.

---

*Furacin dressing, Norden Laboratories, Inc., Lincoln, NE.
†Nitrofurazone solution 0.2%, Tech America Vet. Prod., Kansas City, MO.
‡Garamycin ointment, 0.1%, Schering Corp., Kenilworth, NJ.

Advantages and Disadvantages. Wounds infected with gram-negative bacteria that have not responded to bacitracin-neomycin-polymixin therapy have responded to gentamicin sulfate ointment, particularly when *Pseudomonas* was present. Patients sensitive to neomycin can be treated with gentamicin sulfate. Although gentamicin is effective in controlling bacteria in wounds, some formulations of the drug may temporarily hinder wound healing. When gentamicin sulfate has been applied to wounds in an oil-in-water cream base, the wounds have been noted to enlarge during the first 7 days of treatment, although normal contraction followed. Conversely, wounds treated with an isotonic gentamicin solution began contraction during the first 7 days of therapy. Wound epithelialization was also less after 7 days treatment with the cream preparation than with solution treatment. Gentamicin sulfate ointment is also relatively more expensive than other topical antibacterial drugs.

REFERENCES AND SUGGESTED READING

1. Lee, A.H., Swaim, S.F., Yang, S.L., and Wilken, L.O.: The effects of gentamicin solution and cream on the healing of open wounds. Am. J. Vet. Res. *45*:1487, 1984.
2. Swaim, S.F., and Lee, A.H.: Topical wound medications: A review. J. Am. Vet. Med. Assoc. *190*:1588, 1987.

HYDROPHILIC AGENTS

Copolymer Flakes

Definition and Indications. Copolymer flake dressing* is a dry starch copolymer that forms a hydrophilic gel when water is added. Like other hydrophilic agents, copolymer flakes cause diffusion of body fluids through the wound tissues to bathe the wound from the inside. Copolymer flake dressings are indicated for early treatment of contaminated or infected open wounds.

Technique. A wound should be thoroughly debrided and lavaged before the use of the copolymer flake dressing. Adding sterile water to the flakes at a ratio of 30 cc of water to 5 cc of flakes creates a gel that is placed in the wound. An absorbent bandage should be applied over the gel-filled wound (see Intermediate Bandage Layer, this chapter).

Aftercare. Wound treatment with copolymer flake/gel requires no special aftercare. Bandages should be changed daily.

Advantages and Disadvantages. The gel absorbs tissue fluid by molecular expansion without chem-

ical reaction taking place in the gel or between the wound and the gel. The gel has been used to draw fluids through the wound tissues to help cleanse the tissues with the body's own fluids.

REFERENCES AND SUGGESTED READING

1. Swaim, S.F., Lee, A.H.: Topical wound medications: A review. J. Am. Vet. Med. Assoc. *190*:1588, 1987.
2. Valdez, H.: A hydrogel preparation for cleansing and protecting equine wounds. Equine Pract. *2*:33, 1980.

Dextranomer

Definition and Indications. Dextranomer is a hydrophilic dextran polymer in the form of spherical hydrophilic beads[†] used to cleanse wounds by causing diffusion of fluids through tissues to bathe the wound from the inside. The dextranomer is indicated for treating contaminated or infected open wounds.

Technique. Wounds should be surgically debrided and cleansed with normal saline or Ringer's solution before applying a 3 mm thick layer of dextranomer to the wound. An absorbent bandage is placed over the dextranomer-filled wound.

Aftercare. Wounds treated with dextranomer require no special aftercare. The dextranomer beads change to a gel as absorption takes place. The bandage should be removed daily and the wound washed with normal saline solution or Ringer's solution followed by reapplication of new dextranomer and bandage.

Advantages and Disadvantages. The beads create a "chromatographic-like" separation of discharging wounds. Larger particles such as microorganisms, plasma proteins, fibrinogen and related products, and wound debris are removed from the surface of the wound as capillary flow draws them into the spaces between the beads. The beads themselves also absorb smaller particles. The dextranomer may activate chemotactic factors that attract polymorphonuclear and mononuclear cells, which are necessary for biologic wound debridement. In addition, it has been stated to be superior to gauze for absorbing exudate from wounds with less inflammatory reaction than in gauze-covered wounds. Relief of pain and no allergic reactions have been reported as positive factors. The dextranomer, however, is relatively expensive.

REFERENCES AND SUGGESTED READING

1. Heel, R.C., Morton, P., Brogden, R.N., Speight, T.M., and Avery, G.S.: Dextranomer: A review of its general properties and therapeutic efficacy. Drugs *18*:89, 1979.

---

*Avalon Copolymer Flakes, Summit Hill Laboratories, Avalon, NJ.
[†]Debrisan, Johnson & Johnson, New Brunswick, NJ.

2. Jacobsson, S., Rothmann, U., Arturson, G., Ganrot, K., Haeger, K., and Juhlin, I.: A new principle for cleansing of infected wounds. Scand. J. Plast. Surg. *10*:65, 1976.
3. Lund, C.: Inflammatory reaction and collagen accumulation in an experimental model of open wounds in the rat. Scand. J. Plast. Reconst. Surg. *19*:11, 1985.
4. Oredsson, S.V., Gottrup, F., Beckmann, A., and Hohn, D.C.: Activation of chemotactic factors in serum and wound fluid by dextranomer. Surgery *94*:453, 1983.
5. Swaim, S.F., and Lee, A.H.: Topical wound medication: A review. J. Am. Vet. Med. Assoc. *190*:1588, 1987.

ENZYMES

General Indications, Advantages and Disadvantages

There are two general indications for enzymatic wound debridement. Enzymes may be used to debride wounds in patients who are not considered favorable anesthetic risks for surgical debridement. They are also indicated for debriding wounds in which surgical debridement could result in damage to or removal of healthy tissue. Enzymatic debridement is especially useful for wounds on the limbs and paws, where all available viable tissue is needed for reconstruction. In such instances, the enzyme "decides" which tissues will be removed and which will remain. Thus, the surgeon does not take the chance of removing questionable tissue that may, with time, revitalize and be useful for reconstruction.

The general advantages of enzymatic debridement are related to the indications. First, it allows postponement of surgery until the patient has become a better surgical risk because of improved status. Secondly, enzymatic debridement ensures that healthy tissue and granulation tissue will not be disturbed. Enzymatic debridement may be less expensive than surgical debridement and provides an option for pet owners who are able to change bandages at home or on an outpatient basis.

The general disadvantages of enzymatic debridement include the expense, the time required to remove dead tissue, and possible insufficient debriding action.

Trypsin-Balsam of Peru-Castor Oil*

Definition and Indications. The trypsin of this compound digests necrotic tissue, pyogenic membranes, and crusts. The balsam of Peru serves as a capillary bed stimulant that increases circulation to an area. The castor oil improves epithelialization by reducing premature epithelial desiccation and cornification. It also serves as a protective covering and an analgesic. The authors prefer

---

*Granulex, Beecham Laboratories, Bristol, TN.
†Preparation H, Whitehall Laboratories, Inc., New York, NY.

to use this compound in the early stages of wound therapy.

Technique. The compound should be applied to the wound and covered with an absorbent bandage. The authors prefer a wide-mesh gauze for the contact bandage layer. Bandages ar changed daily.

Aftercare. Wounds treated with this compound require no special aftercare. Once a healthy bed of granulation tissue is established on a wound and epithelialization has started, the authors discontinue use of this compound.

Advantages and Disadvantages. In addition to debriding the wound and favoring the repair processes, this compound has a pleasant odor. Although the pancreatic enzymes do not possess bactericidal properties per se, the bacterial flora of wounds has been found to decrease with use of enzymes such as trypsin. This is attributed to their debriding action which removes the debris that supports bacterial proliferation. In addition, when antibiotics are used in conjunction with enzymes, the coagulum on the wound is liquified by the enzymes. This allows systemic and/or topical antibiotics to contact the bacteria that have been surrounded by the coagulum. Liquifaction of the coagulum also enhances its absorption into a bandage. Trypsin has been reported to cause a stinging sensation when applied topically.

REFERENCES AND SUGGESTED READING

1. Riser, H.G., Patton R., and Roetting, L.C.: Tryptic debridement of necrotic tissue. Arch. Surg. *63*:568, 1951.
2. Shelby, R.W., Taylor L.E., Garnes, A.L., and Prigot, A.: Enzymatic debridement with activated whole pancreas. Am. J. Surg. *96*:545, 1958.
3. Swaim, S.F.: Management and bandaging of soft tissue injuries of dog and cat feet. J. Am. Anim. Hosp. Assoc. *21*:329, 1985.

LIVE YEAST-CELL DERIVATIVE

Definition and Indications. Live yeast-cell derivative, or skin respiratory factor, is a water-soluble extract of Brewer's yeast (*Saccharomyces cerevisiae*) that is available in an over-the-counter hemorrhoid medication.† It has been reported to contain a substance or substances that stimulates early wound angiogenesis, tissue oxygen consumption, epithelialization, and collagen synthesis. It is indicated for treatment of open wounds that are in the repair stage of healing with healthy granulation tissue and epithelium progressing over the granulation tissue.

Technique. A thin coating of live yeast-cell derivative is placed on an absorbent nonadherent dressing pad as the contact bandage layer.

Aftercare. Treatment of a wound with live yeast-cell derivative requires no special aftercare. Bandages should be changed daily.

Advantages and Disadvantages. Live yeast-cell derivative is readily available to veterinarians in the previously mentioned medication. Empirical observation by the authors and controlled studies of others have indicated that the product does stimulate wound epithelialization. Thus, an epithelial covering is supplied for the wound while wound contraction continues to occur, making the wound smaller. A mild stinging sensation has been reported in some human patients on whom the live yeast-cell derivative was used to treat skin graft donor sites. The authors have noted no evidence of discomfort in animals on which the drug has been used.

REFERENCES AND SUGGESTED READING

1. Goodson, W., Hohn, D., Hunt, T.K., and Leung, Y.K.: Augmentation of some aspects of wound healing by a "skin respiratory factor." J. Surg. Res. *21*:125, 1976.
2. Kaplan, G.Z.: Acceleration of healing by a live yeast-cell derivative. Arch. Surg. *119*:1005, 1984.
3. Swaim, S.F., and Lee, A.H.: Topical wound medications: A review. J. Am. Vet. Med. Assoc. *190*:1588, 1987.
4. Wolk, M., and Danon, D.: Promotion of wound healing by yeast glucan evaluated on single animals. Med. Biol. *63*:73, 1985.

4

SPECIFIC TYPES OF WOUNDS

BURN WOUNDS

THERMAL BURNS

Definition and Indications. Common sources of thermal burns in small animals include fires, defective hair driers, electric heating pads, boiling water, steam, hot cooking oil, and the undersides of automobile motors and exhaust systems. Burns have been classified according to their depth. A first-degree (superficial) burn affects only the epidermis (Fig. 4-1A), which becomes thickened and erythematous and ultimately desquamates. A first-degree burn usually heals in 3 to 6 days by re-epithelialization. Hair regrowth is likely. A second-degree (partial-thickness) burn involves the epidermis and varying amounts of dermis (Fig. 4-1B), causing subcutaneous edema and a marked inflammatory response. Second-degree burns heal by re-epithelialization from remnants of deep adnexa; the rate of healing and quantity of hair regrown depend on the depth of the burn. A third-degree (full-thickness) burn destroys the entire skin thickness, forming a dark brown, insensitive, leathery covering (eschar) (Fig. 4-1C). Superficial subcutaneous vessels are thrombosed and deeper vessels are excessively permeable, causing edema of the subcutaneous tissues and gangrene of the damaged tissue. After removal or slough of the eschar, these wounds, if not reconstructed, heal slowly by contraction and re-epithelialization.

---

*Normosol-R, Abbott Hospital Products Div., Chicago, IL.

Burn wounds not only cause local tissue damage, but may also cause severe systemic imbalances, depending on the nature and extent of the burn.

Generally, thermal burn treatment is indicated for all first-degree burns and for second- and third-degree burns that do not cover more than 50% of the total body area. An animal that has received second- and third-degree burns over more than 50% of its body should be euthanized.

Techniques. A burn patient may be sedated to relieve pain and provide restraint if the cardiovascular status is stable. Neuroleptanalgesia in the form of oxymorphone (0.1 mg/kg IM or IV, not exceeding 4 mg total) and acetylpromazine (0.2 mg/kg IM or IV to a maximum dose of 3 mg) for dogs and diazapam (2.5 mg IM or IV) and oxymorphone (0.1 mg/kg IM or IV, not exceeding 4 mg total) for cats is recommended.

Burn Shock Treatment. While physiologic parameters are monitored to determine the type, amount, and rate of administration, fluid administration should be used to treat the shock associated with burns.

Initially, blood samples should be obtained to determine the values for hematocrit, serum protein, hemoglobin, sodium, potassium, and chloride. Catheters are placed in the jugular vein, cephalic vein, and urinary bladder to monitor central venous pressure, administer fluids, and monitor hourly urine output, respectively. Initially, a commercially available replacement type of balanced electrolyte solution* or lactated Ringer's solution is given intravenously.

Urine output and central venous pressure are used to determine the amount of fluid given. Urine production

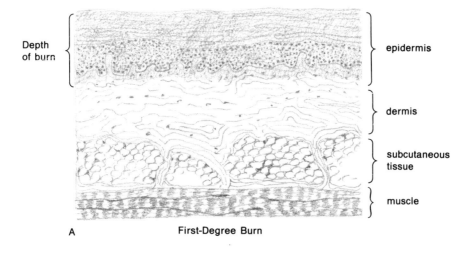

Depth of burn

epidermis

dermis

subcutaneous tissue

muscle

A   First-Degree Burn

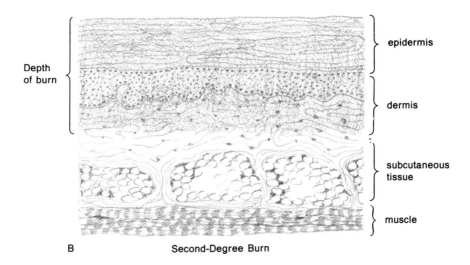

Depth of burn

epidermis

dermis

subcutaneous tissue

muscle

B   Second-Degree Burn

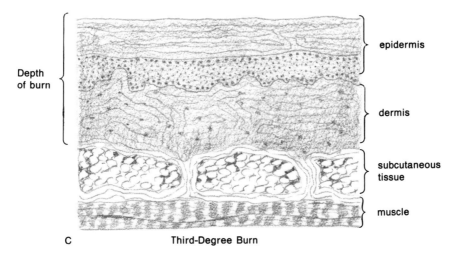

Depth of burn

epidermis

dermis

subcutaneous tissue

muscle

C   Third-Degree Burn

FIG. 4-1. A, First-degree burn involving epidermis. B, Second-degree burn involving epidermis and varying depths of dermis. C, Third-degree burn involving full thickness of skin.

should be kept above 1 ml/kg body weight per hour. Fluid input, however, exceeds urine output by approximately 3 to 4 times during the first 48 hours. During this time, equal volumes of the replacement fluid and a maintenance fluid* are administered at approximately 3 to 4 ml/kg body weight per hour. An increase or decrease in central venous pressure indicates a need to slow or increase the rate of fluid administration.

Control of potassium levels is important in fluid and electrolyte therapy. During the first 24 hours after extensive burn injury, minimal to moderate serum potassium elevation may occur because of thermal destruction of tissue and red blood cells in the presence of reduced kidney function. Because commercially available replacement fluids are low in potassium (4 to 5 m Eq/1), they are indicated during this early period of hyperkalemia. If the animal is severely hyperkalemic (> 8m Eq/1), potassium-free fluids such as 0.9% saline should be given. After the first 24 hours, the return of renal function in the presence of catabolism, the loss of potassium from anoxic heat damaged cells, and increased mineralocorticoid secretion can cause a significant increase in renal potassium excretion and sodium retention. If this condition is untreated, a life-threatening potassium deficit can develop between the third and fifth day postburn. Collection of 24-hour urine samples and measurement of serum potassium levels can be used to monitor potassium loss and establish the need for potassium supplementation.

If kidney function is adequate, supplemental potassium can be given in the presence of hypokalemia. If only replacement fluids are being used, the potassium concentration of these fluids can be raised to 15 to 20 m Eq/1 when the serum potassium is within the range of 3.5 to 4.5 m Eq/1, and 80 m Eq/1 when the serum potassium level is below 2.5 m Eq/1. A safe rate of administering potassium is 0.5 m Eq/kg/hour.

Another means of controlling the potassium levels is by using the potassium concentrations of the commercially available replacement and maintenance fluids used in shock therapy, 4 to 5 m Eq/1 and 13 to 35 m Eq/1, respectively. When each of these fluids is used to replace half of the animal's daily fluid needs, it may be necessary to supplement the potassium if the potassium contents of the fluids are not sufficient.

Severely burned animals are usually acidotic, and blood gas monitoring is advised. Mild to moderate acidosis is usually corrected or controlled by the bicarbonate precursors in electrolyte solutions, (such as the lactate in lactated Ringer's solution). With severe burns, the administration of up to 5 m Eq/kg body weight of

sodium bicarbonate by way of fluids over 30 to 60 minutes is advisable.

Colloid-containing solutions and red blood cells are rarely indicated in the first 2 days postburn. Serum proteins and hematocrit should be monitored, however, and plasma or whole blood given as indicated. Serum protein should be maintained between 3.5 and 6.5 g/dL and red blood cells or whole blood should be administered if the hematocrit falls below 25%. The need for protein and red blood cells is usually greatest after 2 to 5 days.

Respiratory Therapy.   Thermal injury to the respiratory tract should be continuously monitored, and the animal should be turned several times daily to help prevent hypostatic lung congestion. Injury to the tracheal mucociliary clearance apparatus results in mucus accumulation in the trachea and bronchi; suction may be necessary. Congestion and alveolar collapse may require supplemental oxygen-assisted ventilation (mask or intranasal). Upper airway obstruction due to edema or necrosis may necessitate a tracheostomy.

Wound Evaluation and Therapy.   If started soon after injury, 20 minutes of cold applications in the form of towels soaked in ice water or submersion of a burned area in cold water may relieve pain and arrest the progression of the burn (Fig. 4-2A).

If hair remains on burned skin, as with burns caused by steam and electric heating pads, the depth and extent of the burn may be estimated by pulling on the hair (Fig. 4-2B). Hair that epilates easily indicates a deep burn.

Hair should be clipped from the burned surface and the area gently washed with a detergent antiseptic (Fig. 4-2C). If treatment is begun early after a burn, the antiprostaglandin effects of topical aloe vera compounds may preserve a patent dermal vasculature to ensure tissue oxygenation and thus prevent the progression of first-degree burns to second-degree and second-degree to third-degree.

The type of burn is probably better determined by palpation and manipulation of the eschar than by visual observation. Elevating and bending the eschar (Fig. 4-2D) causes first- and second-degree burn eschars to split at the bend, revealing underlying epidermis or dermis. Bending the eschar of a third-degree burn results in either no split in the eschar or splitting down to the subcutaneous tissue. Additionally, third-degree burns are not as painful as first- and second-degree burns.

Loose debris and necrotic tissue on the surface of a first-degree or superficial second-degree burn should be removed while cleansing the wound (Fig. 4-2E). Hydrotherapy may be beneficial in cleansing the wound. Deep second-degree burn eschars should be debrided to the level at which pinpoint dermal bleeding is noticed. A third-degree burn eschar should be removed (Fig. 4-2F)

*Normosol-M, in D 5-W, Abbott Hospital Products Div., Chicago, IL.

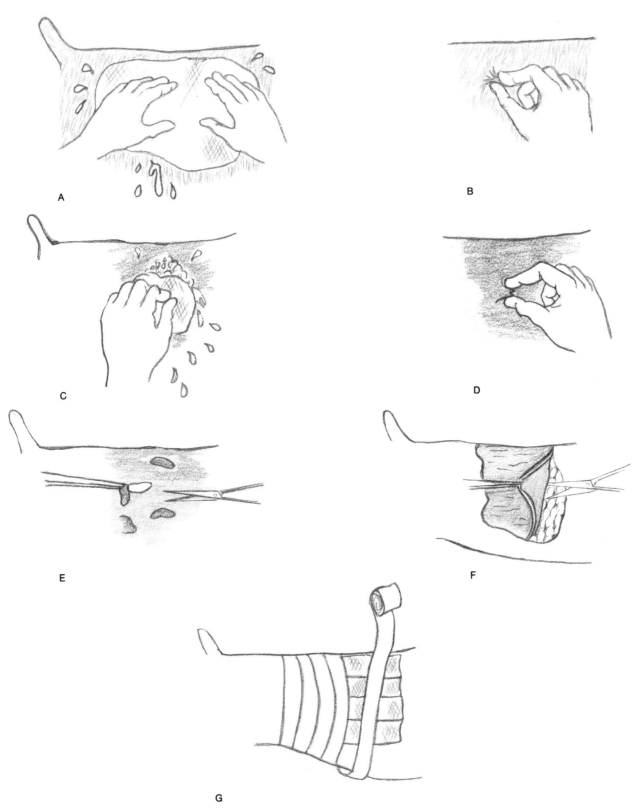

FIG. 4-2. Thermal burn wound management. A, Cold compresses applied soon after burn. B, Attempts to epilate hair to tell depth and extent of burn. C, Area gently washed after hair has been clipped. D, Elevating and bending an eschar can reveal burn depth. E, Loose necrotic tissue removed from surface of a first- or second-degree burn. F, Eschar removed from surface of a third-degree burn. G, Topical medication and bandage applied.

as soon as possible because it may retain infection under it and splint the wound edges, preventing wound contraction. As the eschar separates from underlying tissue, it should be excised with scissors within the limits of the animal's tolerance without anesthesia.

Aftercare. Systemic antibiotics are generally not considered as important in preventing sepsis in first-degree and superficial second-degree wounds as topical silver sulfadiazine* applied under a bandage (Fig. 4-2G). The bandage is removed daily and warm, balanced electrolyte solution is used to cleanse the wound. Surface debris and necrotic tissue are removed from the wound before reapplication of medication and bandage. A first-degree burn may be allowed to heal as an open wound with re-epithelialization of the wound and regrowth of hair on the wound area. If a superficial second-degree burn results in a thinly haired scar after healing as an open wound, it may be more cosmetic to remove the scar tissue and perform a primary closure of the resulting defect if it is not too large. After eschar removal from deep second- and third-degree burns, topical medication and bandages are applied to the wound and changed at least daily. With a deep second-degree burn, the resulting wound may be closed by shifting local tissue or using a flap or graft, allowed to heal as an open wound under a bandage, or allowed to heal partially as an open wound followed by reconstruction once contraction has stopped.

Following eschar removal from a third-degree burn, a decision must be made as to closure of the skin defect. If the tissue is healthy, and there is sufficient healthy surrounding skin, closure by shifting local tissue or using a flap over the wound may be considered. When there is insufficient surrounding healthy skin, a graft is indicated. Allowing the wound to heal by contraction and epithelialization may also be considered.

Advantages and Disadvantages. The advantages and disadvantages of managing dermal injuries associated with thermal burns are those associated with the different techniques used in repairing the defects.

REFERENCES AND SUGGESTED READING

1. Cera, L.M., Heggers, J.P., Robson, M.C., and Hagstrom, W.J.: The therapeutic efficacy of *Aloe vera* cream (Dermaide aloe(R)) in thermal injuries: Two case reports. J. Am. Anim. Hosp. Assoc. *16*:788, 1980.
2. Cera, L.M., Heggers, J.P., Hagstrom, W.J., and Robson, M.C.: Therapeutic protocol for thermally injured animals and its successful use in an extensively burned Rhesus monkey. J. Am. Anim. Hosp. Assoc. *18*:633, 1982.
3. Fox, S.M.: Management of thermal burns—Part I. Compend. Contin. Educ. *7*:631, 1985.
4. Heavner, J.E., and Burga, W.: Burns from an electric heating pad. Vet. Anesth. *5*:14, 1978.
5. Johnston, D.E.: Skin and subcutaneous tissue—Thermal injuries. *In* Pathophysiology in Small Animal Surgery. Edited by M.J. Bojrab. Philadelphia, W.B. Saunders, 1981.
6. Johnston, D.E.: Burns, electrical, chemical and cold injuries. *In* Textbook of Small Animal Surgery. Edited by D.H. Slatter. Philadelphia, W.B. Saunders, 1985.*
7. Muller, G.H., Kirk, R.W., and Scott, D.W.: Small Animal Dermatology. 3rd ed. Philadelphia, W.B. Saunders, 1983.
8. Paddleford, R.P.: Anesthetic management of the critical patient. *In* Veterinary Trauma and Critical Care. Edited by I.M. Zaslow. Philadelphia, Lea & Febiger, 1984.
9. Robson, M.C., Heggers, J.P., and Pineless, G.R.: Myth, magic, witchcraft or fact? *Aloe vera* revisited. Am. Burn Assoc. Abst. *31*:65, 1979.
10. Swaim, S.F., Lee A.H., and Hughes K.S.: Heating pads and thermal burns in small animals. J. Am. Anim. Hosp. Assoc. *25*:156, 1989.

*Primary reference.

ELECTRICAL BURNS

Definition and Indications. Low-tension electrical burns occur when current touches one point on the body with or without points of exit. This occurs most commonly when animals chew on electric cords. The area of contact is usually charred; however, the electric current may flow preferentially along blood vessels, causing thermal damage in the vessel and the tissues they supply. Initially, the tissues appear normal; however, ischemic demarcation and slough occur in 2 to 3 weeks.

When tissues around the mouth are burned, the resulting tissue defects should be reconstructed if adequate tissue is available.

Technique. In an acutely electrocuted animal in shock, fluid administration should be judicious, preferably monitored by CVP and urine output. Electrocution causes acute (neurogenic) pulmonary edema, which may be exacerbated if fluids are administered as would be done in traumatic shock. Pulmonary edema is generally not as severe in cats as in dogs, and cats may recover spontaneously. Although no specific therapy can be recommended in dogs, usual therapy in dogs may include Furosemide† (2.5–5.0 mg/kg once or twice daily at 6 to 8 hour intervals IM, IV, or by mouth for dogs) to decrease plasma volume, with morphine (1 mg/kg IM or subcutaneously) to produce sympatholytic and vasodilatory effects and aminophylline (10 mg/kg every 8 hours IV, IM, or by mouth) to cause vasodilation and bronchodilation. Doses of these drugs should be lower in cats.

---

*Silvidene Creme, Marion Laboratories, Inc., Kansas City, MO.
†Lasix Injectable Solution, National Laboratories Corp., Kansas City, MO.

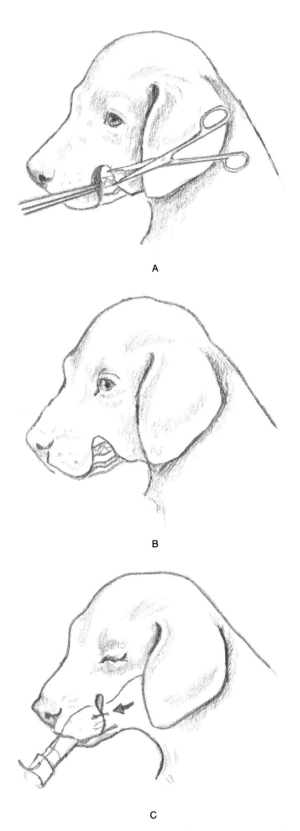

FIG. 4-3. Electrical burns. A, Necrotic tissue removed from lips and other areas over a 2 to 3 week period. B, Lip defect after removing necrotic tissue. C, Closure of lip defect with labial tissue caudal to defect.

Following electrical burns to the mouth and lips, the tissues should be observed regularly over a 2 to 3 week period, with removal of obviously devitalized tissue as necessary (Fig. 4-3A). At the end of the 2 to 3-week period, most devitalized tissue should have separated (Fig. 4-3B).

Aftercare. After the devitalized tissue has separated from the mouth and lips, small lip wounds surrounded by much loose tissue may be allowed to heal as open wounds. Reconstruction of the lip, however, provides a more cosmetic result. Large defects should be sutured (Fig. 4-3C) (See Chronic Lacerations and Tumors of the Lip—Segmental Resection of the Lip, Chapter 6). With some large defects, it may be necessary to create flaps from the tissue caudal to the defect. Oronasal fistulae that may be present should be surgically closed and, when possible, defects in the tongue should be reconstructed.

Advantages and Disadvantages. The advantages and disadvantages of managing lip and mouth injuries associated with electrical burns from chewing on electric cords are those associated with the techniques used in repairing the defects. The reader is referred to the sections of this book associated with labial reconstruction and other texts dealing with reconstructive techniques of the oral and nasal cavities.

REFERENCES AND SUGGESTED READING

1. Johnston, D.E.: Skin and subcutaneous tissue—Thermal injuries. *In* Pathophysiology of Small Animal Surgery. Edited by M.J. Bojrab. Philadelphia, W.B. Saunders, 1981.
2. Johnson, R.: Table of common drugs and approximate doses. *In* Current Veterinary Therapy X. Edited by R.W. Kirk. Philadelphia, W.B. Saunders, 1989.
3. Johnston, D.E.: Burns, electrical, chemical and cold injuries. *In* Textbook of Small Animal Surgery. Edited by D.H. Slatter. Philadelphia, W.B. Saunders, 1985.*

*Primary reference.

CHEMICAL BURNS

Definition and Indications. Chemical burns can be caused by accidental or maliciously induced contact with oxidizing agents, reducing agents, corrosives, protoplasmic poisons, desiccants, and vesicants. In general, these agents cause denaturation and coagulation of tissue protein. Hard or soft eschars or a coagulum may form over the area, with underlying ulcers (Fig. 4-4A). The indications for treating chemical burns are similar to those for treating thermal burns: extent and depth of the burn and availability of skin for reconstruction or allowing open wound healing (see Thermal Burns, this chapter).

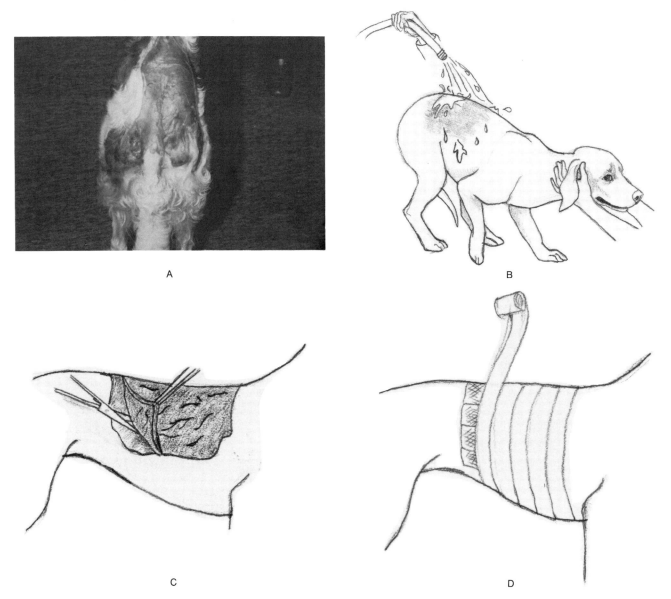

A

B

C

D

FIG. 4-4. Chemical burns. A, Chemical burn over lumbosacral area of a dog. B, Chemical burn lavaged with copious quantities of water, while dog's head is controlled. C, Devitalized tissue removed. D, Topical medication and bandage applied.

Technique. The most important therapy for chemical burns is rapid dilution of the chemical agent by lavage of the burned area with *copious* quantities of water. This removes the chemical agent and dilutes it to reduce its chemical reaction with tissues. It is also important to control the animal's head to prevent it from licking the burned area, which would cause chemical burns of the oropharynx and esophagus (Fig. 4-4B).

After lavage, the wound should be treated as a thermal burn. Devitalized tissue should be removed, followed by (1) topical application of an antibacterial agent and bandage, with daily bandage removal, (2) tissue debridement as necessary, and (3) reapplication of medication and bandage (Fig. 4-4C and D).

Aftercare. After all devitalized tissue has been removed and a healthy bed of granulation tissue is present, the surgeon should decide whether to allow the wound to heal by contraction and epithelialization, perform secondary wound closure over the granulation tissue by shifting local tissue or using a flap, or close the wound with a graft.

Advantages and Disadvantages. The primary disadvantage of treating chemical burns is the uncertainty associated with debridement. If the wound is not debrided early enough after injury, further tissue destruction secondary to continued chemical penetration may occur over 24 to 72 hours. Conversely, aggressive early debridement may result in removal of too much tissue.

REFERENCE AND SUGGESTED READING

1. Johnston D.E.: Burns; Electrical, chemical and cold injuries. *In* Textbook of Small Animal Surgery. Edited by D.H. Slatter. Philadelphia, W.B. Saunders, 1985.

FROSTBITE

Definition and Indications. Frostbite results from exposure of peripheral tissue to freezing temperatures. It is usually restricted to areas where the hair covering is sparse and peripheral circulation is poor, such as the ear, tail tip, scrotum, and mammary glands (Fig. 4-5A). When frozen, the skin is pale, hypoesthetic, and cool to the touch; but when it is thawed, mild hyperemia, pain, and scaliness of the skin may occur. In severe cases, the end result may be dry gangrene and mummification of tissues.

Reconstruction of frostbite-damaged tissue is indicated when a deformity occurs after tissue slough or debridement.

Technique. The accepted method of treating frostbite is rapid rewarming of the affected area. The involved tissues should be warmed at temperatures of 42 to 44° C by means of immersion in warm water or contact with a warm surface rather than by exposure to warm air as with a blowdrier (Fig. 4-5B and C). Twenty minutes of contact with these temperatures is sufficient for rapid rewarming. Because rewarming may be painful, neuroleptanalgesia should be considered, and massage of the tissue should be avoided during rewarming.

To help prevent local vasoconstriction and tissue hypoxia caused by prostaglandins and thromboxane release, aloe vera has been applied topically to frostbitten areas. Pressure bandages should be avoided. If ischemic necrosis develops, the clear-cut line of demarcation between viable and nonviable tissue is usually slow to develop. Thus, there should be no rush in debriding or amputating because tissue initially thought to be nonviable may survive even after periods of 3 to 6 weeks. Once tissue is definitely mummified, however, it should be excised (Fig. 4-5D).

Topical silver sulfadiazine is applied to infected frostbitten tissue.

Aftercare. After amputation of mummified tissue, aftercare may be minor; little or no surgery is required because the surrounding tissue will have already healed under the mummified tissue, (as in the tips of the ears or the tip of the tail.) Aftercare may require some reconstructive procedure such as moving local tissues or use of a flap if the defect is large, as could occur with loss of mammary or scrotal tissue.

Advantages and Disadvantages. The advantage of delaying excision of frostbitten tissue is that more tissue may survive than originally suspected, thus reducing the amount of excision, and in some cases the reconstruction, necessary. Wound management over this longer period could be more costly than acute reconstruction.

REFERENCES AND SUGGESTED READING

1. Christenson, C., and Stewart, C.: Frostbite. Am. Fam. Physician *30*:111, 1984.
2. Johnston, D.E.: Burns; Electrical, chemical, and cold injuries. *In* Textbook of Small Animal Surgery. Edited by D.H. Slatter. Philadelphia, W.B. Saunders 1985.
3. Johnston, D.E.: Skin and subcutaneous tissue—cold injury. *In* Pathophysiology in Small Animal Surgery. Edited by M.J. Bojrab. Philadelphia, Lea & Febiger, 1981.
4. Kirk, R.W., Bistner, S.I.: Handbook of Veterinary Procedures and Emergency Treatment. 4th ed. Philadelphia, W.B. Saunders, 1985.
5. McCauley, R.L., Hing, D.N., Robson, M.C., and Heggers, J.P.: Frostbite injuries: a rational approach based on the pathophysiology. J. Trauma *23*:143, 1983.
6. Muller, G.H., Kirk, R.W., and Scott, D.W.: Small Animal Dermatology. 3rd ed. Philadelphia, W.B. Saunders, 1983.

SNAKEBITE WOUNDS

Definition and Indications. Venomous snakebites may result in tissue necrosis and wounds requiring reconstruction (Fig. 4-6A). In North America, snakes of the *Crotalidae* subfamily (pit vipers), including the copperhead, cottonmouth water moccasin, and rattlesnake, inflict most of these bites. These envenomed wounds vary in severity of both local and systemic signs.

Pit viper venoms cause local myonecrosis and most venoms cause destruction of blood vessel walls, allowing massive leakage of blood into the surrounding tissues. Snake venom may induce coagulation defects, which may be marked. The pain associated with envenomization may subside after 1 or 2 hours, when swelling and tissue necrosis produce an anesthetic effect. Tissue damage varies with the depth of the bite and the amount of venom injected.

Local signs indicating envenomization include the presence of one or two *fang puncture wounds* (often bleeding); immediate and progressive *swelling* with tissue discoloration, including ecchymosis and petechiae formation; and immediate severe *pain*. It should be remembered, however, that the severity of these signs may vary depending on the quantity of venom injected and location (for instance, type of tissue: fat, muscle, or other) in which the venom was injected, and that the severity of envenomization cannot be judged by local signs alone.

The systemic effects of envenomization may include hypotension, shock, lethargy, salivation, painful lymph

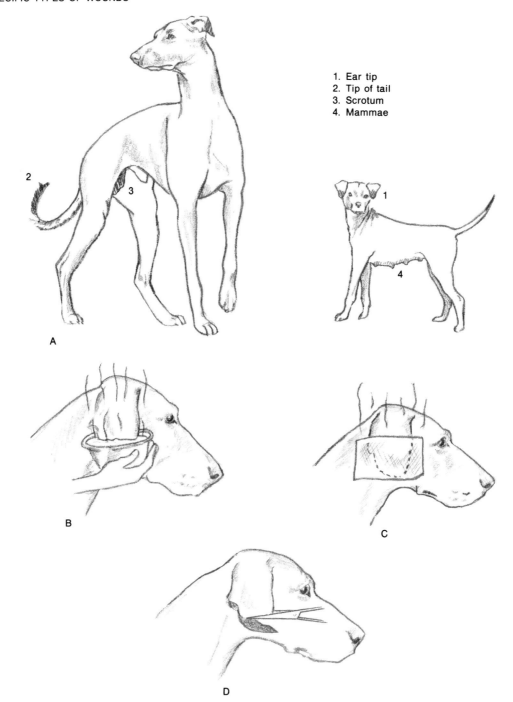

1. Ear tip
2. Tip of tail
3. Scrotum
4. Mammae

FIG. 4-5. Frostbite. A, Areas commonly affected by frostbite. B, Rewarming frostbitten area by immersion in warm water, or C, Contact with warm towels. D, Surgical removal of mummified tissue.

nodes, weakness, muscle fasiculations, and possible respiratory depression. In addition, a myocardial depressant factor has been associated with the venom of eastern and western diamondback rattlesnakes.

The goals in treating venomous snakebites are neutralization of the venom, treatment of the systemic effects of the venom, and in the case of local tissue damage, treatment of wound infection and repair of resulting defects.

Technique. *Initial (Field) Management.* Tourniquets, incision, and suction or manipulation of the bite area are probably of little use in management of snakebite wounds. The most practical early management for snakebite is immobilization of the bitten part (for example, with a bulky bandage or a splint on a limb) and avoidance of excitement or exertion during rapid transport to veterinary facilities (Fig. 4-6B).

Animal Monitoring. When snakebite by a pit viper is suspected, the affected body part should be clipped free of hair and examined for fang puncture wounds, which usually bleed (Fig. 4-6C). Local edema may obscure puncture wounds. Because, in some cases, clinical signs of severe envenomization may take several hours to become evident, and because local tissue reaction may be inadequate for judging the severity of envenomation, snakebitten animals should be hospitalized and observed for 24 hours. Laboratory tests can be valuable in monitoring the degree and progression of envenomization. Initial values should be obtained for CBC, coagulation profile (prothrombin time, partial thrombin time and fibrinogen), platelets, creatine phosphokinase, blood urea nitrogen, serum electrolytes, creatinine, glucose, and urine hemoglobin and myoglobin (Fig. 4-6D). These values should be repeated in 6 hours and as indicated thereafter. The platelet counts and clotting times are often sensitive means of monitoring the severity and progression of envenomization. Decreased platelet counts and prolonged clotting times indicate envenomization severity with most pit viper venoms. A persistent decrease in the platelet count suggests progressive venom activity. Platelet counts and clotting times should be repeated as often as necessary for evaluation (as a minium, initially, at 6 hours, and at 12 hours). Myoglobinuria or hemoglobinuria indicates severe rhabdomyolysis or marked hemolysis, respectively. ECG monitoring should be instituted in severe envenomizations.

The circumference of the affected body part should be measured at, above, and below the bite site (Fig. 4-6E). These measurements should be taken and recorded at 15-minute intervals to quantify the progression of edema. Intervals longer than this may be used after antivenin administration and establishment of clinical stability of the animal.

Laboratory monitoring and quantified measurements of the affected body part allow objective assessment of an animal's response to envenomization and treatment.

Definitive Therapy. Pretreatment with the antihistamine diphenhydramine* (10 mg in small dogs and cats, 25 mg in large dogs) aids in calming fractious patients and provides some protection against any allergic reaction to antivenin that might occur; however, it has no action against the venom itself. Diphenhydramine should be administered with half the dose being given subcutaneously. Following intravenous catherization, the remainder of the dose is given intravenously. Lactated Ringer's solution, physiologic saline, or colloids should be given intravenously (Fig. 4-6 inset).

Because antivenin† prevents systemic reactions and limits tissue necrosis, it should be given as soon as possible to enhance its effectiveness. One vial of antivenin should be reconstituted by adding the diluent and then over several minutes warming it to body temperature and swirling but not shaking it, so that it does not produce a foam.

All animals should be skin-tested before antivenin is administered. Directions on the package insert should be followed when performing this test. The animal should not be left unattended during antivenin administration. Antivenin should be administered *slowly*. With the antivenin mixed into the fluids, 10 to 15 ml. of the mixture is given over 5 to 10 minutes. During this time, the concave surface of the pinna should be observed for hyperemia as an indication of a complement reaction if the administration of the equine foreign protein of the antivenin has been too rapid. If hyperemia occurs, antivenin infusion should be discontinued and diphenhydramine administration repeated. After 15 minutes, antivenin fluid infusion should resume again, but more slowly than initially. If a reaction occurs a second time, consulation with a poison control center should be sought. Epinephrine and resuscitation equipment should be readily available. A minimum of one vial of antivenin has been advocated, with the need for additional vials depending on the patient's clinical signs, the laboratory results, and progression or stabilization of the swelling in the affected part. The willingness of the pet owner to have additional vials administered, based on cost, is another factor governing the total dose of antivenin administered. With a small dog in which an entire container of fluid may result in fluid overload, antivenin may be given slowly through the IV set as fluids are administered (Fig. 4-6 inset). The first 2 to 3 ml of antivenin should be given slowly over 5 to 10 minutes.

Broad-spectrum antibiotic therapy is indicated to help prevent wound infection.

Aftercare. The necrotizing effect of venoms on tissues predisposes to the possibility of tissue loss. As tissues are sloughed, the wound should be managed as an open infected wound. When the slough is complete and healthy granulation tissue is present, it must be decided whether to allow the wound to heal as an open wound by contraction and epithelialization or to perform a reconstructive procedure (such as shifting local tissue, graft, or flap).

---

*Benadryl, Parke-Davis Division of Warner-Lambert Co., Morris Plains, NJ.

†Antivenin (Crotalidae) Polyvalent, Fort Dodge Laboratories, Inc., Fort Dodge, IA.

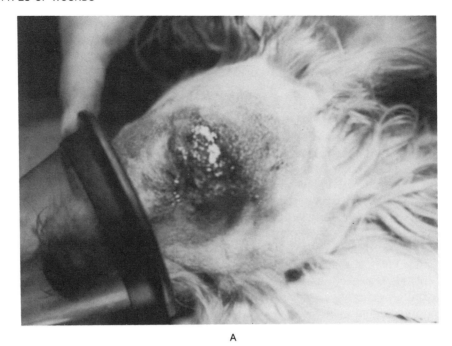

A

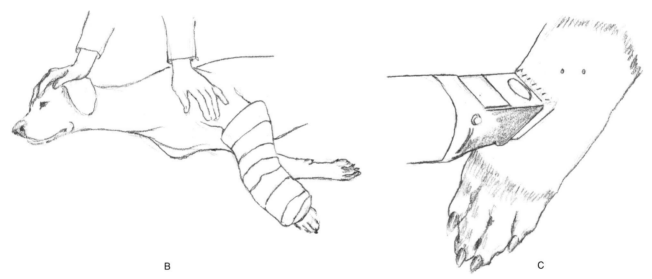

B

C

FIG. 4-6. Venomous snakebite. A, Tissue necrosis above a dog's eye as result of envenomization (Courtesy of M.E. Peterson). B, Bulky bandage to affected limb and avoidance of excitement during transport to veterinarian. C, Clipping hair from affected limb to find fang punctures. Figure continues.

Advantages and Disadvantages. If an animal has a heavy coat and/or rapid swelling of the bitten part, the puncture marks may be obscured. This places the veterinarian at a disadvantage because signs similar to those caused by pit viper envenomization, such as swelling and pain could be associated with envenomization by other species, such as stinging insects. Examination for fang marks is important in deciding whether to use antivenin in treatment. If there is a question as to whether a snakebite has occurred, a platelet count should be performed. A low count increases the suspicion of a snakebite.

Because it is difficult to determine the potential systemic and local response of an animal to envenomization, it is always to the animal's advantage to use antivenin as part of the therapeutic regimen. The cost of the antivenin could be considered a disadvantage; however, if it helps prevent a large tissue slough and averts the greater expense of surgical reconstruction, it is advantageous.

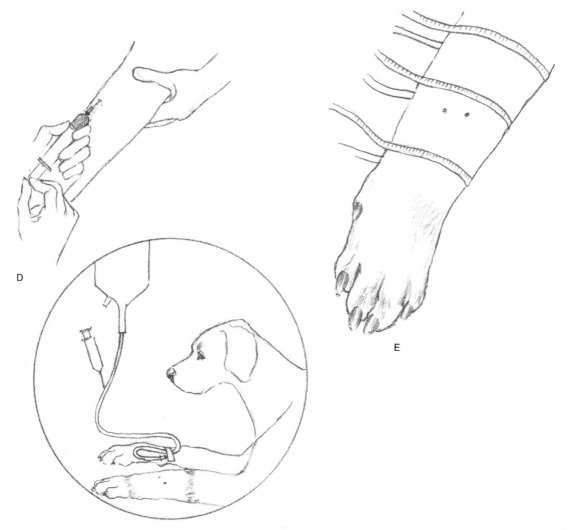

FIG. 4-6. (continued) D, Drawing blood for laboratory evaluations. E, Circumferential measurements at, above, and below bite. Inset, Administration of fluids intravenously, with *slow* administration of antivenin.

REFERENCES AND SUGGESTED READING

1. Peterson, M.E., and Meerdink, G.L.: Bites and stings of venomous animals. *In* Current Veterinary Therapy X. Edited by R.W. Kirk. Philadelphia, W.B. Saunders, 1989.
2. Peterson, M.E.: Venomous snakebite. *In* Proceedings, Critical Care Symposium. Texas A & M University, College Station, TX, June 18–19, 1988.

GUNSHOT WOUNDS

GENERAL DEFINITION AND FACTORS AFFECTING SEVERITY OF INJURY

Gunshot wounds result from penetration (wound of entry) or perforation (wound of entry and exit) of body tissue by some form of missile. The type, size, and severity of a gunshot wound depend on the aerodynamic activity, shape, velocity, mass, and fragmentation of the missile(s) creating the wound. All gunshot wounds are considered contaminated, mandating cleansing and debridement. The specific gravity, water content, and elastic fibers of the injured tissue also influence the nature of the wound.

LOW-VELOCITY GUNSHOT WOUNDS

Definition and Indications. Low-velocity projectiles travel at less than 1000 feet a second. Most handguns fire projectiles of low velocity. As these missiles pass through tissues, they create a permanent tract primarily by crushing and laceration, damaging only tissues contacted by the missile. These wounds generally have a small hole of entry and exit. The tract has bacterial contamination (Fig. 4-7A).

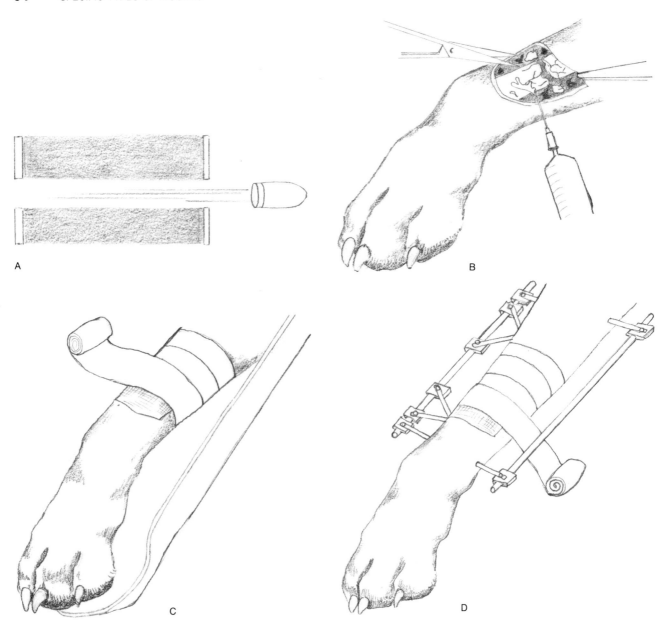

FIG. 4-7. Low-velocity gunshot wounds. A, Low-velocity wounds generally have small holes of entry and exit with damage only to tissues contacted by missile. B, Wound lavage and debridement done on gunshot wound involving soft tissue and bone. C, A splint may be incorporated in bandages for temporary fracture immobilization during treatment of soft tissue wounds. D, An external pin splint may be used to immobilize fracture during treatment of soft tissue wounds.

Treatment of low-velocity gunshot wounds is indicated in the presence of soft-tissue and especially of orthopedic trauma.

If perforation or penetration involves the abdomen, surgical exploration is required. Low-velocity gunshot wounds of the thorax may not need immediate exploration; however, the animal should be observed closely for signs of uncontrollable hemothorax or pneumothorax. Gunshot wounds of the neck may cause esophageal and/or tracheal damage. Therefore, exploration of such wounds with the necessary repair is indicated.

Technique. The animal should be stabilized before undertaking wound management. The involved body part must be thoroughly examined to determine nerve function, vascular disruption, and extent of tissue damage.

At least two radiographic projections are indicated to help locate bullets and bullet fragments. They also help in assessing soft tissue and bone damage and in evaluating missile tracts.

Both high- and low-velocity missiles may leave small holes of perforation. Occasionally the velocity of the wounding missile is unknown. If the holes of perforation are small and the animal shows minimal physical and radiographic signs of tissue damage, the wound has probably been caused by a low-velocity missile. To help ascertain this, limited exploration of the perforations may aid in confirming a diagnosis of low-velocity missile injury.

Low-velocity gunshot wounds are generally small and do not require extensive debridement. The hair is clipped around the wound(s) and the adjacent skin is cleansed. Necessary debridement is completed while intermittently lavaging the wound tract with an antiseptic solution. It is usually unnecessary to remove the bullet or bullet fragments unless they are located intra-articularly, will compromise function, will cause discomfort, or will create further damage if left *in situ*. The wound is generally left open for drainage and covered with a sterile bandage.

Low-velocity missiles may cause fractures with little soft tissue damage. When the wound is debrided and lavaged, bone fragments with soft tissue attachment should be preserved for use in fracture repair. Small unattached fragments should be discarded, but large fragments should remain in place for repair of the fracture (Fig. 4-7B). After debridement, provision should be made for drainage, and exposed tendons and bone should be covered with soft tissue or bandage material. Fractures should be immobilized with external pin splints or dressings and splints while the soft tissue wound is being treated (Fig. 4-7C and D). External pin splints provide optimal fracture fixation for this type of injury because they do not invade the fracture site. With such an external fixation apparatus, pins are placed in healthy tissue above and below the fracture. This gives support to the area for fracture healing while the gunshot wound is treated. If it is anticipated that a secondary fracture fixation may be necessary, the pins of the original external pin splint should be placed as far from the wound as possible to leave enough bone for the secondary fixation. Missile fragments in joints should be removed. Osteochondral fragments are either reattached or removed, depending on their size. The amount of joint damage dictates whether orthopedic reconstruction or arthrodesis is needed. Wounds involving joints should be immobilized for 2 weeks postoperatively. This can be accomplished effectively by a transarticular external pin splint. Return of function should be slow, with splints and soft wraps used for several more weeks or months.

Aftercare. Because gunshot wounds are most likely to be contaminated with gram-positive cocci, an antibi-

otic with appropriate spectrum such as cephalothin* (25 mg/kg IV every 8 hours) is indicated as part of the initial wound treatment. Oral antibiotics may be used after 3 days. The length of time and route of administration of antibiotics depend on the severity of the wound and whether it is treated as an open or closed wound. Good clinical judgment is indicated. Immobilization and rest are indicated, with daily bandage changes as the wound heals. If fractures were associated with the injury and immobilization was temporary by means of a splint incorporated into bandages, definitive fracture repair should be performed after healthy tissue is present in the wound area.

Advantages and Disadvantages. Because low-velocity gunshot wounds do not cause as much tissue damage as high-velocity missile or close-range shotgun wounds, a more conservative approach to management may be followed, unless there is bone involvement. Thus, the healing process is usually shorter in these wounds and may not require the extensive reconstructive procedures needed for high-velocity missile wounds and close-range shotgun wounds. If a splint is incorporated into bandages, movement of the fracture segments may occur when bandages are changed.

REFERENCES AND SUGGESTED READING

1. Adams, D.B.: Wound ballistics: A review. Milit. Med. *147*:831, 1982.
2. Archibald, J., Holt, J.C., and Sokolovsky, V.: Management of Trauma in Dogs and Cats. Santa Barbara, CA, American Veterinary Publications, Inc., 1981.
3. Aron, D.N.: Management of open musculoskeleletal injuries. Semin. Vet. Med. Surg. *3*:290, 1988.
4. Berg, P.: Wound ballistics. *In* Textbook of Small Animal Orthopedics. Edited by C.D. Newton and D.M. Nunamaker. Philadelphia, J.B. Lippincott Co., 1985.
5. Frost, P.A., and Grier, R.L.: Management of gunshot wounds. Iowa State Vet. *47*:133, 1986.
6. Lipowitz, A.J.: Management of gunshot wounds of the soft tissues and extremities. J. Amer. Anim. Hosp. Assoc. *12*:813, 1975.
7. Loden, D., Stickle, R.L., Birchard, S.J.: Conservative management of gunshot wounds. A case report. J. Am. Anim. Hosp. Assoc. *18*:753, 1982.
8. Pavletic, M.M.: A review of 121 gunshot wounds in the dog and cat (abstract). Vet. Surg. *14*:61, 1985.
9. Pavletic, M.M.: Gunshot wounds in veterinary medicine: Projectile ballistics—Part I. Compend. Contin. Educ. *8*:47, 1986.
10. Pavletic, M.M.: Gunshot wounds in veterinary medicine: Projectile ballistics—Part II. Compend. Contin. Educ. *8*:125, 1986.
11. Rendano, V.T., Abdinoor, D.: Management of intra- and extra-articular extremity gunshot wounds. J. Am. Anim. Hosp. Assoc. *13*:577, 1977.
12. Renegar, W.R., and Stoll, S.G.: Gunshot wounds involving the canine carpus: Surgical management. J. Am. Anim. Hosp. Assoc. *16*:233, 1980.

*Keflin, Eli Lilly and Co., Indianapolis, IN.

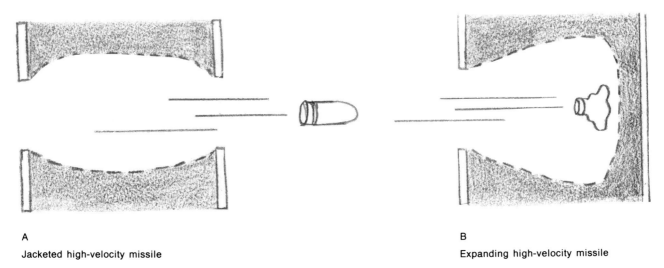

A
Jacketed high-velocity missile

B
Expanding high-velocity missile

FIG. 4-8. High-velocity gunshot wounds. A, Jacketed missile injury generally has a cylindrical tract of extensive damage with deep penetration. B, Expanding missile injury generally has a conical tract of more extensive damage with less penetration.

HIGH-VELOCITY GUNSHOT WOUNDS

Definition and Indications. High-velocity missiles are usually fired from rifles and travel at more than 2000 feet a second. They cause a great amount of tissue damage and transfer considerable energy to adjacent tissues in the form of shock waves and cavitation. The high pulse pressures of the shock waves may create temporary tissue cavitation up to 30 times the diameter of the wounding missile, persisting for 5 to 30 microseconds. This shock wave and cavitation cause blunt contusion of associated tissues. The momentary stretching and tearing of vessels that occurs results in hemorrhage and thrombosis. There is also implosion of debris into the wound. This circulatory insult, resultant tissue necrosis, and presence of imploded foreign debris increase the chance of infection, with the volume of necrosis influenced by the severity of vascular compromise. Fractured bones, bowel ruptures and contusion of heart and lungs may occur as a result of the shock waves without these organs having been directly contacted by the missile. In addition, high-velocity missiles may cause greater tissue destruction if they are tumbling or undergoing some other form of flight instability when they strike the tissue, or if secondary projectiles are formed in the wound as the result of missile fragmentation or shattering of bone. Fractures caused by high-velocity missiles are usually severely comminuted, often with fragments missing. If the hole of perforation is large, it indicates injury by a high-velocity missile. There may, however, be a small hole of perforation associated with a high-velocity fully jacketed missile.

High-velocity bullets are manufactured with a lead core and an outer "jacket" of metal that prevents the lead from melting or the bullet from deforming as it moves through the barrel. If the jacket covers the point of the bullet, it is referred to as a full-metal jacket (FMJ) or metal-case bullet. The design of these bullets does not allow expansion. The damage caused by these missiles is in the form of a cylindrical tract and is less than that caused by expanding bullets (Fig. 4-8A). The bullet, however, can cause sizeable tracts in tissues because of flight instability and fragmentation of bone. If the jacket does not cover the point, the bullet is designated as a soft-point or expanding bullet, which tends to flatten or "mushroom" on contact. This creates a large conical wound tract up to 40 times the diameter of an FMJ wound and transfers more kinetic energy into the tissues than does the FMJ (Fig. 4-8B). The rapid deceleration and instability of expanding missiles in tissue promote fragmentation of the bullet.

Because of the greater tissue damage associated with high-velocity missile wounds, more aggressive debridement is indicated than with low-velocity missile wounds. If perforation or penetration involves the abdomen, surgical exploration is required.

Technique. See Low-Velocity Gunshot Wounds, this chapter. Many of the preliminary procedures and wound management techniques used in managing low-velocity missile injuries apply also to high-velocity missile injuries.

If the velocity of the wounding missile is unknown, a small hole of perforation is present, and the animal shows physical and radiographic signs of severe tissue

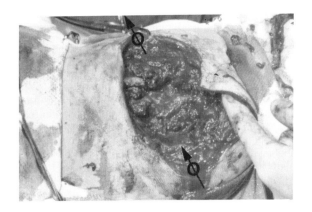

A

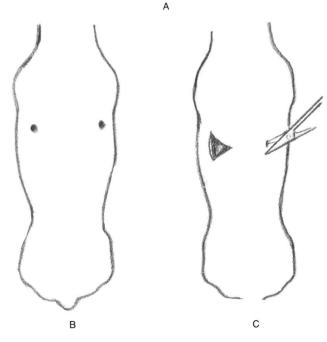

B   C

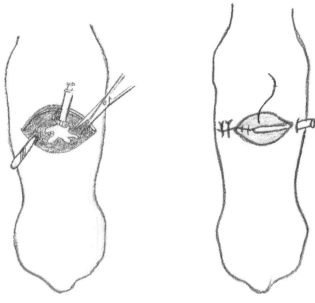

D   E

damage, the wound has probably been caused by a high-velocity fully jacketed missile (Fig. 4-9A and B). Limited exploration of the perforation wounds may confirm the need for aggressive debridement of the wound (Fig. 4-9C).

The wound track is explored, devitalized tissue removed, and hematomas evacuated while the wound is copiously lavaged with an antiseptic solution (Fig. 4-9D). If the wound is to be closed, the dead space is obliterated with interrupted 3-0 absorbable sutures used in as few a number as necessary to close the dead space and cover exposed tendons and nerves. If closure is warranted, a drain is placed in the injury area (Fig. 4-9E). The wound is bandaged and immobilized as necessary. If a large open wound is present with much devitalized tissue, it may be advisable to treat it as an open wound and use delayed primary or secondary closure or let it heal by contraction and epithelialization. Tension should not be used to close a wound because of the increased soft tissue necrosis that will occur. In the presence of fractures, wound management is the same as described for low-velocity gunshot wounds.

Aftercare. See Low-Velocity Gunshot Wounds, this chapter. If a large, deep wound is initially managed as an open wound and delayed primary or secondary closure cannot be effectively performed, skin graft or flap reconstruction may be necessary.

Advantages and Disadvantages. Treatment of high-velocity missile wounds generally has the disadvantage of requiring more extensive debridement and care than that of low-velocity missile injuries. The more extensive debridement leaves a larger tissue defect, resulting in a longer healing time if the wound is allowed to heal as an open wound or requiring more involved reconstructive procedures than those needed for low-velocity missile wounds.

REFERENCES AND SUGGESTED READING

1. Almskog, B.A., Haljamea, H., Hasselgren, P.O., and Nordstrom, G.: Local metabolic changes in skeletal muscle following high energy missile injury. J. Trauma *22*:382, 1982.

FIG. 4-9. Small holes of gunshot perforation of unknown velocity with or without physical and radiographic evidence of severe tissue damage. A, Gunshot wound across lumbar region of a dog. Missile velocity was unknown. Small holes of perforation (arrows). Wound exploration revealed extensive damage. B, Small holes of perforation. C, Limited exploration of the holes reveals severe tissue damage. D, Exposure and debridement of missile tract. E, Wound closure with drain placement.

2. DeMuth, W.E., and Smith J.M.: High velocity bullet wounds of muscle and bone: The basis of rational early treatment. J. Trauma *6*:744, 1966.

3. Livingstone, R.H., and Wilson, R.T.: Gunshot wounds of the limbs. Br. Med. J. *1*:667, 1975.

4. Speer, Omark Industries: Reloading Manual, No. 10. Lewiston, Idaho, Speer, Omark Industries, 1979.

See Low-Velocity Gunshot Wounds, this chapter, for additional references and suggested reading.

SHOTGUN WOUNDS

Definition and Indications. Shotgun injuries occurring within 15 yards of the muzzle of the gun are very destructive because the pellet concentration is dense (Fig. 4-10A). Topical debris such as hair is driven into the wound by the pellets. The wad of felt, paper, cork, or plastic between the powder and pellets may also be driven into the wound. In Type I injuries, subcutaneous tissue and deep fascia have been penetrated. Structures beneath the deep fascia are perforated in Type II injuries, and Type III injuries are at a range of less than 3 yards with an extensive central zone of tissue destruction and a halo of pellet holes peripherally (Fig. 4-10B).

The indication for surgical intervention in shotgun wounds is directly proportional to the closeness at which the injury occurred.

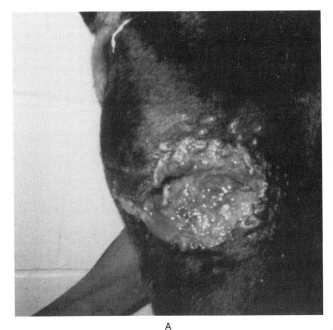

A

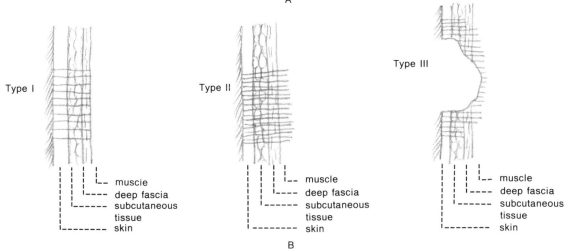

B

FIG. 4-10. Shotgun wounds. A, Type III close-range shotgun injury with extensive tissue damage. B, Types of close-range shotgun wounds. Type I: subcutaneous tissue and deep fascia penetrated. Type II: structures beneath deep fascia penetrated. Type III: extensive central tissue destruction with halo of peripheral pellet holes.

Technique. See Low-Velocity Gunshot Wounds, this chapter. Many of the preliminary procedures used in managing low-velocity missile injuries apply to close-range shotgun injuries. Two radiographic projections are indicated to assess the location and concentration of pellets and the extent of bone damage.

Close-range shotgun injuries with extensive tissue damage require debridement procedures similar to those used for high-velocity gunshot wounds. It is not necessary to remove all the pellets embedded in the soft tissues because they cause little tissue reaction, and attempted removal could cause further tissue damage. Thorough debridement and lavage with an antiseptic solution are necessary, however, to remove the plastic, felt, paper, or cork wadding that may also be in the tissues. Because of the surface expanse and depth of some close-range shotgun injuries, initial management of the injury as an open wound may be indicated. Close-range shotgun injuries that have caused fractures should be managed the same as fracture wounds inflicted by low- and high-velocity missiles.

Aftercare. See Low-Velocity Gunshot Wounds, this chapter. If a large, deep wound is initially managed as an open wound and delayed primary or secondary closure cannot be effectively performed, skin graft or flap reconstruction may be necessary.

Advantages and Disadvantages. Compared to low-velocity missile injuries, close range shotgun injuries generally have the disadvantages of requiring extensive debridement and care, taking longer to heal, and requiring more extensive reconstructive procedures similar to those for high-velocity gunshot injuries.

REFERENCES AND SUGGESTED READING

1. Ledgerwood, A.M.: The management of shotgun wounds. Surg. Clin. North Am. *57*:111, 1977.

2. Sherman, R.T., and Parrish, R.A.: Management of Shotgun Injuries: A review of 152 cases. J. Trauma *3*:76, 1963.

See Low-Velocity Gunshot Wounds, this chapter, for additional references and suggested reading.

BITE WOUNDS

Definition and Indications. Bite wounds result in punctures, crushing, lacerations, or avulsions of flaps of skin or other tissue. Some bite wounds may exhibit the "iceberg" effect with a small surface wound and great underlying tissue damage. Although the wound made by a canine tooth often appears as only a puncture wound, up to 450 psi of crushing force can be transmitted by a dog bite. During the slashing action of a bite, the tooth moves through the underlying subcutaneous and muscular tissues (Fig. 4-11A), but the skin slides with the movement of the tooth. The results are torn muscles, separated fascia planes, and/or severed tendons, arteries, veins, and nerves. Hair from the victim's coat may be embedded into the bite wound, and the wound is innoculated with bacteria from the attacker's mouth, the victim's skin and hair, and soil organisms. These may be aerobic and anaerobic bacteria that interact synergistically. The devitalized tissue, dead space, and serum accumulation provide a good medium in which innoculated bacteria may grow. Occasionally, the skin puncture wound heals but the bacteria continue to grow in the deeper tissues, causing cellulitis or abscess in the area. Intermittent draining sinuses or a large subcutaneous abscess may develop (Fig. 4-11B). With abscess, a large portion of skin may slough (Fig. 4-11C). This problem is more prevalent in cats. Abscesses in cats may cause osteomyelitis of underlying bone, frequently seen in the ilium, sacrum, or coccygeal vertebrae.

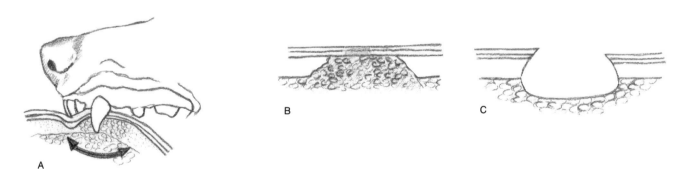

FIG. 4-11. "Iceberg" effect of some bite wounds. A, Skin puncture wound with extensive damage to underlying tissues as tooth moves through tissues. B, Puncture wound heals over damaged tissue, in which an abscess forms. C, Damaged tissue sloughs, leaving a large skin defect.

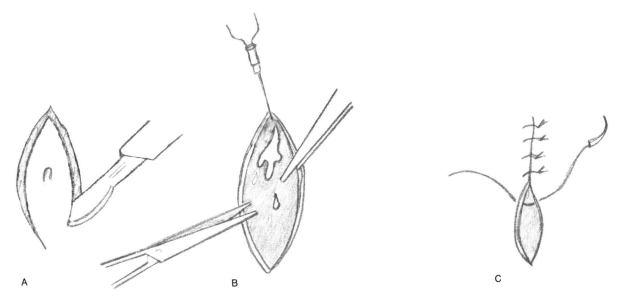

FIG. 4-12. Bite wound management. A, Dorsoventral fusiform excision made around dog bite wound. B, Wound debrided while being lavaged. C, Wound closed.

Major vascular damage may be shown by early excessive swelling of the traumatized part. Animals may exanguinate if large vessels such as the carotid artery or jugular vein are damaged by a neck bite or femoral vessels by a groin bite.

In some instances when a large dog attacks a small dog, there may be numerous puncture wounds over the body with the skin severely contused and separated from severely damaged underlying tissues. Such wounds may also cause thoracic, abdominal, cranial, and spinal punctures and damage.

Surgical exploration, debridement, and lavage are indicated for puncture, laceration, and avulsion bite wounds. Because of the number and extent of some puncture wounds, however, therapy in the form of a subcutaneously placed drain, lavage, and supportive medications is indicated.

Technique.   The area prepared for surgery should be large. Because of the tendency of devitalized tissue to become infected, it is best to open puncture wounds maximally. The wounds should be probed to determine the best direction of incision. In most instances, a dorsoventral incision or fusiform excision is preferable to allow wound debridement and ventral drainage (Fig. 4-12A). Devitalized tissue, especially muscle and fat, should be removed from the wound while it is lavaged with an antiseptic solution (Fig. 4-12B). Care should be taken to maintain intact blood and nerve supply to the remaining tissue.

After debridement of puncture wounds, dead space should be closed or drained. If the wound has been completely debrided, primary closure is indicated, using as few simple interrupted 3-0 absorbable sutures as possible in the deeper tissues and 3-0 monofilament

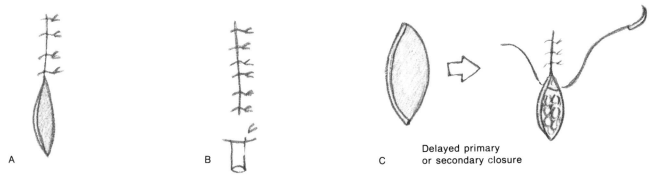

FIG. 4-13. Techniques for drainage of bite wounds. A, Dorsal aspect of wound is closed, leaving ventral aspect open for drainage. B, Penrose drain emerging ventrally. C, The wound is left open, then closed with delayed primary or secondary closure.

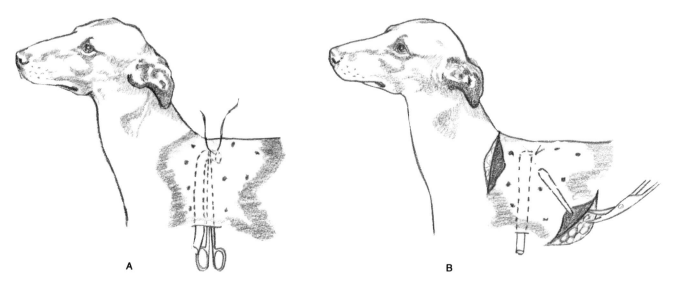

FIG. 4-14. Technique for draining extensive dead space associated with bite wounds. A, Long forceps introduce a Penrose drain from ventral aspect of skin separation. Drain anchored dorsally, with a simple interrupted skin suture. B, As skin becomes obviously devitalized, it is excised.

nonabsorbable skin sutures (Fig. 4-12C). If there is incomplete debridement, contamination, or a compromised blood supply, drainage is definitely indicated. For drainage, the dorsal aspect of the wound may be closed while the ventralmost portion is left open; the wound may be closed with the placement of a Penrose drain; or the wound may be treated as an open wound, followed by delayed primary or secondary closure (Fig. 4-13A through C).

When the animal is in shock because of extensive bite damage, aggressive antibiotic, fluid and steroid therapy are indicated initially. If puncture of the thoracic, abdominal, cranial or spinal areas has occurred, this damage must be initially assessed and treated accordingly. With separation of the skin from the underlying tissues and where extensive debridement would be contraindicated, an alternative or an adjunct to debridement is to establish drainage with a Penrose drain from the ventralmost limit of the subcutaneous separation (Fig. 4-14A). Lavage of the wound(s) during the debridement process or after installation of the drain may be done with an antiseptic solution.

Skin lacerations and avulsion-type wounds should be excised back to healthy tissue and the defect closed primarily or by delayed primary closure. When large amounts of skin have been removed, entire closure of the wound may not be possible. The remaining wound may be closed by a skin graft or flap, moving local skin for closure, or allowing the wound to heal by contraction and epithelialization.

Aftercare. Systemic antibiotics should be used in treatment because of the contaminated/infected state of such wounds. Antibiotics are especially indicated in treating animals with multiple puncture wounds where complete debridement is contraindicated. Numerous organisms have been isolated from dog and cat bite wounds, including *Pasteurella multocida*, *Staphylococcus species*, and *Streptococcus species*, with *Pasteurella multocida* being a major causative organism in bite wound infections, especially cat bites. Although no antibiotic is effective against all organisms present, most organisms are susceptible to penicillin. One regimen of therapy described is procaine penicillin G (200,000 units/kg IM) at the time of wound therapy followed by ampicillin (22 mg/kg every 6 hours by mouth for 3 to 5 days). Another regimen that could be used is cephalothin* (35 mg/kg IV, every 8 hours for 24 hours). This should be followed by intramuscular injection t.i.d. for 4 days with extensive tissue damage. If an oral antibiotic is desired, Amoxicillin[†] (20 mg/kg three times a day by mouth for 5 days) can be given. With massive tissue damage, prolonged antibiotic therapy may be necessary, based on clinical judgement.

In extensive bite wound damage with separation of the skin from the underlying tissue, staged debridement should be performed so that, when the skin becomes obviously nonviable, it is removed along with any underlying nonvital tissue (Fig. 4-14B). The wound may be allowed to heal by contraction and

---

*Keflin, Eli Lilly and Co., Indianapolis, IN.

[†]Amoxicillin film-coated tablets or Amoxi-Drop suspension, Beecham Laboratories, Bristol, TN.

epithelialization. A large defect may require reconstruction through moving local tissues, flaps, or grafts.

Advantages and Disadvantages. Considered from the standpoint of the type of wound, laceration and avulsion-type bite wounds are debrided and lavaged more easily than puncture-type injuries. As a result, the infection rate in such wounds is lower than in puncture wounds, where lavage and debridement may not be as easily accomplished. In addition, the animal with extensive puncture wounds, severely damaged underlying tissues, and separation of the skin from these tissues is difficult to treat successfully because of the severe tissue damage, extensive bacterial contamination/infection, and toxic status of the animal.

REFERENCES AND SUGGESTED READING

1. Archibald, J., Holt, J.C., and Sokolovsky, V.: Management of Trauma in Dogs and Cats. Santa Barbara, CA, American Veterinary Publishers Inc., 1981.
2. Aron, D.N.: Management of open musculoskeletal injuries. Semin. Vet. Med. Surg. *3*:290, 1988.
3. August, J.R.: Dog and cat bites. J. Am. Vet. Med. Assoc. *193*:1394, 1988.
4. Bright R.M., and Probst, C.W.: Management of superficial skin wounds. *In* Textbook of Small Animal Surgery. Edited by D.H. Slatter. Philadelphia, W.B. Saunders, 1985.
5. Callaham, M.L.: Treatment of common dog bites: Infection risk factors. J. Am. Coll. Emerg. Phys. *7*:83, 1978.
6. Callaham, M.L.: Prophylactic antibiotics in common dog bite wounds: A controlled study. Ann. Emerg. Med. *9*:410, 1980.
7. Callaham, M.L.: Dog bite wounds. JAMA *244*:2327, 1980.
8. Kirk, R.W., and Bistner, S.I.: Handbook of Veterinary Procedures and Emergency Treatment. 4th ed. Philadelphia, W.B. Saunders, 1985.
9. Neal, T.M., Key, J.C.: Principles of treatment of dog bite wounds. J. Am. Anim. Hosp. Assoc. *12*:657, 1976.
10. Schultz, R.C., McMaster, W.C.: The treatment of dog bite injuries, especially those of the face. Plast. Reconstr. Surg. *49*:494, 1972.

PSYCHOGENIC DERMATOSES

ACRAL LICK DERMATITIS (LICK GRANULOMA)

Definition and Indications. Clinically, lick granulomas are firm, thickened, ulcerated plaques that may be surrounded by a hyperpigmented halo (Fig. 4-15A). If uncontrolled, they can extend by self-mutilation down through subcutaneous tissue and muscle until bone is exposed. They are the result of continual licking at an area and may occur on any part of the body; however, they occur most frequently on the cranial carpal or metacarpal areas, followed in frequency by the cranial radial, tarsal, metatarsal, and tibial areas (Fig. 4-15B). The lesions may be unilateral or bilateral, with a less favorable prognosis accompanying bilateral lesions.

Positive diagnosis and *early* therapy are indicated for lick granulomas to help establish underlying causes and obtain the best response to therapy before the condition becomes chronic and unresponsive.

Techniques. *Preliminary Procedures.* In the presence of a lick granuloma, the initial history and diagnostic workup should be aimed at determining possible underlying organic factors that may be the cause of continual licking. Diagnostic procedures that may be beneficial include:

Test/Procedure	*Reason*
Thorough history	Ascertain or eliminate any physical reason for licking (previous trauma, foreign body, subcutaneous injection of an irritating substance, etc.). Determine any psychogenic causes of the condition.
Dermatologic examination	Observe for signs and sites of other cutaneous abnormalities.
Skin scraping	Check for demodicosis.
Fungal culture	Check for dermatophytosis.
Biopsy and/or exfoliative cytology	Check for bacterial funiculosis, mycotic or mycobacterial granuloma, or neoplasia (especially mastocytoma or histiocytoma).
Radiographs	Check for underlying osseous pathology (such as arthritis, osteomyelitis, osteosarcoma, periosteal proliferation) or foreign bodies.
Electrodiagnostics (Nerve conduction velocity, electromyogram) if available	Determine if there is abnormal innervation to the area
Intradermal allergy tests	Confirm the presence of atopy or flea allergy
Hypoallergenic dietary trial	Determine the presence of food allergy

If, with the above diagnostic techniques, underlying organic causes are identified as the cause of the lick granuloma, these should be treated. If a cause is not identified, however, three forms of therapy or therapy combinations are used by the authors. These are: (1) topical and intralesional medication, (2) therapy directed toward the psychogenic nature of the condition, and (3) surgical therapy.

Topical and Intralesional Therapy. Topical application of various steriod-antibiotic ointments have been used to treat the condition. Intralesional injections of corticosteriods (triamcinalone acetonide* or methylprednisolone[†]), cobra venom,[‡] and Orgotein[§] have also been described for therapy. Of these, cobra venom is no longer commercially available.

A mixture of 8 ml of fluocinolone acetonide and dimethyl sulfoxide[||] and 3 ml of flunixin meglumine[#] may be applied to the lesion twice daily. A dauber bottle may be used to apply the solution. The lesion is not covered with a bandage. Application of the medication is continued until the lick granuloma is healed.

Radiation therapy has been used to treat lesions and can be considered a form of topical or intralesional therapy.

Therapy Directed at the Psychogenic Nature of the Condition. Environmental Modifications—When the history reveals an environmental factor or factors that causes anxiety or tension in the animal and resulting excessive licking, environmental manipulations are indicated.

Examples of environmental causes of lick granulomas include:

1. Dog left alone all day
2. Long confinement to crate, cage, kennel, or runs
3. New baby in the home
4. New pet in the home
5. Female dog ''in heat'' nearby but not accessible to male dog
6. New dog in the vicinity
7. Loss of a family member
8. Loss of a long-time companion animal

Any management practices, routines, or interaction patterns that are likely to evoke self-mutilation behavior should be avoided. Such changes may include alter-

ing the housing situation for kenneled dogs. Routine exercise and regular periods of individual attention may be necessary. The owner may need to decrease the amount of time away from the animal by going to the animal or keeping it with him or her when possible. Introduction of another pet into the household may be indicated when self-mutilation is induced by loss of a companion animal, prolonged separation from the owners, or boredom because the owner has insufficient time to spend with the animal. The companion animal may be a new puppy or a spayed female for a male dog.

Pharmacologic Behavioral Modifications—This form of therapy may be used in conjunction with topical and systemic therapy or surgical therapy. Phenobarbital (2.2 to 6.6 mg/kg twice a day orally) may be used for long or short-term therapy. Progestogens may be helpful. Repository progesterone[¶] (20 mg/kg injected every 3 weeks) may be successful in some instances. Megestrol acetate[+] (1 mg/kg by mouth daily until improvement is noticed, then tapered to a minimum maintenance dose and frequency) is known for its behavior-modifying effects. The progestogens should not be used on intact female dogs. In some dogs, a beginning dose of the oral progestogens may be at 2.2 mg/kg daily for 1 to 2 weeks, then 1.1 mg/kg daily for 2 weeks, followed by gradual withdrawal.

Nonpharmacologic Behavioral Modification (Physical Restraints)—The use of physical restraining devices to keep a dog from self-molestation should be considered, especially when the dog is unsupervised. Use of these devices should be gradually reduced. Physical restraining measures found to be effective include Elizabethan collars, which can be purchased commercially or made from cardboard (Fig. 4-16A). A plastic bucket can be modified to fit over a dog's head by cutting a hole in the bottom of the bucket just large enough to get the dog's head through (Fig. 4-16B). For added security, lengths of gauze are passed through small holes around the large head hole and affixed to a collar. The length (height) of the bucket should be shortened if necessary so that it does not interfere with drinking or eating.

Wire basket-type muzzles of various sizes can be obtained commercially (Fig. 4-16C). These can be modified, if necessary, by placing a strip of tape or leather from the portion of the muzzle that goes over the nasal area to the strap that goes behind the ears. This prevents the dog from pulling the muzzle off over its nose.

Side braces can be made from aluminum splint rods to help keep dogs from licking the hind limbs. A ring large enough to fit at the base of the dog's neck is bent in the center of the bar. The remaining rod lengths are bent at right angles to the ring, and the ends of the bars are

---

*Vetalog, Solvay Veterinary, Inc., Princeton, NJ.

[†]Depo-Medrol, Upjohn Co., Kalamazoo, MI.

[‡]Cobroxin, No longer available.

[§]Palosein, Diagnostic Data, Inc., Mountain View, CA.

[||]Synotic Otic Solution, Syntex Laboratories, Inc., Palo Alto, CA.

[#]Banamine Solution, Schering Corp., Kenilworth NJ.

[¶]Depo-Provera, Upjohn Co, Kalamazoo, MI.

[+]Megace, Bristol-Meyers Oncology Div., Evansville, IN, and Ovaban, Schering Corp., Kenilworth NJ.

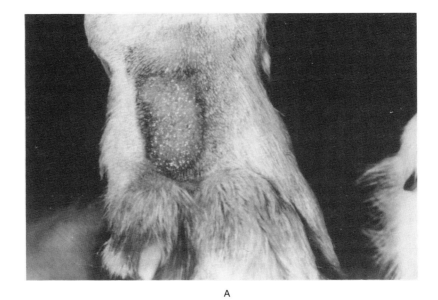

A

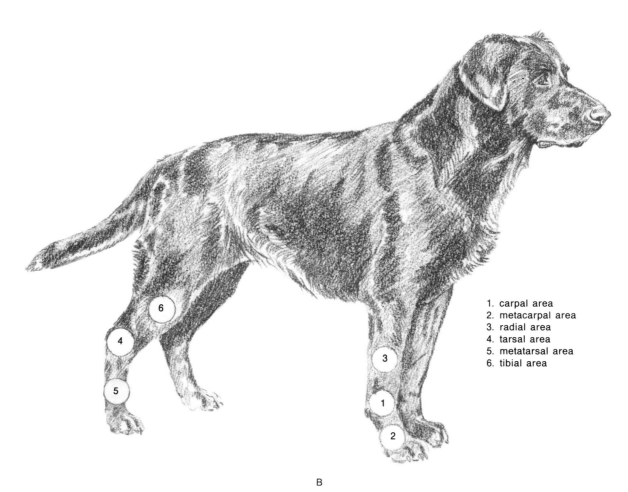

1. carpal area
2. metacarpal area
3. radial area
4. tarsal area
5. metatarsal area
6. tibial area

B

FIG. 4-15. Canine psychogenic dermatosis. A, Typical acral lick dermatitis (lick granuloma) lesion. B, Usual locations of lick granulomas.

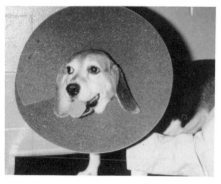
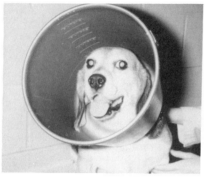
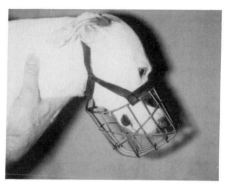

A   B   C

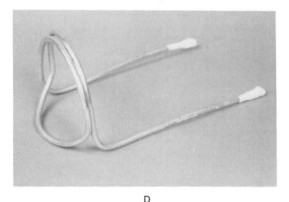
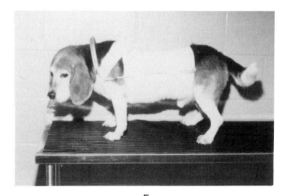

D   E

FIG. 4-16. Physical restraint devices to prevent self-molestation. A, Elizabethan collar. B, Modified plastic bucket over a dog's head. C, Wire basket-type muzzle. D, Aluminum splint rod side braces. E, Aluminum splint rod side braces placed on a dog over a body bandage.

padded (Fig. 4-16D). With the ring at the base of the dog's neck, the two bars extend along the dog's sides to the flank area. Two segments of tape around the body and over the bars keep the bars along the dog's sides. Placing a body bandage around the dog before taping the bars in place makes it more comfortable for the dog than affixing the tape directly to the hair. Two pieces of tape crisscrossed over the brisket of the dog and attached to the body bandage keep the bandage from slipping caudally (Fig. 4-16E).

Topical Chemical Deterrents—The use of bitter-tasting chemicals on or around the lesion or covering bandage may help to prevent self-mutilation. The anticholinergic astringent diphemanil methylsulfate* or other commercially available solutions may be used. For best results, some of the solution should be dabbed on the nose to allow the dog to lick and smell it simultaneously. The lesion or bandage is then sprayed with the solution. Thus, the lingering scent is associated with the bitter taste. Substances such as hot pepper sauce and lemon juice may be harmful to tissue and should be avoided.

No Reinforcement of Excess Grooming and Substitute Behavior—Grooming behavior of the dog should be ignored, not punished. When the dog begins to show an interest in the affected area, it should be distracted and encouraged to perform a substitute behavior which is incompatible with excessive grooming. Such behaviors might be play behavior or assuming a relaxed posture. If done frequently and consistently enough, the animal learns to perform this behavior instead of the excess grooming.

Surgical Therapy. The authors have used three forms of reconstruction after excision of the lesion: (1) primary suturing, (2) skin grafting, or (3) use of a flap. Even large defects may be closed using some form of tension sutures and/or relaxing incision. Mesh grafts, pouch flaps, and axial pattern flaps have been used to close large defects caused by lick granuloma removal. The reader is referred to the sections of the book that deal with these procedures.

Cryosurgery has also been used to treat lick granulomas.

Aftercare. If environmental modifications have been part of the therapy, the dog should be gradually re-exposed to the environmental stimuli that evoke any

*Variton, Schering Corp., Kenilworth, NJ.

anxiety that results in self-mutilation. If the dog performs in an acceptable way, it should be rewarded. An example is leaving the dog alone for increasingly longer periods, with rewards for acceptable behavior when time alone is the anxiety-inducing agent. Gradually reducing the width of an Elizabethan collar or leaving other restraint devices off the dog for increasingly longer times are other examples of aftercare.

Gradual reduction of progestogens to the minimum effective dose and frequency can be considered a form of aftercare when these are used for treatment.

The aftercare of surgical reconstruction is that described for each type of surgery.

Advantages and Disadvantages. Intralesional steroids have been found helpful in lesions smaller than 3 cm in diameter but useless in large chronic lesions. Cobra venom used intralesionally is sometimes beneficial, but it is no longer commercially available. Intralesional Orgotein has been helpful, but is painful and requires general anesthesia for injection. Radiation therapy has been found rarely, or at best 50%, effective. Cryosurgery has been described as a last resort for large lesions that have not responded to other therapies. It results in a slough that occurs over 2 to 3 weeks, but has been claimed to destroy nerve endings in the area to block the itch-lick cycle. It may need to be repeated 2 to 3 times.

The relative success of topical fluocinolone acetonide, dimethyl sulfoxide, and flunixin meglumine mixture make it a good therapeutic choice.

Environmental modifications and subsequent re-exposure require time and effort on the part of the pet owner, as does teaching the dog a substitute behavior. Addition of another pet to the environment may be beneficial. The dogs may not be compatible, however; they may compete for attention from the owner and occasionally may both lick at the lesion.

Though progestogens may be effective, their use should be undertaken with adequate warning to the owner. They are not approved for behavioral therapy in dogs. These drugs are expensive and should not be used on intact females. In addition, they may eliminate one behavioral abnormality and induce another.

The use of physical restraint devices may be beneficial; however, these require periodic adjustment and removal. If improperly fitted or padded, they may cause abrasions such as those caused by a wire basket muzzle. They may also further frustrate a psychotic dog. Topical chemical deterrents may be initially effective, but the animal may eventually develop a taste for the chemical or learn to tolerate the taste so that it can remove bandages and continue licking.

When surgical treatment is performed, owners should always be informed that it is possible to obtain a good reconstruction and uneventful healing with the aid of bandages and restraint devices; however, at some point after removal of restraint devices, the animal may severely damage or destroy the area. Gradual removal of restraints and use of other forms of therapy may be helpful.

REFERENCES AND SUGGESTED READING

1. Krahwinkel, D.J., and Bone, D.L.: Surgical management of specific skin disorders. *In* Textbook of Small Animal Surgery. Edited by D.H. Slatter. Philadelphia, W.B. Saunders, 1985.
2. Muller, G.H., Kirk, R.W., Scott, D.W.: Small Animal Dermatology. 3rd ed. Philadelphia, W.B. Saunders, 1983.
3. Scott, D.W., Walton, D.K.: Clinical evaluation of a topical treatment for canine acral lick dermatitis. J. Am. Anim. Hosp. Assoc. *20*:565, 1984.
4. Walton, D.K.: Psychodermatoses. *In* Current Veterinary Therapy IX. Edited by R.W. Kirk. Philadelphia, W.B. Saunders, 1986.
5. Young, M.S.: Psychogenic dermatoses. Dermatol. Repts. (Vet. Learning Syst.) *3*:1, 1984.*

*Primary reference.

PRESSURE SORES

Definition and Indications. *Decubital Ulcers.* Decubital ulcers are open wounds that develop over bony prominences as the result of pressure in animals that have been recumbent for long periods due to paralysis, multiple fractures, or convalescence from other severe injuries or illnesses. In general, decubital ulcers are caused by pathologic changes occurring in the soft tissues because of their compression between a bony prominence and the surface on which the animal has been resting.

Decubital ulcers may be classified according to the severity of the lesion (Fig. 4-17A through D) and as follows:

Ulcer Type	Characteristics
Grade I	1. Dark reddened area that does not blanch on pressure. 2. Epidermis and upper dermis may slough.
Grade II	1. Full-thickness skin loss down to the subcutaneous fat.
Grade III	1. Ulcer extends through the subcutaneous fat down to the deeper fascia. 2. Wound edges may be undermined.
Grade IV	1. Ulcer extends through the deep fascia down to the bone. 2. Osteomyelitis or septic arthritis may be present.

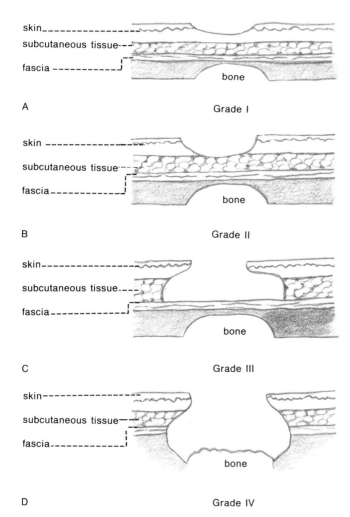

skin

subcutaneous tissue

fascia

bone

A   Grade I

skin

subcutaneous tissue

fascia

bone

B   Grade II

skin

subcutaneous tissue

fascia

bone

C   Grade III

skin

subcutaneous tissue

fascia

bone

D   Grade IV

FIG. 4-17. Decubital ulcer types. A, Grade I: Epidermis and upper dermis slough. B, Grade II: Full-thickness skin loss down to subcutaneous tissue. C, Grade III: Ulcer extends to deep fascia. May be undermining of wound edges. D, Grade IV: Ulcer extends to bone. Osteomyelitis is present.

Areas of skin that are subject to pressure sores are those over the ischiatic tuberosity, greater trochanter, tuber coxae, acromion of the scapula, lateral epicondyle of the humerus, lateral condyle of the tibia, lateral malleolus, lateral aspects of the fifth digits, olecranon, calcaneal tuber, and sternum (Fig. 4-18A).

Cast and Bandage Pressure Sores. Another form of pressure sore develops over bony prominences within a cast or bandage as a result of inadequate or loose padding within the cast, leading to pressure and friction. A more severe type of pressure injury occurs from applying a cast or bandage too tightly, with resultant avascular necrosis of the more peripheral portions of the limb.

In dealing with potential decubital ulcer patients, the primary indication is to prevent the occurrence of such

wounds. If a decubital ulcer does develop, early therapy and preventive measures are indicated to help prevent the wound from becoming more severe. Likewise, with cast and bandage pressure sores, the primary indication is prevention by proper cast or bandage application and investigation if there is any indication of impending pressure necrosis.

Technique. The following factors are beneficial management practices in preventing decubital ulcers:

1. Bedding the animal on a well-padded surface such as a water mattress, air mattress, or artificial fleece.
2. Changing the animal's position frequently.
3. Checking skin over the bony prominences often for signs of an impending decubital ulcer:
   A. Hyperemia
   B. Moisture
   C. Easily epilated hair
4. Keeping the skin clean and dry.
5. Feeding the animal a well balanced, high-protein diet.

Regardless of the type of therapy used, the main factor in therapy is preventing pressure over the ulcer or ulcer repair area. This can be accomplished by use of some form of pressure relief bandage, such as a donut-shaped bandage or a pipe insulation bandage. For a donut-shaped bandage, towels may be rolled and taped together and formed into a "donut" shape just large enough to fit around the ulcer, impending ulcer, or repair area (Fig. 4-18B and C). The "donut" is affixed to the area with tape (Fig. 4-18D). Relatively firm foam rubber (such as pipe insulation) can be cut to form a pressure relief bandage to place over the olecranon area. Pipe insulation of the proper length and diameter is cut lengthwise, and a hole is cut in its center to accommodate the ulcer (Fig. 4-18E). Two or three pieces may be stacked and taped together to help provide sufficient thickness so that the material does not compress when pressure is placed over the area. The cranial aspect of the radial-humeral area is *well* padded with cast padding before taping the pressure relief bandage in place with the hole over the olecranon (Fig. 4-18F). This padding helps to prevent the dog from flexing the joint, which would be necessary for the dog to lie in sternal recumbency and place pressure over the olecranon. Impaired flexion also helps keep the olecranon below the outer surface of the bandage. It may be difficult to secure the bandage so that it does not slip distally on the limb, especially on an obese dog with a relatively short segment of limb proximal to the radial-humeral joint to which the bandage can be affixed. A spica-type bandage may be required to hold the pressure relief bandage up. Placing a bandage with additional padding over an ulcer should be avoided because additional padding over a convex surface actually increases the pressure over the area.

The pipe insulation pressure relief bandage is also effective in the treatment or prevention of decubital ulcers

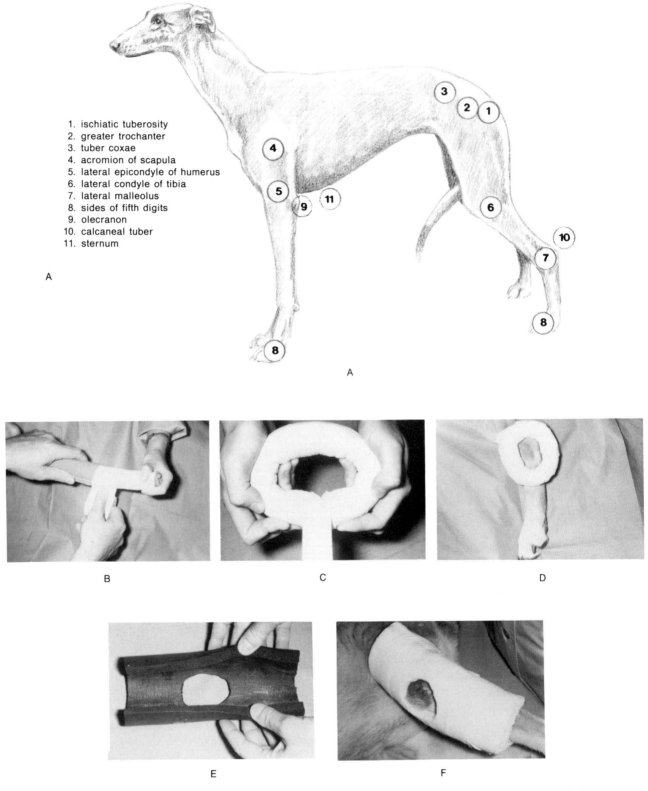

1. ischiatic tuberosity
2. greater trochanter
3. tuber coxae
4. acromion of scapula
5. lateral epicondyle of humerus
6. lateral condyle of tibia
7. lateral malleolus
8. sides of fifth digits
9. olecranon
10. calcaneal tuber
11. sternum

A

A

B

C

D

E

F

FIG. 4-18. Decubital ulcer prevention. A, Areas to observe for decubital ulcers. B, A rolled towel is taped. C, After towel is cut to proper length, ends are taped together to form a "donut." D, "Donut" taped in position over an impending decubital ulcer, ulcer, or repair site. E, Pipe insulation split lengthwise with a hole cut in its center to fit over impending decubital ulcer, ulcer, or repair site. F, Two pieces of pipe insulation stacked and taped together and affixed over the olecranon area after the cranial surface of the radial-humeral joint has been *well* padded.

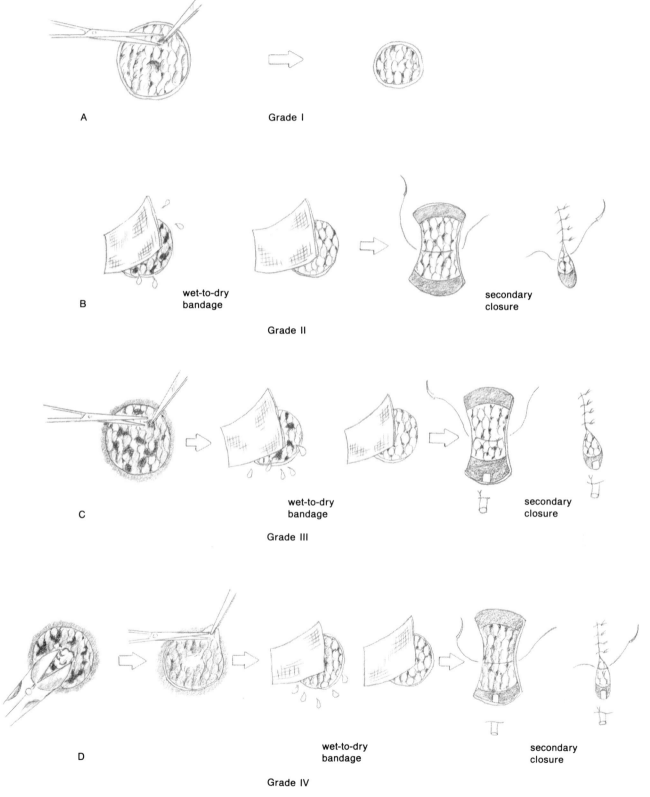

FIG. 4-19. Decubital ulcer therapy. A, Grade I: Cleansing wound and removing sloughing tissue periodically. Heals as open wound. B, Grade II: Wet-to-dry dressings followed by secondary closure. C, Grade III: Debridement, use of wet-to-dry dressings, drainage of dead space, and secondary closure. D, Grade IV: Removal of infected bone, debridement of pockets and tracts, wet-to-dry dressings, drainage of dead space, and secondary closure.

over the sternum because it prevents the dog from assuming a sternal recumbent position. Other effective means of keeping an animal from lying in sternal recumbency are a Schroeder-Thomas splint and a full-length forelimb bandage incorporating some form of splinting material in its lateral aspect that extends from the proximal scapular area to the paw with the bandage affixed to the limb and body in a spica-like fashion.

Treatment of decubital ulcers depends on the grade of the ulcer. A Grade I ulcer may be treated by periodic wound cleansing and removal of any surface tissue that is sloughing. It is allowed to heal as an open wound (Fig. 4-19A).

Grade II ulcers may also be treated as open wounds by keeping them clean. Wet-to-dry dressings may be used to help cleanse and debride the wound of necrotic tissue. Secondary closure may be considered once the wound has formed a bed of healthy granulation tissue (Fig. 4-19B). As with all decubital ulcer closures, there should be no suture lines directly over the bony prominences.

Grade III ulcers with undermining should be debrided of nonviable tissue and treated as open wounds until a healthy bed of granulation tissue has formed. Wet-to-dry bandages may be used. If drainage is copious, however, dry-to-dry bandages may be necessary. If pockets are present in the undermined skin, a 1/4" diameter Penrose drain or a small length of rubber cut from such a drain may be placed at the most dependent area to allow drainage. Secondary closure may be performed as soon as a bed of healthy granulation tissue has formed (Fig. 4-19C).

Grade IV ulcers require removal of infected tissue, including infected cortical bone (removal of the bony prominences). Sinus tracts and pockets should be excised or opened and debrided. Wet-to-dry or dry-to-dry bandages should be used to aid in finishing the debridement process. If pockets are present in the undermined skin, a 1/4" diameter Penrose drain may be placed in the most dependent area to allow drainage. As soon as a bed of healthy granulation tissue has formed, secondary closure should be undertaken (Fig. 4-19D). Because of the size of the wound, a skin flap may be necessary to close it. Such flaps should have as much subcutaneous tissue as possible on their undersides to provide padding over the area of repair.

As with decubital ulcers, pressure sores should be prevented by properly applying casts or bandages. The cast or bandage should be removed to investigate the area when the animal shows signs of undue pressure, such as licking and chewing at the cast or bandage, swelling or hypothermia of digits, malodorous cast or bandage, or staining of the cast or bandage over a bony prominence. When a pressure sore is the result of a cast or bandage causing pressure or friction over a bony prominence, treatment is similar to that described for decubital ulcers.

Aftercare. The aftercare of a surgical repair site for a decubital ulcer entails keeping pressure off the area by using a pressure relief bandage and bedding the dog on sufficient padding. The area should also be kept clean and dry, and an immobile animal's position changed often. If it is necessary to retain a cast on a limb with a pressure sore, sutured or not, a window should be cut in the cast over the pressure sore to relieve the pressure and allow treatment.

Advantages and Disadvantages. The veterinarian is at a disadvantage when dealing with an animal with the potential for developing decubital ulcers because the animal's coat may obscure the early signs of a developing ulcer. If the skin over bony prominences is not observed closely by separating the hair to examine it, a patch of skin may necrose and slough before the veterinarian is aware of an impending problem.

In a paralyzed animal with decubital ulcers, the denervated tissues may heal, but are more subject to trauma and wound disruption. Therefore, care and protection of the ulcer or repair site are especially important.

Constructing and maintaining a pressure relief bandage over some areas of the body may be difficult in some cases, for example, over the hock of a dachshund—maintaining a "donut" bandage, or over the olecranon of an obese dog—maintaining a pipe insulation bandage.

REFERENCES AND SUGGESTED READING

1. Betts, C.W., and Crane, S.W.: Manual of Small Animal Surgical Therapeutics. New York, Churchill Livingstone, 1986.
2. Swaim, S.F., and Votau, K.: Prevention and treatment of decubital ulcers in the dog. Vet. Med. Small Anim. Clin. *65*:1069, 1975.
3. Swaim, S.F., and Wilhalf, D.: The physics, physiology, and chemistry of bandaging open wounds. Compend. Contin. Educ. *7*:146, 1985.

CHRONIC WOUNDS, SINUS TRACTS, AND FISTULAE

Definition and Indications. Chronic wounds, sinus tracts, and fistulae are forms of nonhealing or slow-healing wounds. Chronic wounds are generally full-thickness defects that, regardless of the usual antibacterial therapy and bandaging, do not heal. They may have an edematous unhealthy granulation tissue base with or without sinus tracts in it (Fig. 4-20A). A sinus is a tubular ulcer lined with granulation tissue that does not heal, or that heals after medical therapy and reforms at a later date at the same location or adjacent to it. A purulent, serous, or serosanguineous discharge from the sinus is present. Fistulae are similar to sinus tracts; however, they connect the skin with a mucous surface or one mucous surface to another. They may be lined with either granulation tissue or epithelium from the mucous surface(s).

Some locations, causes, and characteristics of specific sinus and fistulous tracts are:

may heal, only to recur when the administration is discontinued.

Grass awns that migrate in the tissues are a major cause of sinus tracts. They cause problems in certain localities and during certain seasons and are commonly

Sinus Tracts

Location	Cause	Characteristics
Rostroventral to eye	Abscess of fourth premolar tooth	Swelling with subsequent drainage
Rostral muzzle	Abscess of canine tooth	Swelling with subsequent drainage
Intermandibular space	Abscess of mandibular teeth	Swelling with subsequent drainage
Dorsal neck or back (Rhodesian Ridgebacks)	Dermoid or pilonidal cyst	Extends from skin to supraspinous ligament or vertebral dorsal spine, lined with hair follicles and sebaceous glands
Ventral neck	Tracheocutaneous	Occurs after removal of tracheostomy tube
External ear	Middle ear abscess	Draining sinus tract
Sublumbar or precrural area	Migrating grass awn	May be associated with osteomyelitis of vertebrae
Flank in ovariohysterectomized female	Reaction to ovarian pedicle ligature	Draining sinus tract, may adhere to kidney pole and entrap ureter
Inguinal region or precrural fold	Reaction to uterine pedicle ligature	Sometimes bilateral, may not occur simultaneously, may not be on same side as ligature, may adhere to bladder, ureters, and colon
Extremities	Chronic osteomyelitis from bite wounds, surgical intervention with implants, extension from soft tissue infections	Presence of foreign bodies (hair, broken tooth, bone sequestrum, orthopedic implant), instability of fixation implant
Interdigital spaces	Foreign bodies (grass awns, thorns, glass, gravel)	Draining sinus tracts
Perianal area	Anal sac abscesses	Draining sinus tracts that do not communicate with anus

Fistulous Tracts

Location	Cause	Characteristics
Umbilical area	Patent urachus	Tract between bladder and umbilicus. Urine expelled through umbilicus
	Patent vitellointestinal duct	Tract between jejunum and umbilicus. Ingesta expelled through umbilicus
Perianal area	Fecaliths in anal crypts with abscess, necrosis, and erosion through skin	Tracts between anus and skin, may coalesce and form ulcers

Chronic nonhealing wounds or sinus tracts may develop at any place on the body. Sinus tracts may be associated with bacterial and fungal infections. In addition, sinus tracts commonly result from the presence of foreign bodies deep in the tissues (for example, twigs, small branches, grass awns). Pain, swelling, and a serous or purulent discharge are characteristic. With antibiotic therapy, these signs may subside and the lesion

seen in hunting dogs. Awns may penetrate the skin or any of the body orifices. With migration, they may gain access to a variety of sites. They may penetrate the skin to cause an abscess or lodge in the ear canal and rupture the tympanic membrane. Interdigital penetration with a subsequent draining tract is common. Penetration of the oral mucosa may cause head and neck abscesses or periorbital or retrobulbar abscesses if they migrate into these areas. Entry through the conjunctiva may cause abscesses in these areas. Swallowed awns may result in penetration of the gastrointestinal tract and peritonitis.

Chronic wounds may be the result of neoplasms. In cats, such wounds may indicate feline leukemia virus infection and immunosuppression. These wounds may also be the result of infections by bacterial or fungal organisms, which require special diagnostic procedures such as culture techniques and biopsy examination. Such bacterial infections include cutaneous bacterial granulomas, atypical mycobacterial granulomas, actinomycosis, actinobacillosis, and nocardiosis. Subcutaneous fungal infections include eumycotic mycetomas, sporotrichosis, and phaeohyphomycosis.

Chronic wounds may also be secondary to immunosuppression (such as prolonged glucocorticoid therapy), hypothyroidism, and underlying metabolic or neoplastic disease.

The primary indication associated with chronic wounds, sinus tracts, and fistulae is to establish the cause of the lesion so that appropriate surgical and/or medical therapy may be undertaken.

Techniques. *Diagnostic Procedures.* For sinus tracts and chronic wounds, smears of the discharge, samples for bacterial culture/sensitivity, and samples for fungal culture should be obtained to help ensure proper medical therapy (Fig. 4-20B and C). A sinus tract should be carefully and aseptically probed to determine whether it is superficial or has an extensive tract system. Organisms that may cause such lesions may require special diagnostic techniques, including culture techniques, to identify the causative organism. Tissue biopsies are also essential in diagnosing neoplasias and helpful in culturing true causative organisms rather than surface contaminants (Fig. 4-20D).*

Radiographs are indicated to ascertain whether skeletal or organ involvement exists when there is a history of previous trauma (such as fracture or penetrating wound) or surgery is indicated if the physical exam reveals pain associated with deep structures (Fig. 4-20E).

Fistulography with a positive contrast medium is indicated to outline foreign bodies with a sinus tract or to determine the direction and extent of the sinus tract(s). The contrast medium should be injected after cultures have been taken because the media are iodinated and therefore potentially germicidal. For large sinus tracts, injection may be by means of a Foley bulb catheter with the inflated bulb helping to prevent backflow (Fig. 4-20F). With small-diameter tracts, injec-

*The reader is referred to other texts for more specific information on the diagnostic technique for microorganisms.

tion through a plastic catheter while manually occluding the sinus opening works well (Fig. 4-20G). Radiographs should be taken immediately after injection because of the rapid absorption of most media and the possibility of backflow onto the skin to obscure the tract.

Surgery. Surgery on a sinus tract should be planned at a time when the wound is relatively quiet, yet actively draining. Because of the potential for extensive exploration, the area around a sinus tract should be widely clipped. Meticulous hemostasis and anatomic closure of all surgical wounds are important in preventing seromas. Placement of a Penrose drain in the wound is indicated if a potential for fluid accumulation exists.

In one technique for sinus tract removal, 1% methylene blue is injected into the tract(s) 24 hours before exploration for better visualization. Sinus tract incisional dissection entails opening each fibrous tubular tract and following it to its point of origin (Fig. 4-21A). The stained tissues are removed.

A second technique for sinus tract removal involves excisional dissection of the tract to its point of origin. An elliptical excision is made around the sinus opening and blunt and sharp dissection are used to isolate the tract(s). This technique may be performed using low blended cutting/coagulation electrosurgical current for dissection. This helps in attaining hemostasis for better identification of structures. Insertion of a plastic catheter in the tract may facilitate in following its course (Fig. 4-21B).

A third technique for dealing with sinus tracts may be used when the cause is known. For instance, when osteomyelitis is associated with metal implants or bone sequestra or an abscessed tooth is present, routine techniques are used to remove the nidus without removing the sinus tract (Fig. 4-21C).

If a chronic nonhealing wound is the result of neoplasia, adequate excision of the involved tissue followed by some form of reconstruction (such as moving local tissue, flaps or graft) is necessary. With some bacterial infections, complete surgical excision of the wound followed by open wound healing is indicated (for example, in cutaneous bacterial granuloma, mycobacterial granuloma caused by *M. lepraemurium*, or atypical mycobacterial granuloma). Likewise, chronic nonhealing wounds caused by fungal infections may require complete surgical removal of the affected tissue or even amputation of a badly infected limb (as in eumycotic mycetoma and phaeohyphomycosis).

Treatment of some infections requires surgical debridement and drainage combined with specific medication for the causative organism. In actinomycosis, penicillin (100,000 U/kg/day IM) is the drug of choice, given over a long period of time, usually for several months until the animal is free of signs and cultures are

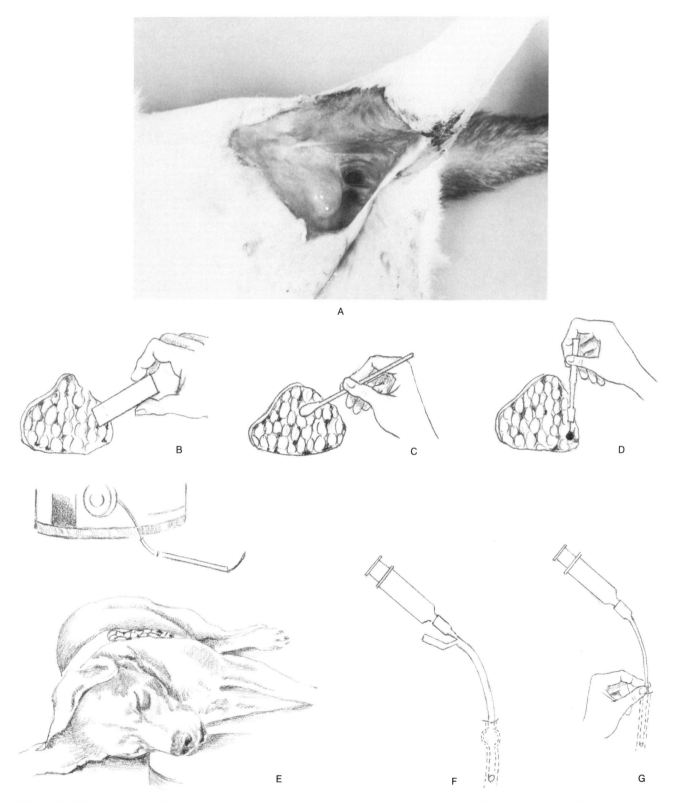

FIG. 4-20. Diagnostic techniques for chronic wounds and sinus tracts. A, Chronic nonhealing wound with sinus tracts. Nocardiosis. B, Impression smear taken for examination. C, Sample taken for bacterial culture/sensitivity and fungal culture. D, Tissue biopsy taken for histopathology and culture. E, Radiographs taken to determine deep tissue involvement. F, Fistulography of a large sinus tract with Foley bulb catheter, to occlude fistula opening. G, Fistulography of small sinus tract with a small catheter and digital occlusion of fistula opening.

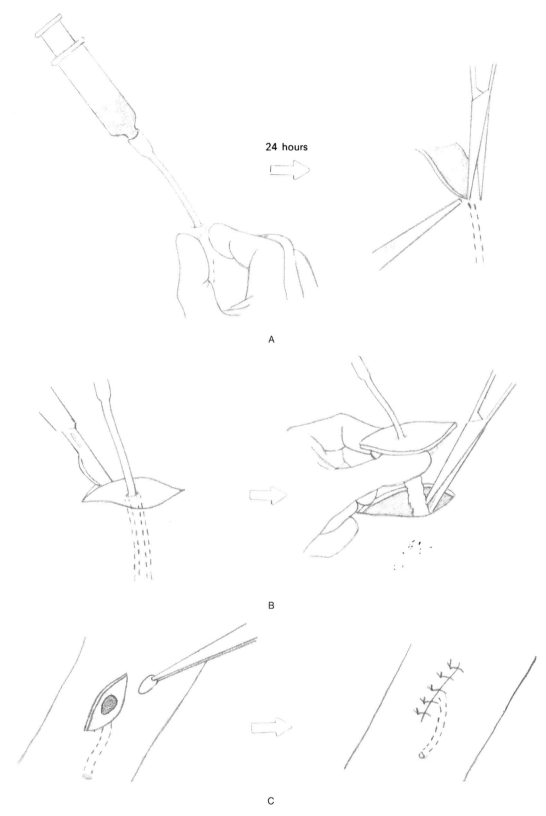

FIG. 4-21. Surgery on a sinus tract. A, Technique 1 (incisional dissection): methylene blue injected into sinus tract 24 hours before surgery, sinus tract incised and dissected. B, Technique 2 (excisional dissection): catheter insertion into tract, elliptical incision around opening, and blunt excisional dissection around tract. C, Technique 3 (nidus removal): Removal of the known nidus (sequestrum) without removing the tract.

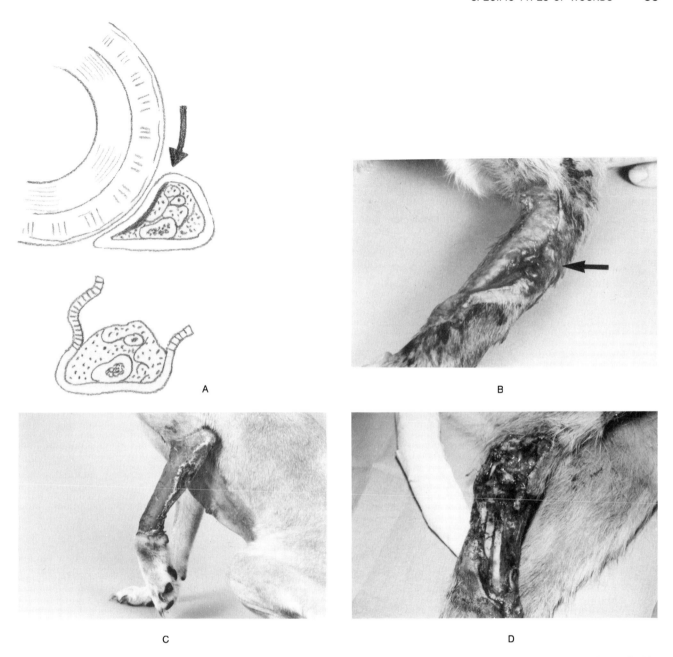

FIG. 4-22. Degloving Wounds. A, Dynamics of automobile tire causing a degloving injury. B, Wound with a flap of skin (arrow) attached by a broad pedicle. C, Wound with skin missing. D, Abrasion associated with wound with exposed tarsal bones. (A, from McGregor, I.A.: Fundamental Techniques of Plastic Surgery, 7th ed. Edinburgh, Churchill Livingstone, 1980. p. 195; D, from Swaim, S.F.: Management and bandaging of soft tissue injuries of dog and cat feet. J. Am. Anim. Hosp. Assoc. *21*:331, 1985).

negative. Topical application of iodine preparations to localized lesions may be helpful. In addition to surgical extirpation and drainage, actinobacillosis infections are treated with sodium iodide (0.2 ml/kg of 20% solution orally twice a day). The course of therapy is long. Nocardiosis may be treated with high doses of penicillin and sulfadiazine. Equal parts of sulfadiazine and trimethoprim (not the 20:1 ratio) are effective against

the organism. The course of therapy may be several months; it should not be stopped until 4 weeks after clinical remission. All tissues removed should be submitted for histopathologic examination.

Aftercare. General observation of the wound closure site and area of drain exit, if a drain has been used, are indicated. Drains should generally be removed 3 to 5 days after surgery. Wounds left to heal as open wounds following excision should be bandaged, with periodic bandage changes. Daily wound lavage with an antiseptic solution may be beneficial.

Advantages and Disadvantages.   If a sinus tract has been explored previously without finding its cause, subsequent explorations are significantly more difficult and often unproductive. Fistulography may be unsuccessful if the contrast medium is too dilute, if the amount injected is inadequate, or if there is a delay in taking radiographs following injection.

The veterinarian should be aware and the pet owner warned of the difficulty, frustration, prolonged treatment and unsuccessful results that may accompany the treatment of some chronic nonhealing wounds and sinus tracts. Excisional dissection of tracts has the advantage of reduced healing time in comparison to incisional dissection and open packing of the wound.

REFERENCES AND SUGGESTED READING

1. Archibald, J., Holt, J.C., and Sokolovsky, V.; Management of Trauma in Dogs and Cats. Santa Barbara, CA, American Veterinary Publications, Inc., 1981.
2. Attleberger, M.H.: Actinomycosis, nocardiosis, and dermatophilosis. *In* Current Veterinary Therapy VIII. Edited by R.W. Kirk. Philadelphia, W.B. Saunders, 1983.
3. Brennan, K.E., and Ihrke, P.J.: Grass awn migration in dogs and cats: A retrospective study of 182 cases. J. Am. Vet. Med. Assoc. *182*:1201, 1983.
4. Johnston, D.E.: Skin and subcutaneous tissue—Cutaneous ulcers, sinuses, and fistulas. *In* Pathophysiology in Small Animal Surgery. Edited by M.J. Bojrab. Philadelphia, Lea & Febiger, 1981.
5. Muller, G.H., Kirk, R.W., and Scott, D.W.: Small Animal Dermatology. 3rd ed. Philadelphia, W.B. Saunders, 1983.
6. Nichols, F.R., and Horne, R.D.: Grass awn penetration in the dog. Auburn Vet. *29*:59, 1973.
7. Wykes, P.M.: Cutaneous sinus tracts of the dog. Compend. Contin. Educ. *4*:293, 1982.

DEGLOVING WOUNDS

Definition and Indications.   Degloving wounds generally occur on the limbs. They result from shearing forces applied to the skin and subcutaneous tissue which separate them from underlying muscle and fascia. These injuries are often caused by an automobile tire passing over the limb of an animal (Fig. 4-22A). The skin is avulsed from the underlying tissue, producing a flap attached by a pedicle of varying widths (Fig. 4-22B). In some cases, the skin is completely detached (Fig. 4-22C). Many degloving injuries are associated with a crushing type of injury in which single or multiple fractures and damage to major blood vessels and nerves may also have occurred. Abrasion may also be a part of the degloving injury, with skin and underlying tissue being ground away by the pavement. Such injuries often expose bones and joints in the carpal/metacarpal and tarsal/metatarsal areas (Fig. 4-22D).

Initial wound management is indicated for such injuries, followed by reconstruction of the area.

Techniques.   See Wound Management, Chapter 2; Wound Dressing Materials and Topical Medications, Chapter 3; Low-Velocity Gunshot Wounds, this chapter (for fracture management); and Wounds on the Limbs, Chapter 9.

Aftercare.   See Wound Management, Chapter 2; Wound Dressing Materials and Topical Medications, Chapter 3; Low-Velocity Gunshot Wounds, this chapter (for fracture management); and Wounds on the Limbs, Chapter 9.

Advantages and Disadvantages.   See Wound Management, Chapter 2; Wound Dressing Materials and Topical Medications, Chapter 3; Low-Velocity Gunshot Wounds, this chapter (for fracture management); and Wounds on the Limbs, Chapter 9.

REFERENCES AND SUGGESTED READING

1. Swaim, S.F., and Pope, E.R.: Early management of limb degloving injuries. Semin. Vet. Med. Surg. *3*:274, 1988.
See Wound Management, Chapter 2; Wound Dressing Materials and Topical Medications, Chapter 3; Low-Velocity Gunshot Wounds, this chapter (for fracture management); and Wounds, on the Limbs, Chapter 9, for additional references and suggested readings.

MANAGEMENT OF SKIN TENSION

5

TENSION LINES AND WOUND TENSION

INCISION AND SUTURE LINES

Definition and Indications. All portions of a dog's skin are not equally pliable in different directions. Tension lines in the skin of dogs are formed by the predominant pull of fibrous tissue within the skin. Tension lines allow motion of a part while providing support and thus differ in different areas of the body. There is general agreement regarding the main direction of tension lines in the skin of the "average dog" (Fig. 5-1). However, breed, sex and age affect tension lines. Some breeds, such as the bassett hound, have relatively more skin than others (Fig. 5-2), and in these breeds skin tension lines are less important in planning a surgical procedure. Other breeds, such as the greyhound, have much less loose skin (Fig. 5-3), and consideration of the effects of tension lines may be important in operative planning.

There are two general rules related to skin tension lines and skin tension. Application of these rules is indicated when planning incisions and closing pre-existing wounds. First, whenever possible, it is best to make incisions that run parallel to tension lines to avoid wound tension. Second, pre-existing wounds should be closed in a direction that will avoid or minimize skin tension.

Technique. Incision lines made across tension lines tend to gape widely (Fig. 5-4A). Incisions made at an angle to tension lines will take a curvilinear shape (Fig. 5-4B). The ideal is to make incisions parallel to tension lines because they gape minimally (Fig. 5-4C).

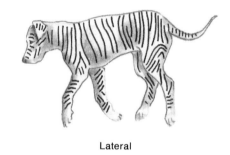

Lateral

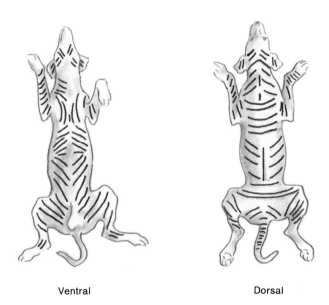

Ventral

Dorsal

FIG. 5-1. Skin tension lines of dog (after Irwin, D.H.G: Tension lines in the skin of the dog. J. Small Anim. Pract. *7*:595, 1966).

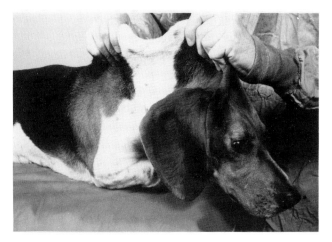

FIG. 5-2. Great abundance of skin on a bassett hound.

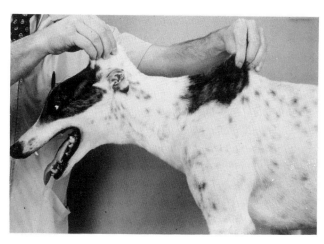

FIG. 5-3. Less abundance of skin on a greyhound.

When preparing to close an irregular-shaped wound, the surgeon should manipulate the wound edges to ascertain in which direction the suture line should run to have the least amount of tension on it. In some instances, this may be in the direction of tension line pull. Noting the long axis of the wound, an attempt should be made to appose the wound edges so that the suture line will be in the direction of this axis. This axis *may* indicate the direction of tension line pull, and closure would thus be parallel to the tension lines. This may not always be the case, however. The long axis may be across tension lines, but closure along this axis may still cause less wound tension than trying to close the wound parallel to tension lines (Fig. 5-4D and E).

Another factor to consider in closing irregular-shaped wounds is the formation of puckers ("dog ears") of extra skin at the ends of the closure. Ideally, the direction of closure should be such that "dog ears" are avoided or minimized. In general, the direction of closure with the least amount of tension also has small or no "dog ears" (Fig. 5-4D and E).

When closing wounds on limbs under tension, the surgeon should be aware of the possibility of creating a "biologic tourniquet." In such instances, the defect is so large and the skin is closed so tightly around the limb, with or without tension-relieving techniques, that it creates a tourniquet.

Aftercare. Closed incisions that have been made parallel to skin tension lines and wounds closed to avoid tension generally require no special aftercare. Limb wounds that have been closed under tension should be observed for signs of a "biologic tourniquet"—edema and hypothermia distal to the wound closure site. If these are present, the surgeon should *seriously* consider removing the skin sutures and consider letting the

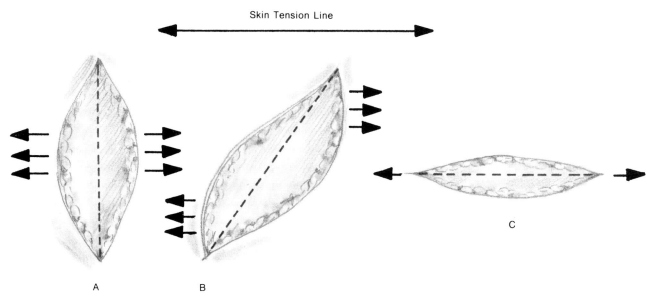

FIG. 5-4. Legend on facing page.

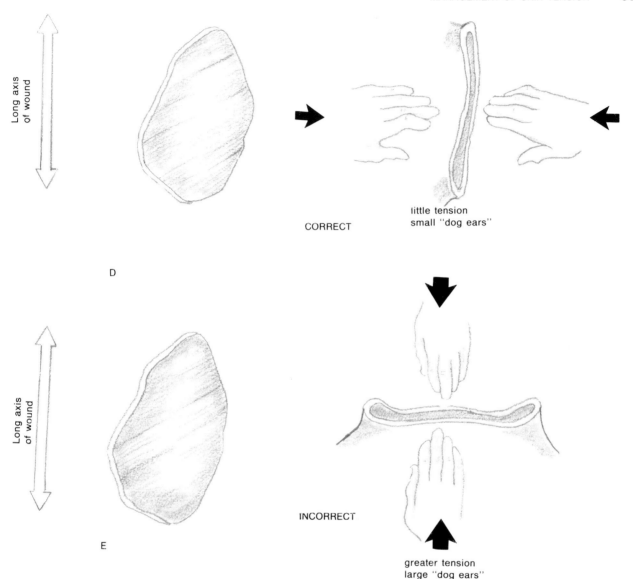

FIG. 5-4. Skin tension line–incision line relationships. A, Incision perpendicular to tension lines results in a widened wound. B, Incision at an angle to tension lines results in a curvilinear wound. C, Incision parallel to tension lines results in minimal gap (after Borges, A.F.: Elective Incisions and Scar Revision. Boston, Little, Brown and Co., 1975, p. 14). D, Correct wound closure to avoid tension (small arrows)—closure along wound's long axis with small "dog ears." E, Incorrect wound closure results in tension (larger arrows)—closure against wound's long axis with large "dog ears."

wound heal by second intention or using a skin graft or flap for closure. The main point is *not to jeopardize the distal portion of a limb because of insufficient circulation merely to close a wound.*

Advantages and Disadvantages. Incisions made across tension lines require more sutures for closure, including tension sutures, and are more likely to disrupt. Incisions made parallel to tension lines require fewer sutures for closure and are less likely to disrupt. Similarly, wounds closed in a direction that avoids suture line tension are less likely to disrupt than those closed without attention to direction.

Although it is possible to close a limb wound under tension, the circulatory embarrassment that may result can lead to loss of tissue if the tension is not relieved.

REFERENCES AND SUGGESTED READING

1. Irwin, D.H.G.: Tension lines in the skin of the dog. J. Small Anim. Pract. 7:593, 1966.
2. Swaim, S.F.: Management of skin tension in dermal surgery. Compend. Contin. Educ. 2:758, 1980.

UNDERMINING

Definition and Indications. Undermining is the use of scissors or a scalpel to separate the skin or skin and panniculus muscle from underlying tissue. This allows the full elastic potential of the skin to be used as it is stretched to cover a wound.

Techniques. Blunt undermining may be performed by advancing closed scissor blades beneath the tissues and then opening them after they have reached the desired limit of undermining (Fig. 5-5A). For general undermining, blunt-blunt scissors (such as Metzenbaum's) are best. For meticulous dissection around specific structures, sharp-sharp scissors are preferred. The points delicately engage the connective tissue with much less pressure applied, and the blades, when opened, bluntly separate the tissue. Blunt dissection may also be accomplished by moving the blunt end of a scalpel handle back and forth in the subcutaneous tissue (Fig. 5-5B).

Sharp undermining may be performed by snipping the tissue with the scissor blades as they are advanced through the tissue (Fig. 5-5C). This is commonly combined with blunt scissor undermining. Sharp undermining may also be performed by cutting the connective tissue with a scalpel blade held parallel to the undersurface of the skin (Fig. 5-5D).

When undermining, the surgeon should try to preserve the blood supply to the skin, which is furnished by direct cutaneous vessels. These vessels run parallel to the skin surface and supply the subdermal plexus of the skin. On areas of the body which have one of the panniculus muscles (platysma, sphincter colli superficialis, cutaneous

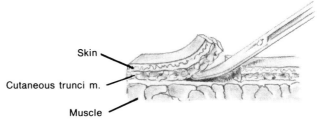

FIG. 5-6. Undermining on trunk deep to cutaneous trunci muscle.

trunci, supramammaricus, or preputialis muscles) under the skin, undermining should be deep to the muscle because the blood supply to the skin lies both superficial and deep to these muscles (Fig. 5-6).

Undermining of skin with no underlying panniculus muscle should be done in the loose areolar fascia deep to the dermis. With skin closely associated with underlying fascia (such as on the ventral thorax or the caudolateral aspect of the pelvic limbs), undermining should include a portion of the subcutaneous fascia with the dermis. When undermining on the face, damage to nerves, vessels and salivary ducts should be avoided by undermining in the fascia just under the dermis (Fig. 5-7).

The surgeon should use good judgment in the manipulation of recently traumatized skin. Added insult to the skin vasculature could result in a slough. When the integrity of skin vasculature is in question, a delay in wound closure is indicated.

Aftercare. If undermining has created considerable dead space between the skin and underlying tissues, or if sharp dissection has resulted in hemorrhage in the area, a Penrose drain or drains should be placed under the skin to help prevent formation of a seroma or hematoma. Absorbent bandages should be placed over the area to help protect both wound and drain from injury and contamination and to absorb any drainage from the wound. The drain should be removed in 3 to 4 days or when drainage has become minimal.

Advantages and Disadvantages. Undermining releases the skin from underlying attachments so that its

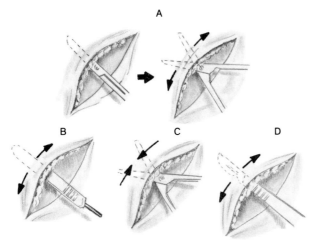

FIG. 5-5. Undermining techniques. A, Blunt undermining with scissors. B, Blunt undermining with scalpel handle. C, Sharp undermining with scissors. D, Sharp undermining with scalpel blade.

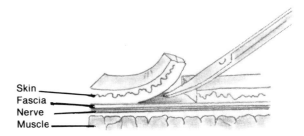

FIG. 5-7. Undermining on face within the areolar fascia deep to the dermis.

elasticity can be taken advantage of in moving it to cover a wound. In some instances, the procedure may provide enough laxity for closure of a wound without additional incisions of the skin such as relaxing incisions, flaps or grafts. The procedure creates a dead space or potential dead space that could lead to seroma or hematoma formation.

REFERENCES AND SUGGESTED READING

1. Braden, T.D.: Plastic and reconstructive surgery of the canine torso. Vet. Clin. North Am. *9*:285, 1979.
2. McGuire, M.F.: Studies of the excisional wound: I. Biomechanical effects of undermining and wound orientation on closing tension and work. Plast. Reconstr. Surg. *66*:419, 1980.
3. Pavletic, M.M.: Undermining for repair of large skin defects in small animals. Mod. Vet. Pract. *67*:13, 1986.
4. Swaim, S.F.: Management of skin tension in dermal surgery. Compend. Contin. Educ. *2*:758, 1980.

TENSION SUTURES

"WALKING" SUTURES

Definition and Indications. "Walking" sutures are interrupted sutures of absorbable suture material placed from the deeper portion of the dermis to underlying fascias. They are combined with undermining and flaps to move skin from around a wound to cover the wound, and thus serve as tension sutures (Fig. 5-8A through C).

Technique. The skin around the wound is undermined; care is taken to leave intact any large direct cutaneous blood vessels coming from underlying tissues to the dermis. With 2-0 or 3-0 *absorbable* suture material with a swaged needle, the first "walking" suture is placed near the junction of the undermined skin with the underlying tissue. The first portion of the suture is placed by passing the needle through the deep portion of the dermis but not through the full thickness of the skin. With careful observation of the deep portion of the dermis in areas where a panniculus muscle is absent, incorporation of large vessels into the suture can be avoided, and adequate blood supply to the skin ensured. The second "bite" of the suture is taken toward the center of the wound (Fig. 5-9A). As the suture is tied, skin is advanced slightly toward the center of the wound because of its elasticity (Fig. 5-9B). "Walking" sutures are placed in rows (Fig. 5-9C), thereby moving skin across the defect. After two or three rows of sutures have been placed, the skin is usually halfway across the wound. Repeating the same procedure on the opposite side of the wound results in almost complete closure of the wound. When the wound is adjacent to a body

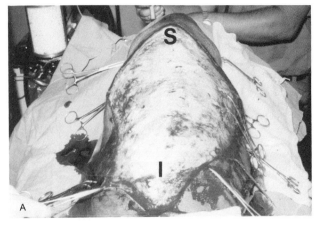
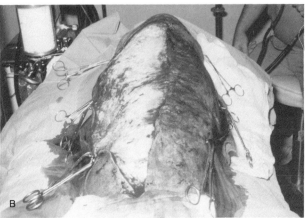
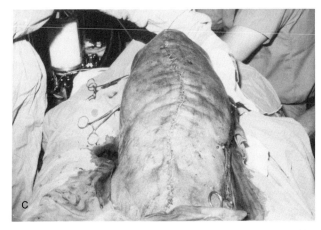

FIG. 5-8. "Walking" sutures. A, Large open wound on dog's back. S = Area between scapulae; I = Area between ilial wings. B, Skin from one side has been walked halfway across defect. C, Skin from opposite side has been walked halfway across defect.

structure or orifice (such as the eye or anus), "walking" sutures advance skin from only one side of the wound to prevent distortion of the structure or orifice. A simple continuous subcuticular suture of 3-0 or 4-0 *absorbable* suture material is placed along the wound edge to

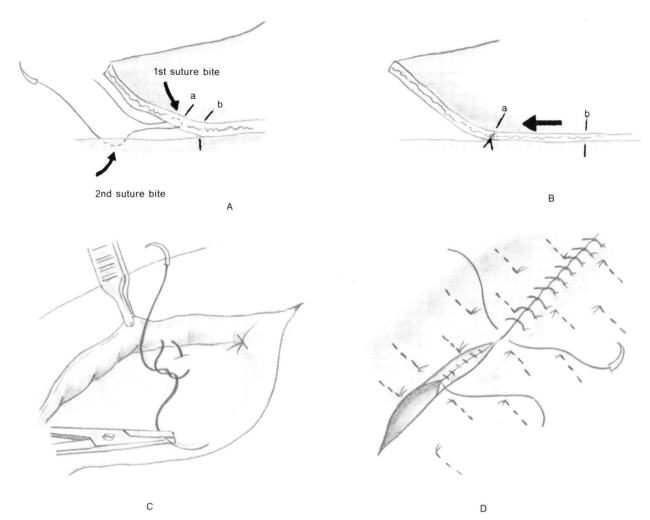

FIG. 5-9. "Walking" sutures. A, Placing first and second suture bites. Segment of skin to be stretched (a to b). B, Tying a walking suture advances skin toward center of wound (a to b increased). C, Walking sutures placed in rows. D, Placing a simple continuous subcuticular suture along wound edge, and simple interrupted skin apposition sutures. Broken lines are buried "walking" sutures. (C, D after Swaim, S.F.: The repair of the skin: Techniques of plastic and reconstructive surgery. *In* Atlas of Canine Surgical Techniques. Edited by P.G.C. Bedford. Oxford, Blackwell Scientific Publications, 1984. p. 49.)

approximate the tissues. Final skin closure is accomplished with simple interrupted 3-0 or 4-0 nonabsorbable sutures, with no tension on these sutures (Fig. 5-9D).

Aftercare. Every other skin suture is removed 10 days postoperatively, with the remaining skin sutures being removed at 14 days.

Advantages and Disadvantages. Most large skin defects on dogs and cats can be closed with "walking" sutures. These sutures advance local skin to close large defects, distribute tension around a wound, and obliterate dead space. "Walking" sutures create temporary ties between the skin and underlying tissues; however, these disappear in 2 to 3 weeks if absorbable suture materials have been used.

REFERENCES AND SUGGESTED READING

1. Swaim, S.F.: A "walking" suture technique for closing of large skin defects in the dog and cat. J. Am. Anim. Hosp. Assoc. *12*:597, 1976.
2. Swaim, S.F.: Management of skin tension in dermal surgery. Compend. Contin. Educ. *2*:758, 1980.

SIMPLE INTERRUPTED SUTURES

Definition and Indications. Each suture is a single loop of suture material passed perpendicular to the plane of the tissue, with the ends emerging on opposite sides of the wound. These are indicated for suturing

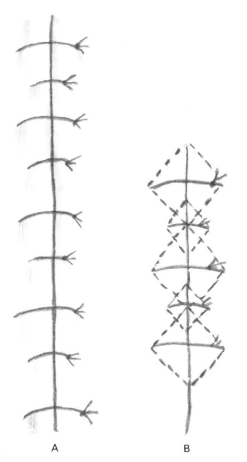

FIG. 5-10. Alternating wide and narrow bites with simple interrupted sutures. A, Suture placement. B, Zone of wound supported by each suture is within square associated with that suture (broken lines). Note overlap of squares.

wounds that have *minimal* tension associated with closure.

Technique. See Secondary Management, Closed Wounds, Primary Closure, Skin Suture Patterns, Chapter 2.

When used as tension sutures, simple interrupted sutures are placed by alternating wide and narrow bites using 2-0 or 3-0 nonabsorbable material. The sutures, placed widely, serve as tension sutures (Fig. 5-10A and B). If the skin edges cannot be brought into close apposition with thumb forceps and mild tension, there may be too much skin tension to use simple interrupted sutures.

Aftercare. Sutures should be removed 7 to 10 days after surgery.

Advantages and Disadvantages. These sutures supply simple effective closure of wounds that have minimal tension associated with their closure. As with other types of interrupted tension sutures, the surgeon can adjust the tension of each suture at each segment of

the wound according to the spreading forces present. If too much tension is applied in tying the sutures, however, the wound edges may invert when slight eversion would be more desirable. If these sutures are used on wounds where tension is too great, the sutures may tend to cut through the skin, leaving an uncosmetic effect.

REFERENCES AND SUGGESTED READING

1. Bellenger, C.R.: Sutures, Part II: The use of sutures and alternative methods of closure. Compend. Contin. Educ. *4*:587, 1982.
2. Braden, T.D.: Plastic and reconstructive surgery of the canine torso. Vet. Clin. North Am. *9*:285, 1979.
3. Swaim, S.F.: Management of skin tension in dermal surgery. Compend. Contin. Educ. *2*:758, 1980.

INTERRUPTED HORIZONTAL MATTRESS SUTURES

Definition and Indications. A horizontal mattress suture is a loop of suture material placed interruptedly in the same plane as the tissue with both ends of the suture emerging on the same side of the wound. The sutures are indicated for closure of wounds where tension is necessary to appose the wound edges.

Technique. An interrupted horizontal mattress suture of 2-0 or 3-0 nonabsorbable material is placed by inserting the needle approximately 5 mm from the edge of one side of the wound. The needle is passed angularly through the tissue below the edge of the tissue plane to prevent excessive eversion of the tissues. It crosses the incision and exits in an angular pattern on the opposite side of the wound. The suture is then advanced 8 mm along this side of the wound, reintroduced into the skin,

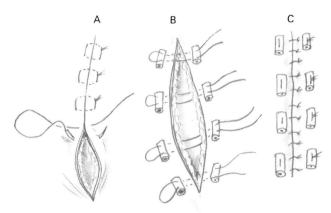

FIG. 5-11. Horizontal mattress tension sutures. A, Placing sutures. B, Placing sutures through segments of rubber tubing. C, Sutures tied and simple interrupted sutures placed for final wound closure.

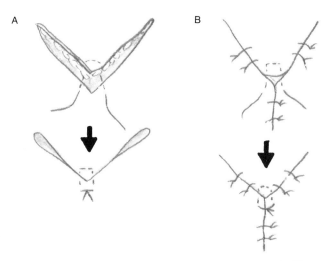

FIG. 5-12. Half-buried horizontal mattress sutures. A, Placing at point of a V-shaped wound. B, Placing at juncture of three suture lines.

passed back across the wound as previously described, and tied (Fig. 5-11A). These sutures are usually placed 4 mm apart; however, the width of the sutures and the distance between them depend on the thickness of skin being sutured and the intended use of the suture. When considerable tension is required for wound closure, segments of rubber tubing or buttons may be placed as stents under the sutures to help prevent them from cutting into the tissue (Fig. 5-11B and C). Simple interrupted sutures may be used in conjunction with horizontal mattress tension sutures to obtain final skin edge apposition.

A half-buried horizontal mattress suture has been found effective in closing the point of a V-shaped wound (Fig. 5-12A) or for closing the junction of three suture lines (Fig. 5-12B). The portion of the suture that passes through the point of the V or one of the skin segments formed by two of the three suture lines is buried in the dermis and runs in the same plane as the skin.

Aftercare. Horizontal mattress tension sutures should be removed on the third or fourth postoperative day. If a bandage is placed over the sutures that have rubber tubing or buttons under them, the bandages should be loosely applied because pressure bandages tend to increase the incidence of pressure necrosis under the tubing or buttons.

Advantages and Disadvantages. Horizontal mattress sutures can be effective in relieving tension on wounds. Because of their conformation, horizontal mattress sutures tend to interfere with circulation at the skin edges and to cut through the skin and become embedded (Fig. 5-14A). These sutures concen-

trate pressure on the skin near the wound edges, where pressure could be the most detrimental to wound healing.

REFERENCES AND SUGGESTED READING

1. Bellenger, C.R.: Sutures, Part II: The use of sutures and alternative methods of closure. Compend. Contin. Educ. *4*:587, 1982.
2. Braden, T.D.: Plastic and reconstructive surgery of the canine torso. Vet. Clin. North Am. *9*:285, 1979.
3. Grabb, W.C.: Basic techniques of plastic surgery. *In* Plastic Surgery. 3rd ed. Edited by W.C. Grabb, and J.W. Smith. Boston, Little, Brown & Co., 1979.
4. Knecht, C.D., Allen, A.R., Williams, D.J., and Johnson, J.H.: Fundamental Techniques in Veterinary Surgery. 3rd ed. Philadelphia, W.B. Saunders, 1987.
5. Stashak, T.S.: Reconstructive surgery in the horse. J. Am. Vet. Med. Assoc. *170*:143, 1977.
6. Swaim, S.F.: Management of skin tension in dermal surgery. Compend. Contin. Educ. *2*:758, 1980.

INTERRUPTED VERTICAL MATTRESS SUTURES

Definition and Indications. A vertical mattress suture is a loop of suture material inserted perpendicular to the plane of the tissue with both suture ends emerging on the same side of the wound. The sutures are indicated for closure of wounds where tension is necessary to appose the wound edges.

Technique. An interrupted vertical mattress suture of 2-0 or 3-0 nonabsorbable material is placed by inserting the needle approximately 8 mm from the skin edge and passing it across the wound to exit at a

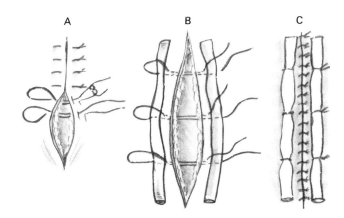

FIG. 5-13. Vertical mattress tension sutures. A, Placing sutures. B, Placing sutures over segments of soft rubber tubing. C, Sutures tied and simple interrupted sutures placed for final wound closure.

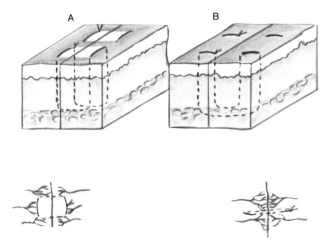

FIG. 5-14. Horizontal versus vertical mattress sutures. A, Horizontal mattress sutures tend to interfere with circulation at skin edges. B, Vertical mattress sutures do not interfere with circulation at skin edges.

corresponding point on the opposite side. From this point, the needle is advanced 4 mm toward the skin edge. It is reinserted through the skin and passed back across the wound to a point 4 mm from the skin edge on the original side. An alternative to the second bite is to split the thickness of the skin with the needle. The sutures are usually placed 5 mm apart, but this varies with the subject and the thickness of the skin being sutured (Fig. 5-13A). Simple interrupted sutures may be used with vertical mattress sutures for final skin edge apposition. In the presence of considerable wound tension, firm (intravenous) or soft (Penrose drain) tubing may be placed under vertical mattress sutures to help prevent them from cutting into the tissue (Fig. 5-13B and C).

Aftercare: Vertical mattress tension sutures should be removed on the third or fourth postoperative day. If a bandage is placed over sutures with rubber tubing under them, the bandage should be applied loosely because pressure bandages tend to increase the incidence of pressure necrosis under the tubing.

Advantages and Disadvantages. Vertical mattress sutures can be effective in relieving tension on wounds. They do not tend to interfere with circulation at the skin edges as do horizontal mattress sutures (Fig. 5-14A and B). These sutures, however, concentrate pressure on the skin near the wound edges where pressure could be the most detrimental to wound healing.

REFERENCES AND SUGGESTED READING

See Interrupted Horizontal Mattress Sutures, this chapter.

FAR-NEAR-NEAR-FAR SUTURES AND FAR-FAR-NEAR-NEAR SUTURES

Definition and Indications. Far-near-near-far and far-far-near-near sutures are combinations of tension and approximating sutures placed in the order that their names indicate. The far component supplies the tension while the near component apposes the skin edges. These sutures are indicated for closure of wounds in which tension within the tissues must be overcome to appose the wound edges or in which tension on the wound edges cyclically increases and decreases during movement, such as a flexion surface or lacerated paw pad.

Techniques

Far-near-near-far. With 2-0 or 3-0 nonabsorbable suture material, the first bite of a far-near-near-far suture is placed 5 to 7 mm from the skin edge. The needle is passed through the skin and subcutaneous tissue, crosses the wound, and exits through the skin on the opposite side of the wound about 1 to 3 mm from the edge. The needle is returned externally across the wound and inserted through the skin 1 to 3 mm from the wound edge. It then passes through the skin and subcutaneous tissue and advances across the wound, exiting 5 to 7 mm from the wound edge. All entrance and exit points of the suture in the skin are in a straight line (Fig. 5-15A).

The distance for placing these sutures may vary based upon the location and tissue being sutured.

Far-far-near-near. The far-far-near-near suture is placed by inserting the needle at a point 5 to 7 mm distant from the skin edge and passing it across the wound to a corresponding point on the opposite side of

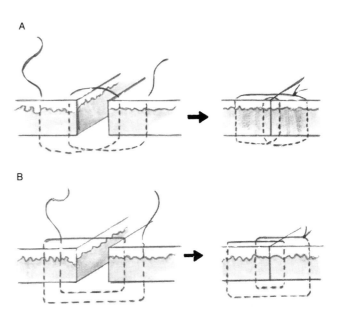

FIG. 5-15. Combination tension and approximating sutures. A, Far-near-near-far sutures. B, Far-far-near-near sutures.

the wound. After the needle is returned across the wound externally, it is passed from a point 1 to 3 mm from the wound edge on the original side to a similar close point on the opposite side of the wound. All entrance and exit points of the suture in the skin are in a straight line (Fig. 5-15B).

Aftercare. The sutures can be removed 7 to 10 days after surgery except in areas where tension caused by tissue movement is a factor, such as in the paw pads. In such areas, sutures should be left in place for at least 14 days or longer if warranted based on clinical judgment.

Advantages and Disadvantages. Both of these types of suture supply apposition and tension relief in one suture. If they are tightened too much, however, they may invert the skin and impair healing. They place a large amount of suture material in one area, with double sutures in the wound and an overlapping pattern on the skin.

REFERENCES AND SUGGESTED READING

1. Bellenger, C.R.: Sutures, Part II. The use of sutures and alternative methods of closure. Compend. Contin. Educ. *4*:587, 1982.
2. Braden, T.D.: Plastic and reconstructive surgery of the canine torso. Vet. Clin. North Am. *9*:285, 1979.
3. Knecht, C.D., Allen, A.R., Williams, D.J., and Johnson, J.H.: Fundamental Techniques in Veterinary Surgery. 3rd ed. Philadelphia, W.B. Saunders, 1987.
4. Stashak, T.S.: Reconstructive surgery in the horse. J. Am. Vet. Med. Assoc. *170*:143, 1977.
5. Swaim, S.F.: Management of skin tension in dermal surgery. Compend. Contin. Educ. *2*:758, 1980.

STENT SUTURES

Definition and Indications. A stent suture is a suture placed deeply in the tissues. After closure of the deep and superficial wound tissues, the stent sutures are tied over a rolled towel or gauze laid over the closed wound. They serve as tension sutures and are also effective for obliterating dead space and reducing postoperative edema and hemorrhage. They are also a method of bandaging difficult sites.

Techniques. A large curved suture needle and 2-0 or 3-0 nonabsorbable monofilament suture material are used to place the sutures 12 to 17 mm apart along the wound, with the needle entering the skin 7 to 12 mm from the wound edge. The needle is passed deep into the underlying tissues and emerges 7 to 12 mm from the opposite wound edge (Fig. 5-16A). The sutures are left untied. The wound is closed; buried sutures are placed to appose deep tissues and skin sutures are placed for final closure. Simple interrupted, simple continuous, or lock

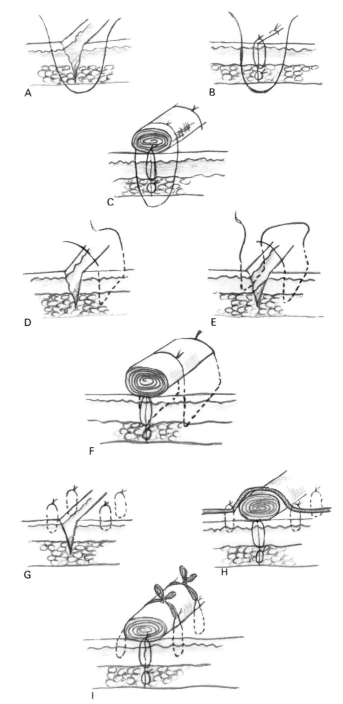

FIG. 5-16. Stent sutures. A, Placing a stent suture. B, Closure of deep and superficial wound tissues. C, Sutures tied over a gauze roll. D, Placing first bite of a double stent suture parallel to wound axis. E, Placing second bite of a double stent suture parallel to wound axis on opposite side of wound. F, Double stent suture tied over gauze roll. G, Placement of paired simple interrupted suture loops at intervals along wound. H, After wound closure, umbilical tape segments or segments of other sutures are placed through loops. I, Umbilical tape or suture segments tied over gauze roll.

sutures can be used to close the skin (Fig. 5-16B). A roll of gauze or towel 12 mm in diameter is placed over the skin suture line, and the preplaced sutures are tied firmly over the roll (Fig. 5-16C).

As an alternate technique, a double stent suture is placed by passing the needle into the skin 7 to 12 mm from the wound edge, and passing it parallel to the wound's long axis in the deep tissues. The needle emerges on the same side of the wound 12 to 17 mm from its entry point and 7 to 12 mm from the wound edge (Fig. 5-16D). It is then advanced across the wound and passed in the same manner on the opposite side of the wound back toward the area of the suture's origin (Fig. 5-16E). After the wound is closed, a 12 mm diameter gauze or towel roll is placed over the suture line and under the loops of suture crossing the wound. The ends of the stent sutures are tied over the roll (Fig. 5-16F).

A third type of stent suture is placed by inserting a series of paired simple interrupted loops of suture material 7 to 12 mm from the wound edge at 12 to 17 mm intervals along the wound (Fig. 5-16G). After the wound is closed, a 12 mm diameter gauze or towel roll is placed over the wound and segments of suture material or umbilical tape are passed between adjacent loops and tied over the roll with bow knots (Fig. 5-16H and I).

Aftercare. With the first two types of stents, the stent bandage should be covered longitudinally with strips of 1″ adhesive tape applied to the gauze roll to help keep the external surface of the bandage clean. With the third type of stent, the segments of suture or umbilical tape between the loops may be untied and the roll removed, and replaced with a fresh roll. The bandage should be examined daily to ascertain that no areas of drainage are developing along the suture line. Seven days postoperatively, the sutures of the bandage are cut and the bandage removed. Three days later, skin sutures are removed.

Advantages and Disadvantages. Stent bandages exert even pressure between the wound edges and underlying tissues. They eliminate dead space and act as self-retaining bandages. Stent bandages also help prevent the animal from molesting the wound and provide a means of bandaging wounds that would be difficult to bandage by other means. With the first two types of bandages, if the gauze or towel roll becomes wet and/or contaminated, it may become a source of infection to the wound, whereas the third type of stent can be replaced if it becomes soiled. If the sutures are tied too tightly, the stent may cause skin necrosis.

REFERENCE AND SUGGESTED READING

1. Swaim, S.F.: Management of skin tension in dermal surgery. Compend. Contin. Educ. *2:*758, 1980.

INTRADERMAL TENSION SUTURES

Definition and Indications. Although not exactly synonymous, the terms intradermal sutures and subcuticular sutures are often used interchangeably to describe a simple interrupted or continuous suture placed either at the lower portion of the dermis or in the area where the dermis blends into the subcuticular tissue. They serve as tension sutures to help prevent wound disruption and scar widening and also help to control skin capillary hemorrhage and obliterate dead space caused by closing skin over a subcutaneous defect. They should be used in combination with skin apposition sutures in wounds where tension is not excessive, or in combination with other types of tension sutures (such as walking sutures) to close wounds where considerable tension exists.

Techniques

Simple interrupted. Strong 3-0 or 4-0 absorbable or monofilament nonabsorbable suture material may be used for these intradermal sutures. If nonabsorbable suture is used, it should be undyed, especially if used on a thin-skinned area with a thin haircoat, so that it does not show under the skin. A simple interrupted intradermal suture is placed by inserting the needle into the deeper portion of the dermis first, incorporating a small amount of subcutaneous tissue and the deeper portion of the dermis (Fig. 5-17A). On the opposite side of the wound, the direction of needle passage is reversed so the needle passes through the dermis first, then the subcutaneous tissue (Fig. 5-17B). When the suture is tied, the knot is buried deep in the subcutaneous tissue rather than being close to the skin's surface (Fig. 5-17C).

Continuous. A continuous 3-0 or 4-0 monofilament nonabsorbable suture can be placed so that it can be removed at a later time. The suture can be anchored at one end of the wound by placing a simple interrupted suture just beyond the commissure of the wound and

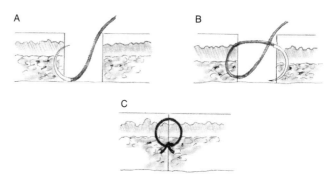

FIG. 5-17. Interrupted intradermal suture (absorbable). A, Needle passed from deep to superficial on one side of wound. B, Needle passed from superficial to deep on opposite side of wound. C, Suture tied.

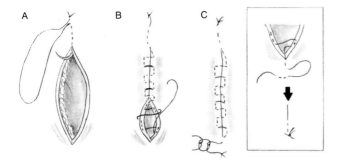

FIG. 5-18. Continuous intradermal suture (nonabsorbable). A, Anchoring suture beyond one end of wound and passing it into wound commissure. B, Placing suture, passing an occasional loop over skin. C, Ending suture by passing it beyond other commissure, cutting it, and tying it to a simple interrupted suture in skin. Inset: Alternate ending for suture. Passing suture out through commissure, taking a bite in adjacent skin, and tying free suture end to resultant loop.

passing the needle from this point through the wound commissure (Fig. 5-18A). Suturing is continued by passing the needle horizontally through the dermis. Small bites, the size of the arc of the needle, are taken alternately from each side of the wound. To facilitate suture removal, each needle entrance point should be opposite the last exit point on the apposing side of the wound (Fig. 5-18B). Removal may be further facilitated by passing the suture through the skin to the outside at 3 to 7 cm intervals along its length. At removal, these loops are cut to produce suture ends that can be pulled. To end the suture, the needle passes out through the other wound commissure. The suture is cut, a simple interrupted suture is placed in line with the wound, and the cut end of the running suture is tied to it (Fig. 5-18C). A similar pattern can be placed without cutting the suture to tie it at its end; instead, a bite is taken through the skin from the outside, and the suture is tied back onto itself (Fig. 5-18 Inset).

Absorbable or nonabsorbable 3-0 or 4-0 continuous intradermal sutures may be left in place. If a nonabsorbable suture is to be left in place, it should be undyed for the reason stated previously for interrupted intradermal sutures.

When continuous intradermal sutures are to be left in place, the beginning knot is buried by placing the first suture in the same manner as described above for placing a simple interrupted absorbable intradermal suture (Fig. 5-19A and B).

The method used to complete suturing depends on the type of needle. When a swaged needle is used, it is inserted from superficially to deeply in the subcutis; following this, a loop of suture is lifted from the wound (Fig. 5-20A). The needle is then inserted from deeply to superficially in the subcutis on one side of the wound (Fig. 5-20B). It is passed across the wound and inserted in the subcutis from superficially to deeply toward the previously created loop (Fig. 5-20C). Tying the suture end to the loop (Fig. 5-20D) results in a buried knot.

When an eyed needle is used, the next-to-last suture bite near the end of the wound is placed in the subcutis from deeply to superficially (Fig. 5-21A). A double-stranded loop of suture is drawn outside of the wound, and the needle is then inserted in the subcutis on the opposite side of the wound from superficially to deeply, and the doubled strand of suture with the needle is withdrawn from beneath the skin (Fig. 5-21B). The single strand of suture protruding from the wound at the next-to-last suture bite is held while the needle in the double strand coming from the last suture bite is pulled. This pulls the previously created loop beneath the skin (Fig. 5-21C). The double strand is tied to the single strand (Fig. 5-21D). The suture ends are cut near the knot, resulting in a buried knot.

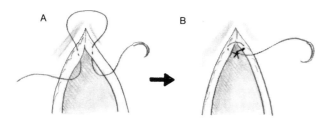

FIG. 5-19. Beginning a continuous intradermal suture (absorbable). A, Placing suture from deeply to superficially on one side of wound and superficially to deeply on opposite side. B, Tying suture buries knot.

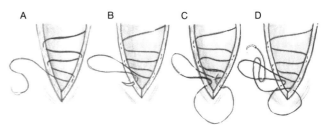

FIG. 5-20. Ending a continuous intradermal suture (absorbable—swaged needle). A, Loop of suture is lifted from wound. B, Needle passed from deeply to superficially on one side of wound. C, Needle passed from superficially to deeply on opposite side of wound. D, Tying free end of suture to previously created loop.

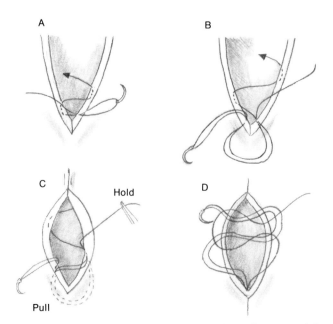

FIG. 5-21. Ending a continuous intradermal suture (absorbable—eyed needle). A, Placing next-to-last suture bite from deeply to superficially. B, A double-stranded loop of suture is drawn from wound, and needle is inserted from superficially to deeply on opposite side of wound. C, Single strand of suture is held while needle is pulled to pull double-stranded loop beneath skin. D, Double strand tied to single strand.

Aftercare. Continuous nonabsorbable intradermal sutures may be removed 10 to 14 days after wound closure or left in place permanently to help prevent scar widening if there was considerable tension at wound closure. If the suture is to be removed, it should be cut at the ends and at any loops that were left exposed, and the segments gently removed.

Advantages and Disadvantages. Intradermal tension sutures are much less prone to animal molestation than other types of exposed tension sutures. They help to prevent widening of scars after skin apposition sutures are removed and may be combined with other tension sutures. When knots on absorbable intradermal sutures are large and not buried sufficiently, however, they may cause pressure and local necrosis of the skin. Removal of a nonabsorbable intradermal suture may be painful for the animal as the suture is pulled through the skin. If any portion of a braided suture is near the skin surface and exposed to bacterial contaminants, a suture line abscess may occur.

REFERENCE AND SUGGESTED READING

1. Swaim, S.F.: Management of skin tension in dermal surgery. Compend. Contin. Educ. *2:*758, 1980.

RELAXING INCISIONS

BIPEDICLE FLAP AND SIMPLE RELAXING INCISION

Definition and Indications. A bipedicle flap is created by making an incision in the skin adjacent to a wound to allow the skin between the incision and the wound to be advanced to cover the wound. The defect left after closing the original wound is closed because it is located in loose elastic skin. A simple relaxing incision is made adjacent to a wound to allow the skin between the relaxing incision and the wound to be advanced to cover the wound. Because of the lack of loose elastic skin in the area, however, the relaxing incision defect is left to heal as an open wound.

These relaxing procedures are indicated for closing defects that are: (1) chronic and surrounded by fibrotic, immovable skin, such as a chronic decubital ulcer (bipedicle flap); (2) near structures such as an eye or around the anus, which would be distorted by closure under tension (bipedicle flap); or (3) in areas where a lack of skin does not allow wound closure such as on the lower limb (simple relaxing incision). Simple relaxing incisions are indicated for closing wounds that are too large to close by using extensive skin undermining and yet are not of a nature or size that warrants more involved reconstructive procedures.

Techniques. When a bipedicle flap is to be made adjacent to a chronic fibrotic lesion or a body structure, the skin edge on the side of the wound from which the flap is planned should be freed from underlying tissue. The skin is then undermined bluntly on that side of the defect (Fig. 5-22A). If the undermining does not provide sufficient relaxation for wound closure (Fig. 5-22B), a bipedicle flap should be created by making an incision in the skin that is basically parallel to the long axis of the wound. If the incision is slightly curved so that the concave side is toward the wound, however, movement of the flap may be facilitated (Fig. 5-22C). Because the incision is made in loose elastic skin, the width of the flap is not as critical as it would be if a simple relaxing incision were made in an area of sparse skin. A rule of thumb, however, would be to make the width of the flap equal to the width of the skin defect to be covered (Fig. 5-22C). A few 3-0 or 4-0 absorbable tacking sutures may be placed under the flap to help close dead space. The wound is closed with some form of tension suture, if it is deemed necessary, and simple interrupted 3-0 nonabsorbable skin apposition sutures (Fig. 5-22D). After the wound is closed, the defect left from moving the flap can be readily closed because the incision was made in loose elastic skin (Fig. 5-22E). If bilateral bipedicle flaps are to be used to close a chronic wound, each flap

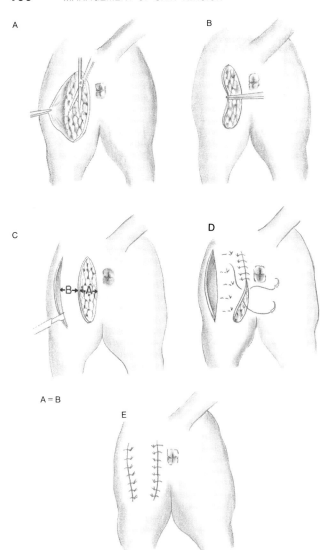

FIG. 5-22. Bipedicle flap. A, Undermining skin on side of defect from which flap will come. B, Checking to see if undermining provided sufficient skin for wound closure. C, Making incision to create bipedicle flap. Wound and flap width are equal (A = B). D, Flap sutured into position. E, Donor site sutured.

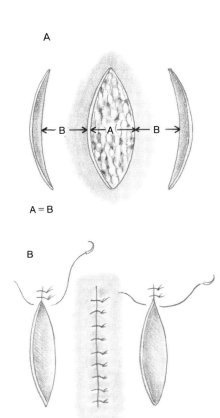

FIG. 5-23. Bipedicle flaps to close a wound surrounded by fibrotic inelastic skin (shaded skin). A, Flap incisions made in supple skin (unshaded) with each flap being at least as wide as defect (A = B). B, Closure of wound followed by closure of two flap donor sites.

Aftercare. Adequate tacking sutures should eliminate the chance of seroma or need for drains; however, the flap(s) should be observed for accumulation of serum or blood. If such accumulation occurs, Penrose drains should be placed under the flap(s) through stab incisions made at the dependent base of the flap(s).

The suture line and open donor site wounds left from relaxing incisions should be bandaged with a nonadherent wound contact material, absorbent wrap, and adhesive tape. Bandages should be changed daily during the early stages and less often in the later stages of healing of the relaxing incision sites. Clinical judgment should be used as to when to discontinue bandaging.

Advantages and Disadvantages. The two procedures provide a means of closing wounds that would have tension on them. The surgeon must realize, however, that these procedures entail creating wounds to close wounds and should be reserved for instances when simple undermining and tension suture techniques are not effective. When the incision is made to create a bipedicle flap, it may be discomforting to the surgeon to notice that there are now two large wounds rather than one. Likewise, relaxing incisions may cause concern after

should be as wide as the defect to be covered. This helps prevent tension on the suture line closing the wound (Fig. 5-23A and B). If the incisions would still be in fibrotic tissue, however, the flaps should be made wider so that the incisions are in supple skin, which generally allows closure of the donor sites.

When a simple relaxing incision(s) is/are to be used to close a wound that is not surrounded by loose elastic skin, the procedure is like that for a bipedicle flap(s); however, the defect(s) left after closing the original wound is/are left to heal as open wounds. These are generally healed within 21 to 30 days.

closure of the original wound because there is a new wound the same size as the original wound on another surface of the limb. It should be realized that such wounds usually heal uneventfully in time because they are in healthy skin.

REFERENCES AND SUGGESTED READING

1. Braden, T.D.: Plastic and reconstructive surgery of the canine torso. Vet. Clin. North Am. *9*:285, 1979.
2. Swaim, S.F.: Management of skin tension in dermal surgery. Compend. Contin. Educ. *2*:758. 1980.

V-TO-Y PLASTY

Definition and Indications. V-to-Y plasty is a form of relaxing incision that provides an advancement flap of skin to cover a defect. The indications are the same as for a bipedicle flap, namely, closing defects that are chronic and surrounded by inelastic skin and closing wounds near structures that would be distorted by closure under tension.

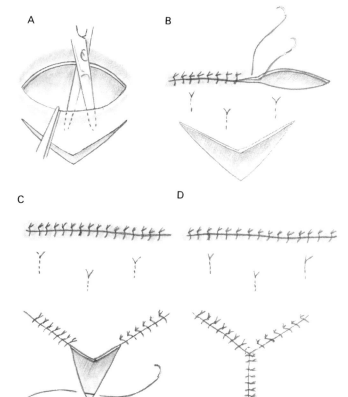

FIG. 5-24. V-to-Y plasty relaxing incision. A, A V-shaped incision made adjacent to defect with point of V away from defect. Skin between defect and incision undermined. B, Closure of defect. C, Closure of V-shaped incision beginning at ends. D, Closure of stem of Y.

Technique. A V-shaped incision is made in the skin adjacent to the defect, with the point of the V away from the defect. The skin between the V and the defect is undermined (Fig. 5-24A) and advanced over the defect. A few simple interrupted 3-0 or 4-0 absorbable tacking sutures may be placed under the advanced tissue to help close dead space. The defect is closed with an appropriate tension suture if deemed necessary and simple interrupted 3-0 nonabsorbable skin apposition sutures (Fig. 5-24B). The remaining defect is closed in the shape of a Y. Suturing is started at the ends of the V and continued until tension starts to develop. The remainder of the defect is closed as the stem of the Y (Fig. 5-24C and D).

Aftercare. As with bipedicle flaps, the use of tacking sutures should obviate the need for a drain in the area around the surgical site. The area, however, should be observed for development of a seroma or hematoma under the undermined tissue. A Penrose drain should be placed in the area if either develops.

Advantages and Disadvantages. The procedure provides a means of tension relief for closing wounds in which tension could be a problem. Like bipedicle flaps, V-to-Y plasty entails creating a wound to close a wound.

REFERENCES AND SUGGESTED READING

1. Grabb, W.C.: Basic techniques of plastic surgery. *In* Plastic Surgery, 3rd ed. Edited by W.C. Grabb, and J.W. Smith. Boston, Little, Brown and Co., 1979.
2. Stashak, T.S.: Reconstructive surgery in the horse. J. Am. Vet. Med. Assoc. *170*:143, 1977.
3. Swaim, S.F.: Management of skin tension in dermal surgery. Compend. Contin. Educ. *2*:758, 1980.

Z-PLASTY

Definition and Indications. Z-plasty is composed of a central limb, two arms, and two angles where the arms join the central limb. The central limb and arms are of equal length. The angles can be any size between 30 and 90 degrees. They may be of equal size or any combination of sizes; however, the most workable angle in skin is 60 degrees, with both angles of this size (Fig. 5-25). The dynamics of a Z-plasty involve transposition of two interdigitating triangular flaps of skin (Fig. 5-26A through C). With these dynamics, the Z-plasty can be used to relieve tension along a bowstring scar that restricts joint extension or to provide skin relaxation for closing wounds. In both instances, the principle involved is *gaining length or relaxation in the direction of the original central limb of the Z after the flaps of the Z are transposed.*

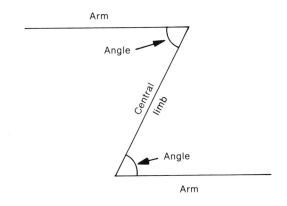

Central Limb Length = Arm Length
Angles = From 30° to 90° (60° is most common)

FIG. 5-25. Components and rules of Z-plasty.

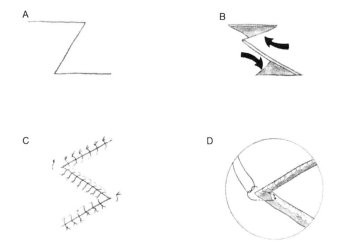

FIG. 5-26. Dynamics of a Z-plasty. A, Incision of Z. B, Undermining and transposition of Z flaps. C, Flaps sutured in their new positions. Inset: Half-buried horizontal mattress suture at flap tips.

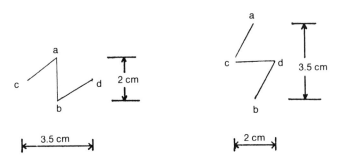

FIG. 5-27. Principle of Z-plasty as a relaxing incision: a gain in length in direction of original central limb of Z after flap transposition. Gain in length is due to shortening of skin along opposite sides of Z-plasty. Distance from a to b lengthens as distance from c to d shortens.

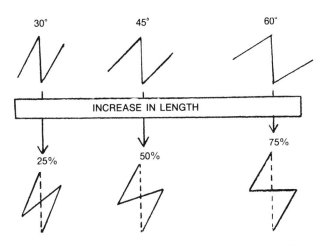

FIG. 5-28. Percentage of increase in length in direction of original central limb with various angle sizes (after Grabb, W.C.: Basic techniques in plastic surgery. *In* Plastic Surgery. 3rd. ed. Edited by W.C. Grabb and J.W. Smith. Boston, Little, Brown and Co., 1979. p. 60).

The gain in length (relaxation) in one direction is caused by shortening of the skin along the opposite sides of the Z-plasty (Fig. 5-27).

The gain in length in the direction of the original central limb can be governed by the size of the angles of the Z-plasty (larger angles give more length gain) (Fig. 5-28) or the length of the central limb (longer length gives more length gain) (Fig. 5-29).

Techniques. Before using a Z-plasty as a relaxing incision, the surgeon should manipulate the skin around

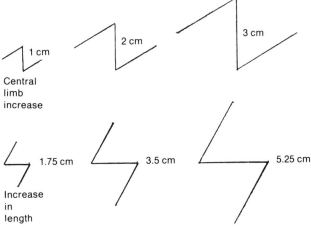

FIG. 5-29. Amount of increase in length in direction of original central limb with various lengths of central limb and 60 degree angles (after Grabb, W.C.: Basic techniques in plastic surgery. *In* Plastic Surgery. 3rd ed. Edited by W.C. Grabb, and J.W. Smith, Boston, Little, Brown and Co., 1979. p. 61).

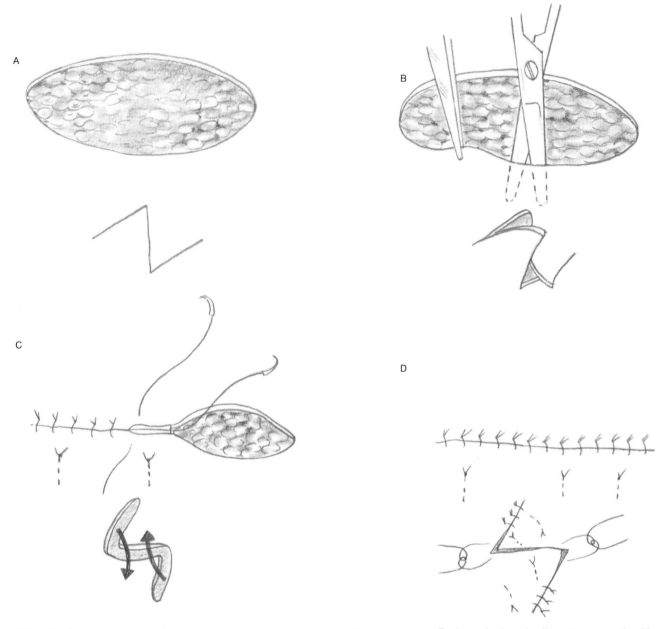

FIG. 5-30. Z-plasty as a relaxing incision for wound closure. A, A 60 degree angle Z-plasty designed adjacent to wound, with central limb in direction relaxation is needed. B, Z-plasty has been cut. Z-plasty flaps and adjacent skin undermined. C, Closure of defect. D, Suturing Z-plasty flaps into their new positions.

the defect to determine if there will be sufficient skin in one plane to allow the needed relaxation in the perpendicular plane. When relaxation is needed to close a wound, a Z-plasty with all limbs of equal length and angles of 60 degrees is designed adjacent to the lesion, with the central limb of the Z in the direction where relaxation is needed (Fig. 5-30A). After the Z is incised, its flaps and the skin between the Z and the lesion are undermined (Fig. 5-30B). This skin can be advanced toward the center of the defect because of the relaxation

provided by the Z-plasty. As the skin is advanced over the defect, underlying tacking sutures of 3-0 absorbable suture may be used to help close dead space. The flaps of the Z-plasty transpose themselves and tend to lie in their new position for final suturing (Fig. 5-30C). The defect is closed with some form of tension suture, if necessary, and 3-0 nonabsorbable simple interrupted skin sutures. The Z-plasty defect is sutured. A few 3-0 absorbable interrupted tacking sutures may be placed under large thick Z-plasty flaps to close dead space, and

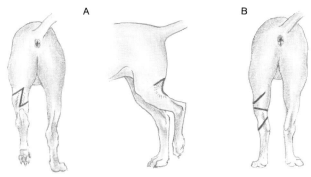

FIG. 5-31. Z-plasty to lengthen a bowstring scar. A, Caudal and lateral views of a Z-plasty designed over a bowstring scar that limits stifle extension. B, Increased length after transposition of Z-plasty flaps allows stifle extension.

the tips of the flaps are sutured with half-buried horizontal mattress sutures of 3-0 to 4-0 material (Fig. 5-30D).

To relieve the tension of a bowstring scar across a flexion surface, the Z is constructed with the central limb of the "Z" along the scar. The arms are directed from either end of the central limb at 60 degrees and are equal in length to the central limb (Fig. 5-31A). After the flaps of the Z are incised and undermined, they are transposed and sutured into place. A few 3-0 interrupted absorbable tacking sutures may be placed under the Z-plasty flaps to help immobilize them in place. Half-buried horizontal mattress sutures of 3-0 or 4-0 nonabsorbable material are used at the flap tips (see Fig. 5-26). Simple interrupted nonabsorbable 3-0 skin sutures are placed. After completion of the procedure, relaxation has been gained in the direction of the central limb of the Z and the tension of the bowstring scar is relieved (Fig. 5-31B). If a restricting scar across a flexion surface is thick and wide, total excision followed by reconstruction with a flap or graft is indicated rather than a Z-plasty relaxing procedure.

Aftercare. When Z-plasty is used as a relaxing procedure to close a wound, the area around the wound and Z-plasty where undermining was performed should be observed for accumulation of serum or blood beneath the skin. If this occurs a Penrose drain should be placed to allow drainage. When Z-plasty has been used to relieve the tension of a bowstring scar over the flexion surface of a joint, the limb should be placed in an immobilization bandage for 7 to 10 days to help prevent movement in the area, which could interfere with suture line healing.

Advantages and Disadvantages. Z-plasty provides tension relief for wound closure, but it also requires creating a wound to close a wound. When used to relieve the tension of a simple bowstring scar, the technique has the advantage of not requiring the removal of any tissue for correction. There is, however, a

possibiltiy of wound disruption if the joint over which surgery was performed is not immobilized for 7 to 10 days following surgery.

REFERENCES AND SUGGESTED READING

1. Grabb, W.C.: Basic techniques of plastic surgery. In Plastic Surgery. 3rd ed. Edited by W.C. Grabb, and J.W. Smith. Boston, Little, Brown and Co., 1979.
2. McGregor, I.A.: Fundamental Techniques of Plastic Surgery. 7th ed. Edinburgh, Churchill Livingston, 1980.
3. Stashak, T.S.: Reconstructive surgery in the horse. J. Am. Vet. Med. Assoc. *170*:143, 1977.
4. Swaim, S.F.: Management of skin tension in dermal surgery. Compend. Contin. Educ. *2*:758, 1980.

MULTIPLE PUNCTATE RELAXING INCISIONS

Definition and Indications. Multiple punctate relaxing incisions are multiple small parallel staggered incisions made in the skin adjacent to a wound to relieve the tension associated with wound closure.

Technique. The skin around a wound is undermined. If it is not possible to appose the skin edges after undermining, multiple punctate relaxing incisions may be considered. Wound closure is begun with a continuous intradermal tension suture with 3-0 or 4-0 absorbable suture material. This suture is preplaced and not tightened or tied at its end (Fig. 5-32A). With tension held on the free end of the suture, a pair of closed hemostats is slipped under a loop near the beginning of the suture and pulled up. If the skin edges do not appose in the area, one or two punctate incisions are made on either side of the wound in the area of tension approximately 1 cm from the wound edge. These incisions are about 1 cm long and 0.5 cm apart (Fig. 5-32B). If the skin edges still do not appose or if they appose with considerable tension, a second row of punctate incisions may be started 0.5 cm lateral to the first row; they are parallel to the first row but staggered with it (Fig. 5-32C).

The hemostats are moved a short distance down the suture line and placed under another loop of suture. Again, tension is applied to the free suture end as the loop is pulled upward, and punctate incisions are made as previously described to allow wound edges to appose in the area (Fig. 5-32D). The procedure is continued until the wound edges can be apposed along their entire length by tightening the intradermal suture. The intradermal suture is then tied. Simple interrupted 3-0 nonabsorbable sutures are placed in the skin for final closure (Fig. 5-32E). No more punctate incisions are made than

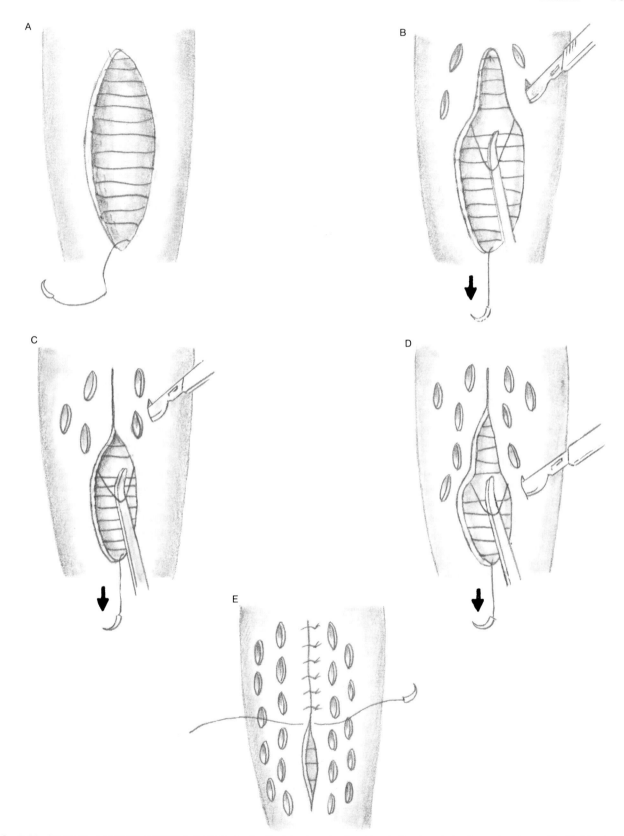

FIG. 5-32. Multiple punctate relaxing incisions. A, Preplacing a simple continuous intradermal suture. B, Tightening a section of suture while making punctate incisions. C, Making more punctate incisions for relaxation. D, Tightening another section of suture while making more punctate incisions. E, Final closure with simple interrupted sutures.

are necessary to allow wound closure without excess tension because the more incisions made, the greater are the chances of interfering with the blood supply to the skin adjacent to the wound and thus jeopardizing wound healing.

Aftercare. The suture line and open punctate wounds should be bandaged with a nonadherent wound contact material, an absorbent wrap, and adhesive tape. Bandages should be changed daily during the early stages of healing and less often as healing progresses. The punctate incisions should be healed in 21 to 30 days. Clinical judgment should be used as to when to discontinue bandaging.

Advantages and Disadvantages. Compared to a single relaxing incision, multiple punctate incisions have the advantage of being more cosmetic and healing faster than one large open wound, and are thus more acceptable to the animal owner. They require making wounds to close a wound, however. The amount of relaxation may not be as great as that attained with one large relaxing incision.

REFERENCES AND SUGGESTED READING

1. Bailey, J.V., and Jacobs, K.A.: The mesh expansion method of suturing wounds on the legs of horses. Vet. Surg. *12*:78, 1983.
2. Vig, M.M.: Management of integumentary wounds of extremities in dogs: An experimental study. J. Am. Anim. Hosp. Assoc. *21*:187, 1985.
3. Bailey, J.V., Caron, J.P., and Lees, M.J.: Wound closure by mesh-expansion technique in 2 equine skin wounds. Mod. Vet. Pract. *67*:355, 1986.

6

WOUNDS OF THE HEAD

FULL-THICKNESS LIP LACERATION

SUTURE REPAIR

Definition and Indications. By definition, lacerations of tissues result from trauma, but other conditions may cause a full-thickness defect. Lip laceration repair is accomplished by using sutures to appose individual layers of the lip. Suture repair may not be needed for full-thickness puncture wounds, but is nearly always necessary when the laceration penetrates the margin of the lip, forming two flaps.

Technique. The tissues should be protected and cleansed (see Chapter 2, Wound Management). After surgical preparation, devitalized tissue should be trimmed until blood oozes from the wound margin (Fig. 6-1A). If the laceration is caudal to the fourth premolar, the integrity of the parotid salivary duct should be affirmed by identifying the intraoral papilla and inserting a thin wire loop into the duct. The wire loop should remain in place during reconstruction if the laceration is near the duct. The lip margin should be perfectly aligned for optimum healing, function, and appearance. Therefore the margin is apposed and sutured first with a 3-0 monofilament in a "figure-of-8," vertical mattress, or near-far suture pattern. The "figure-of-8" suture begins by penetrating the skin away from the lip margin. The suture then angles through the subcutis, crosses the wound space, and engages the dermis of the opposite margin. The suture crosses the wound at the margin a second time to engage the dermis of the other wound border and then crosses the wound space again, at which time it engages and exits the skin on the side of the wound opposite which it began. The suture is then tied (Fig. 6-1B).

The lip is sutured in four layers: the submucosa, muscle fascia, subcutis, and skin. The first layer to be sutured is the fibro-elastic submucosa (Fig. 6-1C). A 4-0 or 3-0 absorbable suture is placed in a simple continuous pattern. Selection of small-sized suture, monofilament construction, and use of fewer knots in the sutured wound provoke less tissue reaction. The mucous membrane is slightly everted into the oral cavity when proper submucosal sutures have been placed. Note that the mucosa is not sutured, although it may be, but from within the oral cavity and only after the submucosa has been apposed to prevent inversion of the mucosa.

The (buccal) muscle fascia and subcutaneous tissue are sutured with the same absorbable suture as used in the submucosa, in a simple interrupted or continuous pattern. The bulkiness of the suture should be reduced by accurately tied square knots rather than multiple throws.

Subcutis and skin are the final layers sutured. Although the skin may be sutured in a single layer, the authors prefer to appose and reinforce the skin with 4-0 absorbable, subcuticular (Guard) sutures, especially when slight tension is present. Loosely tied 4-0 monofilament sutures are placed in the skin for final alignment (Fig. 6-1D).

A common error in suturing mucous membrane is the full-thickness suturing of the mucosa and submucosa as a unit, which decreases the wound surface contact area and is likely to cause the mucosa to invert (Fig. 6-1E), predisposing the wound to dehiscence.

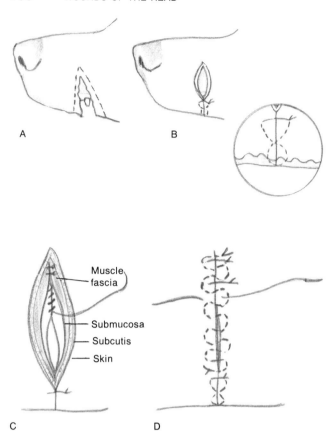

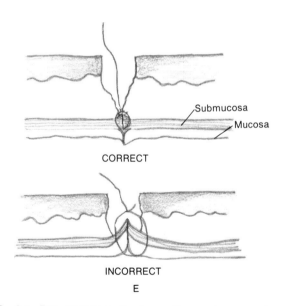

FIG. 6-1. Full thickness lip laceration: suture repair. A, Devitalized tissue to be debrided (broken line). B, Placement of "Figure-of-8" suture at lip margin with detail view (inset). C, Layer by layer closure of lip: continuous suture of submucosa and interrupted suture of buccinator muscle. D, Subcuticular Guard and "Figure-of-8" sutures with simple interrupted sutures in the skin. E, Correct and incorrect apposition of submucosa and mucosa.

Aftercare. Antibiotics are indicated if a lip laceration is infected at the time of reconstruction.

Self-mutilation by the animal is uncommon if sutures have been placed with proper tension, but an Elizabethan collar may be used if needed.

Advantages and Disadvantages. It is an advantage for the surgeon to repair a lip laceration as soon after injury as possible because the wound margins begin to retract immediately, making reconstruction more difficult. Failure to reconstruct a wound that involves the margin of the lip produces structural and functional defects because healing by contraction and epithelialization enlarges the defect and epithelium covers the injured tissue. Cosmetically, if the defect is not closed, the teeth may be revealed, and functionally, mastication and retention of a food bolus may be difficult.

REFERENCE AND SUGGESTED READING

1. Swaim, S.F., Henderson, R.A., and Sutton, H.H.: Correction of triangular and wedge shaped skin defects in dogs and cats. J. Am. Anim. Hosp. Assoc. *16*:225, 1980.

CHRONIC LACERATIONS AND TUMORS OF THE LIP

SEGMENTAL RESECTION OF THE LIP

Definition and Indications. Wide debridement of infected lip lacerations and excision of lip tumors frequently create variously shaped defects. Segmental resection is the intentional creation of a wedge-shaped defect, indicated because the wound edges possess a good blood supply to all parts and this shape is one of the easiest to close cosmetically. The quantity of tissue removed depends on the shape of the lesion and the nature of the ongoing disease process.

Technique. The reason for using a wedge-shaped segmental lip excision is that it easily creates wound margins of nearly equal length. The relationship of the parotid salivary duct and papilla to the area of tissue being excised must be considered. If the resection is to be near the parotid papilla, parotid duct cannulation with a wire loop before incision is prudent. The incisions used must take into consideration the blood supply to the wound edges and the quantity of tissue that must be removed. The arborizations of the infraorbital and facial arteries supply blood to the upper lip (Fig. 6-2A). Although extensive collateral circulation exists, debridement or excisions that produce flaps at the lip margin should be avoided because they may predispose to dehiscence (Fig. 6-2B). Incisions should be perpendicular

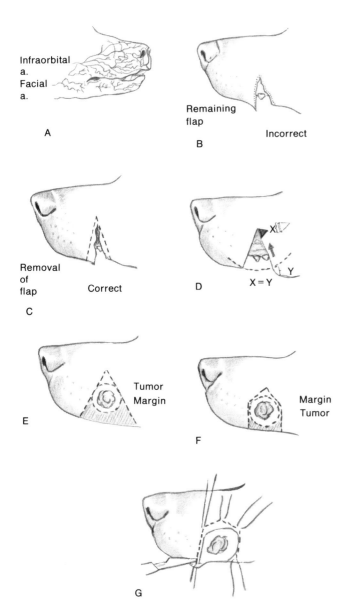

Although incisions of identical length are ideal, they are not always used because of the elasticity of the skin and mucous membrane. Significant disparity of length between wound edges may be corrected by removal of a triangle of tissue from the long side of the defect near the apex of the wedge (Fig. 6-2D).

When potentially malignant tumors are excised, an additional margin of "normal" tissue, usually a minimum of 1 to 2 cm, must also be removed (see Excision Biopsies and Principles of Tumor Excision, Chapter 10). If the primary tumor is small or near the lip margin, excision is not difficult if an isosceles triangle is used. As the tumor size increases or the tumor is situated farther from the lip margin, a straight-sided isosceles triangle excises too much normal skin at the margin (Fig. 6-2E). A pentagon-shaped excision spares excessive skin loss (Fig. 6-2F).

The lip is difficult to incise because of its flexibility and free margin. The margin of normal tissue to be removed with the tumor and thus the proposed line of incision, may be roughly scribed with a splintered wooden applicator stick and sterile new methylene blue. Straight incisions are then made by holding the line of incision under tension with skin hooks, towel clamps, or tension sutures (Fig. 6-2G). The tissue is then incised to full thickness with a No. 11 blade. The lip is sutured in layers (see Full-Thickness Lip Laceration, Suture Repair, this chapter).

Aftercare. See Full-thickness Lip Laceration—Suture Repair, this chapter.

Advantages and Disadvantages. Pentagonal excisions have an obvious advantage over triangular excisions when a lesion is located increasingly farther from the lip margin. Pentagonal excisions require only a little more time for placement of traction sutures to make accurate, straight incisions.

FIG. 6-2. Segmental resection of lip. A, Arborization of infraorbital and facial arteries. B, Incorrect debridement (dotted line) leaves flap. C, Correct debridement (broken line) leaves no flap. D, Compensation for unequal wound edge length by removing Burow's triangle (x = y) and shifting skin (arrow). E, Excessive normal tissue removal (cross-hatched area) with triangular excision of a lip tumor and "margin." F, Pentagonal incision for lip tumor and "margin": removal of less normal lip margin (cross-hatched area). G, Traction sutures to tense skin during full-thickness pentagonal excision.

(or slightly oblique) to the lip margin, removing any tissue that would remain as a flap. This ensures an adequate blood supply and facilitates approximation of the lip margin (Fig. 6-2C). See Full-Thickness Lip Laceration, Suture Repair, this chapter.

REFERENCE AND SUGGESTED READING

1. Swaim, S.F., Henderson, R.A., and Sutton, H.H.: Correction of triangular and wedge-shaped skin defects in dogs and cats. J. Am. Anim. Hosp. Assoc. *16*:225, 1980.

FACIAL AND LIP FOLD DERMATITIS

EXCISION OF FOLDS

Definition and Indications. Facial folds and lip folds, made up of skin or skin and mucous membrane, may become pathologic in certain instances. When the hair stubble of one skin surface rubs the other surface in the creases of folds (intertriginous zone) and the area is

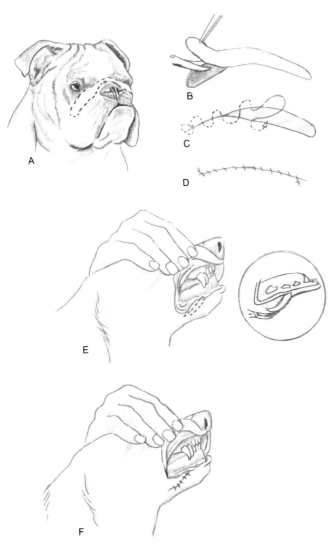

FIG. 6-3. Facial and lip fold excision. A, Correct incisions for facial fold excision (broken line). B, Fusiform excision of facial fold. C, Placement of subcuticular Guard suture. D, Continuous suture placed to avoid knots near the eyes. E, Correct incision for lip fold removal (broken line). Inset: Removal of lip fold. F, Sutured wound after lip fold excision.

management of the dermatitis. Another indication for removal of facial folds is when the hair of the fold contacts the cornea and produces chronic keratitis. Excision of facial folds is frequently timed to coincide with another operation such as caudectomy (for ingrown tail), blepharoplasty, nasopharyngeal reconstructive procedures, or neutering.

Technique. Acute inflammation should be controlled before surgery. The sutured wound may dehisce or the scar may be excessive if the tissues are excised while acutely inflamed. Most inflammation may be controlled initially by cleansing and the use of topical antibiotics. Occasionally, systemic antibiotics and topical steroids are required. Recurrent infections should be cultured and bacterial sensitivity obtained before medical therapy is instituted again. Before surgery, the surgical site is clipped, cleansed, and surgically prepared, especially in the recesses of the folds.

Facial Folds. The quantity of tissue to be removed is assessed by pinching the base of the fold(s) together to determine the probable tension after excision. The base of the fold to be removed is incised with a scalpel, one recess at a time, and each end of the wound is tapered to a point to prevent "dog ears." The fold is removed with sharp, curved scissors (Fig. 6-3A and B). This creates a basically fusiform wound over the bridge of the nose (Fig. 6-3B). The wound edges are undermined if necessary to achieve closure without tension. Hemorrhage is controlled with fine ligatures or pinpoint electrocoagulation. The wound edges may be initially aligned by applying towel forceps or a skin hook to each end of the wound and placing the wound in traction. Several simple interrupted 4-0 subcutaneous sutures are used to align the skin edges, and the skin is initially apposed with a 3-0 or 4-0 subcuticular Guard suture (Fig. 6-3C). Short-haired breeds are more likely to have residual surgical scars if subcuticular support is not used. Skin sutures are then placed for final wound alignment. Because the suture line is close to the eyes, no suture ends should be placed where they could irritate the cornea. The authors prefer 4-0 silk for use around the eye. A continuous suture pattern with a 3-0 or 4-0 monofilament suture, tied at each end, also protects the eye (Fig. 6-3D).

Multiple folds which may be present in some dogs may be excised with the same incision, but it may not be necessary to excise all folds. Removing only one pathologic fold sometimes reduces the effect of a second fold.

Lip Fold. The offending fold(s) is (are) excised with sharp, heavy, curved scissors (Fig. 6-3E and inset). The edges of the wound are undermined if necessary, and the wound is sutured in two layers. The buccinator muscle is apposed with 4-0 absorbable suture, and the skin is

chronically moistened by tears or saliva, the environment may encourage proliferation of secondary pathogens such as bacteria or yeast. Facial folds are most frequently seen over the bridge of the nose in brachycephalic breeds of dogs (Fig. 6-3A). Folds of the lower lips in some dogs, especially the spaniel breeds, may direct saliva onto the skin, causing cheilitis (see Fig. 6-3E).

Removal of either the ridge or trough of the fold is termed fold excision. Excision of facial and lip folds is indicated in chronic intertriginous infections when cleansing alone has not resolved the inflammation. Excision prevents intertriginous contact and facilitates apposed with interrupted or continuous 4-0 silk sutures (Fig. 6-3F).

Aftercare. The postoperative wound is cleansed and antiseptic is applied to the suture line. Sutures are usually removed in 7 days because the capillarity of silk predisposes to suture abscesses if they are left longer.

Advantages and Disadvantages. Although heavy, sharp scissors may be used to excise facial folds, the use of scissors is discouraged. If scissors are used, the resulting incision edge is not perpendicular to the skin surface, especially at the ends of the wound which may pose problems when attempting to obtain cosmetic alignment. Owners should be informed that excision of facial folds may change the appearance of the dog. Removing too much skin with the facial fold may produce tension on the wound, scarring, or ectropion.

REFERENCES AND SUGGESTED READING

1. Harvey, C.E.: The oral cavity and pharynx. In Textbook of Small Animal Surgery. Edited by D.H. Slatter. Philadelphia, W.B. Saunders, 1985.
2. Krahwinkel, D.J.: Correction of specific skin diseases. In Surgery of Traumatized Skin: Management and Reconstruction in the Dog and Cat. Edited by S.F. Swaim. Philadelphia, W.B. Saunders, 1980.
3. Krahwinkel., D.J., and Bone, D.: Surgical management of specific skin disorders. In Textbook of Small Animal Surgery. Edited by D.H. Slatter. Philadelphia, W.B. Saunders, 1985.
4. Smeak, D.D.: Anti-Drool Cheiloplasty: Clinical Results in Six Dogs. Am. Anim. Hosp. Assoc. 25:181, 1989.

LOWER LIP AVULSION

TRANSOSSEOUS SUTURES

Definition and Indications. Lower lip avulsion is the traumatic disruption of the labial or gingival mucosa and subcutaneous tissue from the mandible (Fig. 6-4A). The shearing force generated when the lower lip impacts the ground (as when an animal is struck by a car) may disrupt the soft tissues along the base of the teeth and may also cause grade III mandibular fractures. The possibility of concomitant fractures of the spine or pelvis must also be considered (Fig. 6-4C).

Reattachment of the lip to the mandible with transosseous sutures is essential to healing (Fig. 6-4B). Merely attempting to suture the avulsed gingiva is futile and contraindicated because of gingival friability and the weight of the edematous avulsed tissue.

Technique. Proper healing requires simultaneous reduction and stabilization of fractures, reattachment and immobilization of the avulsed tissue, and drainage of dependent recesses. The initial wound is of traumatic

origin and must be considered dirty or infected. Systemic antibiotics are administered and the wound is treated on the basis of duration, blood supply, degree of infection, and amount of foreign debris present (see Chapter 2, Wound Management). When the condition of the treated wound is suitable, the mandibular fracture(s), if present, is (are) reduced and stabilized and the injured tissues are reattached with transosseous tension sutures followed by gingival sutures. The reattachment procedure is started by making stab incisions at the caudal recess of the flap to allow the emergence of flat drainage tubes (if they are to be used). The wound is frequently irrigated with 1:40 chlorhexidine diacetate during surgery.

Transosseous tension sutures are placed by drilling through the mandible between the teeth from lateral to medial with a 1.1 mm (0.045 inch) Kirchner wire or small bit while attempting to avoid the tooth roots (Fig. 6-4D). The lip is approximated into normal position, and a 20-gauge hypodermic needle is inserted through the skin at the intended emergence of the suture. The needle is guided through the drilled hole in the mandible to emerge on the medial aspect of the mandible. One end of a 2-0 monofilament nonabsorbable suture is threaded through the tip of the hypodermic needle until it emerges through the hub of the needle. The same maneuver is repeated for the other end of the suture so that the suture midpoint is medial to the manidible (Fig. 6-4E). The suture is loosely tied, approximating the soft tissues of the lip and the mandible (Fig. 6-4F). The process is repeated until the lip is secured.

The gingival surface is then apposed with simple interrupted sutures of 4-0 absorbable suture (Fig. 6-4G). A swaged, taper-cut needle benefits the surgeon by reducing the tendency of the tissues to tear. The drainage tubes are secured to the skin at their points of emergence.

The entire lip may not be available for reconstruction because of loss through abrasion or slough. Lip defects may be reconstructed at the time of initial repair or delayed until most of the wound is healed. In severe cases, the skin of the neck combined with mucous membranes may be advanced or the mandibles may be shortened. An exposed mandible must not be allowed to dry because, if it dries, the mandibular periosteum will die and a portion of the exposed cortex may also die.

Aftercare. The drain tubes are removed when the quantity of drainage is reduced, usually on the fourth to fifth day. The transosseous sutures are removed after 10 to 14 days. Mucosal sutures are not removed. Antibiotic administration is usually continued in these cases because the initial wound is often heavily contaminated or infected.

Advantages and Disadvantages. Compared to techniques in which only the mucosa is repaired, the described technique accommodates the tension which

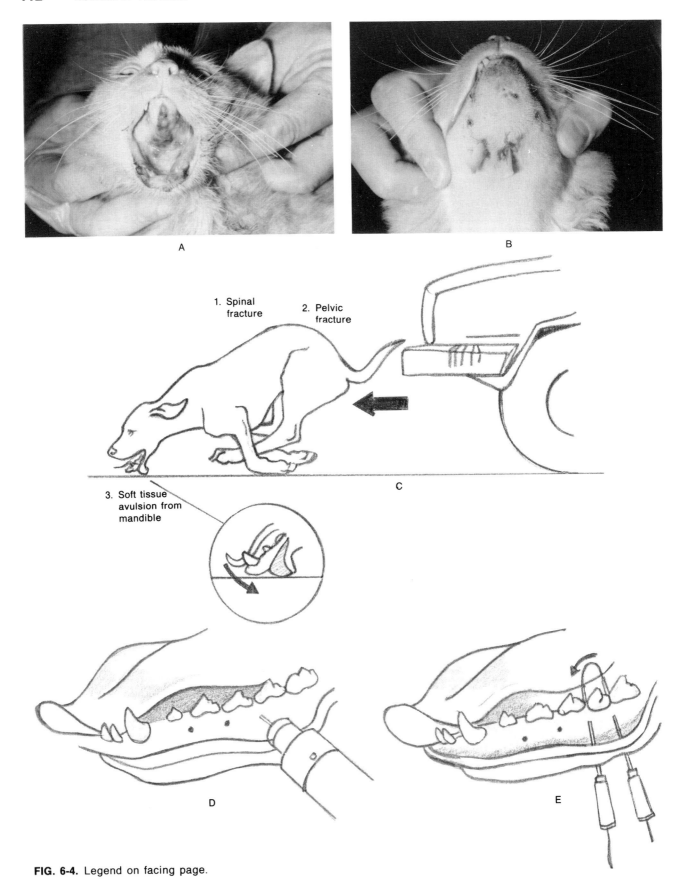

1. Spinal fracture
2. Pelvic fracture
3. Soft tissue avulsion from mandible

A

B

C

D

E

FIG. 6-4. Legend on facing page.

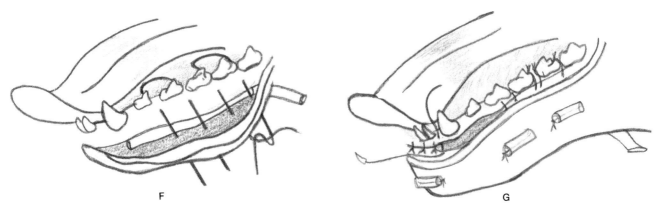

FIG. 6-4. Lower lip avulsion. A, Lower lip avulsion on a cat. B, Same cat 5 days after surgical repair. C, Injury potential: 1) spinal fracture, 2) pelvic fracture, and 3) labial avulsion from mandible. D, Drilling holes between teeth for transosseous tension sutures. E, 20 guage hypodermic needles through skin and mandible for passing 2-0 transosseous suture. F, Two transosseous sutures placed. Flat latex drain in place. G, Additional transosseous tied over rubber tube stents. Interrupted gingivolabial sutures being placed.

may arise secondary to swelling, seroma, and other problems. Mucosal sutures alone are inadequate to support complete avulsions.

REFERENCES AND SUGGESTED READING

1. Miller, W.W., Swaim, S.F., and Pope, E.R.: Labial avulsion repair in the dog and cat. Am. Anim. Hosp. Assoc. *21*:435, 1985.
2. Richardson, D.C.: Fracture first aid: The open (compound) fracture. *In* Textbook of Small Animal Surgery. Edited by D.H. Slatter. Philadelphia, W.B. Saunders, 1985.

AURICULAR HEMATOMA

DRAINAGE VERSUS OBLITERATION

Definition and Indications. Auricular hematoma is the collection of blood and/or serum in the pinna. The hematoma usually forms secondary to a longitudinal planar fracture of the auricular cartilage or separation of the cartilage and perichondrium. The cause is usually traumatic. Resorption is slow, and untreated hematomas may cause persistent head shaking and deformity of the pinna.

Drainage is an established method to provide release of accumulated blood and serum, usually through one or more puncture wounds. Obliteration is a method whereby the hematoma is incised and curetted to cause the wound surface to unite, followed by the use of sutures to appose the walls of the hematoma cavity, which prevents its refilling. Pressure is the application of

external force to assist gravitational drainage and immobilization of the ear.

Acute hematomas respond to simple drainage and pressure wraps better than hematomas of longer than 7 days' duration. After 7 to 10 days, the fibrin clot begins to be replaced with fibroblastic contractile elements, and the likelihood of the pinna being deformed increases. Long-standing hematomas should be treated by obliteration of the space with sutures. The mature collagen found lining, long-standing hematomas may not unite when simply pressed together or sutured. Recreation of the wound inflammation stage of healing seems important to promote union of the tissues lining the cavity of the chronic hematoma.

Technique. The cause of the hematoma should be investigated and treated. Common causes include parasites, bacteria, fungi, neoplasia, and trauma. These cause the animal to scratch the ears and shake the head and ear flap, initiating and sustaining a hematoma. The exudate in the ear should be examined by direct smear for arachnids and yeast. Chronic conditions should be cultured. Redness of the entire pinna should prompt examination of other body sites such as the feet and muzzle for evidence of atopy. The owner should also be questioned as to the possible seasonal occurrence of the problem.

Drainage and Pressure. The concave (hairless) aspect of the ear is surgically prepared. A small incision is made in the most distal aspect of the hematoma (Fig. 6-5A) and a self-retaining teat tube* is placed into the cavity (Fig. 6-5B). The tube is secured with a suture. The contents of the hematoma are expressed through the drain, the cavity irrigated with saline, and the contents expressed again. This step may be repeated to remove as

---

*Dr. Larsen's Plastic Teat Tube, Haver-Lockhart, Shawnee, KS.

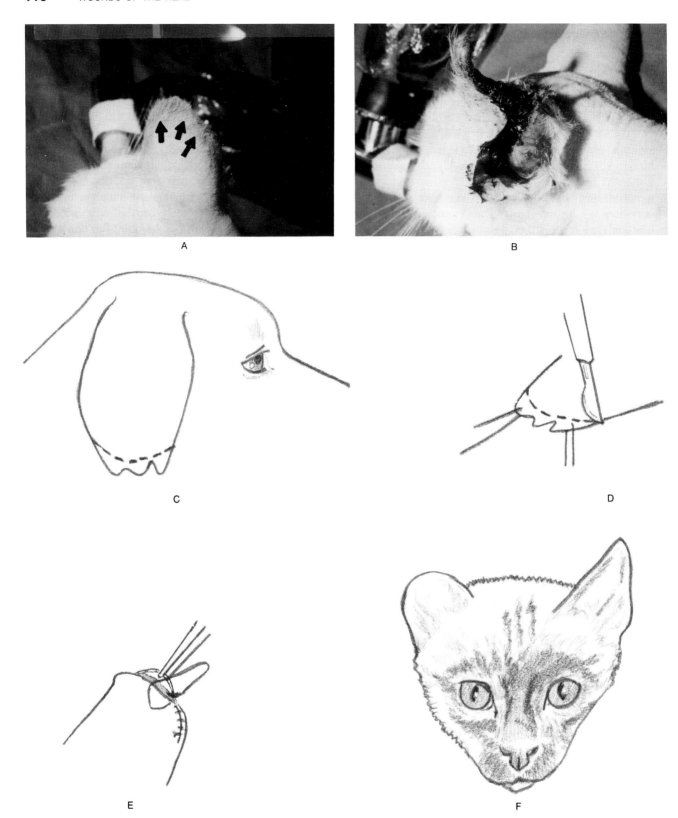

FIG. 6-7. Correction of marginal defect, excision. A, Cat's ear affected with mild actinic keratosis (arrows). B, Opposite ear of cat in Fig. 6-7A affected by squamous cell carcinoma. C, Ear fissures indicating partial amputation area (broken line). D, Pinna tensed with suture to assist incision. E, Ear margin being sutured. F, Resultant cosmetic appearance of cat with partial amputation of the pinna.

DEFECTS OF THE MARGIN OF THE PINNA

PARTIAL AMPUTATION

Definition and Indications. Excision of, or trauma to, the skin and cartilage of the margin of the pinna frequently results in defects that cannot be closed cosmetically by moving local skin. The inelasticity of the cartilage sandwiched between the skin surfaces prevents all but the smallest defects from being undermined and sutured directly. Partial amputation is the removal of a portion of the ear flap to remove a disease process.

Small defects of the margin of the pinna, such as ear fissures from chronic head shaking or bite wounds, as well as larger lesions involving major portions of the margins such as ulcers from biting flies, chronic actinic keratosis (Fig. 6-7A), or squamous cell carcinoma (Fig. 6-7B) may be excised by partial amputation. Larger segmental defects may be reconstructed by transferring skin from the head or neck as flaps (see Defects of the Margin of the Pinna, Reconstruction with Flaps, this chapter).

Technique. Both surfaces of the ear are surgically prepared by clipping, scrubbing, and applying an antiseptic. The quantity of ear to be removed depends on the biologic behavior of the lesion being treated. Ear fissures may be cosmetically reconstructed by excision of a 1 to 2 mm zone of normal tissue (Fig. 6-7C), but squamous cell carcinoma should have a measured margin of normal appearing tissue of at least 1 cm (see Excision Biopsies and Principles of Tumor Excision, Chapter 10). In addition, the final shape of the ear must be taken into consideration, and this may change the margin of normal ear removed along the line of excision. The intended line of incision may be lightly scribed with the back side of the scalpel or with a sterile splintered applicator stick and new methylene blue stain. The amputation should be performed with a scalpel rather than scissors because of the crushing effect of scissors on the skin. The ear margin must be tensed with hooks, suture, or forceps during amputation to assist in making a smooth incision (Fig. 6-7D). Neoplastic tissue should be covered and should not be touched with surgical gloves or instruments, which could transfer tumor cells to the fresh wound and cause recurrence. After amputation of the affected part, the skin retracts and the cartilage may be shaped and smoothed with finely serrated scissors. After excision, the skin edges are sutured with a simple continuous 4-0 monofilament suture (Fig. 6-7E). The edges of the wound are optimally apposed when wrapped (rolled) around the edge of the cartilage and are directly abutted.

Aftercare. Bandages may be necessary to protect a pendulous ear flap after partial amputation. No other special care is required.

Advantages and Disadvantages. Partial amputation usually requires excision of more of the ear flap than is needed to achieve a smooth ear margin. Cosmetically, the ear flaps will not match after partial amputation. The quantity of amputation will govern the cosmetic distortion (Fig. 6-7F). Partial amputation of the pinna is a rapid, inexpensive method to manage defects and diseases of the margin of the pinna.

REFERENCES AND SUGGESTED READING

1. Henderson R.A.: Reconstructive ear surgery. *In* Surgery of Traumatized Skin: Management and Reconstruction in the Dog and Cat. Edited by S.F. Swaim. Philadelphia, W.B. Saunders, 1980.
2. Horne, R.D., and Henderson R.A.: The pinna. *In* Textbook of Small Animal Surgery. Edited by D.H. Slatter. Philadelphia, W.B. Saunders, 1985.

RECONSTRUCTION USING FLAPS

Definition and Indications. Excision of, or trauma to, the skin and cartilage of the pinna may result in defects that cannot be closed cosmetically by moving local skin, and when partial amputation is undesirable (see Defects of the Margin of the Pinna, Partial Amputation, this chapter). Large segmental defects may be reconstructed by transferring skin flaps from the head or neck.

Technique

Three-stage Flap. Correction of a large margin defect of the ear, especially of the tip, is performed in three stages (Figs. 6-8 and 6-9). The ear and the side of the head and neck are surgically prepared. During the first stage, the defect edges are debrided and the ear is positioned on the donor skin of the cheek/neck. The donor skin is incised parallel to the edges of the defect and the edge of the resulting flap is sutured to the skin edge on the convex (lateral) surface of the ear with simple interrupted 4-0 monofilament material (Fig. 6-8A and inset). The surgical site is protected by a bandage for 2 weeks.

The second stage of correction is performed 2 weeks after the first. The flap pedicle is incised in the shape of the new pinna margin needed or slightly larger to allow for contraction (Fig. 6-8B). The pinna is transferred to the dorsum of the head, where another flap is prepared to provide a medial surface for the stage 1 flap. A traction suture may be used to place and secure the recipient site under the flap (Fig. 6-8C). The flap is sutured in place. This second flap is also protected for 2 weeks.

The procedure is completed in the third stage,

during which, the pedicle of the second flap is incised to match the first (Fig. 6-8D). The edges of convex surface flap and concave surface flap are sutured together to create the edge of the ear (Fig. 6-8E). The two-flap technique can also be used on the straight margins of

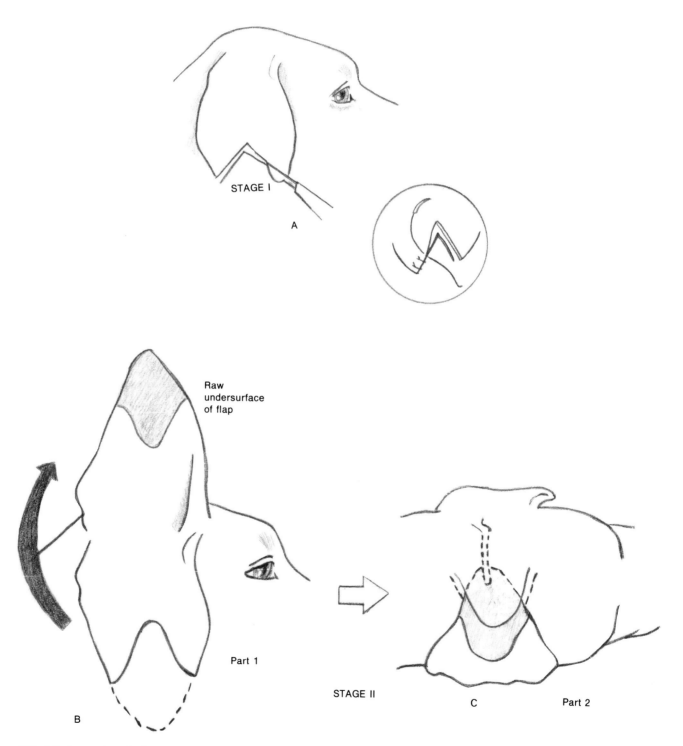

FIG. 6-8. Legend on facing page.

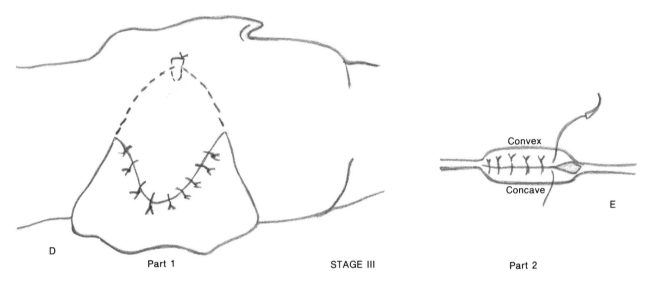

FIG. 6-8. Correction of marginal defect with three stage cranial and cheek/neck flaps. A, Stage I. Incising cheek/neck skin for flap to fill a lateral ear tip defect. Inset: Suturing flap edge to skin edge on *lateral* side of ear. B, Stage II, Part 1. Incisions of flap base (broken line) and dorsal rotation of pinna (arrow). C, Stage II, Part 2. Pinna defect slipped under donor flap on dorsum of head, secured with suture. D, Stage III, Part 1. Incision of cranial (second) flap's base (broken line). E, Stage III, Part 2. Suturing edges of concave and convex flaps together.

rostral or caudal defects as shown in Figure 6-9A through G.

Two-stage Flap. Large margin defects along the straight borders of the pinna may be reconstructed in two stages. The first stage is the same as described for the three-stage flap. The second stage is different in that the incision of the flap pedicle must be a mirror image of the undersurface to allow the flap to be *loosely* folded to form the medial coverage of the flap rather than using a second flap (Fig. 6-10A through D).

Aftercare. Bandages are necessary to protect the pedicles from injury during the interoperative periods. Initially, bandages are changed daily and the wound is gently cleansed. As the flaps heal, bandage changes become less frequent. No other special care is required.

Advantages and Disadvantages. The principal disadvantage of both of these techniques is the increased thickness of the skin of the neck and head compared to that of the ear, especially the medial surface of the pinna. The reconstructed tissues lack cartilage to give the ear shape, which limits the usefulness of these techniques to filling defects as opposed to creating a new pinna.

Two-stage repairs require less time; however, in two-stage repairs, the blood supply to the folded portion of

the flap is easily jeopardized if the fold is too acute. Also, the flattened edge created by folding the flap restricts this technique to a straight edge of the ear. If folding the flap causes avascular necrosis, the third stage of a three-stage flap can be used to fill the defect after debridement.

The three-stage technique is required for reconstruction of the tip or for other curved surfaces; however, it can be used on the rostral and caudal edge equally well, and the authors prefer this technique. The length and direction of hair growth may be more noticeable on some dogs than others, depending on the length of hair on the ear and the donor sites (Fig. 6-9).

REFERENCES AND SUGGESTED READING

1. Henderson, R.A.: Reconstructive ear surgery. *In* Surgery of Traumatized Skin: Management and Reconstruction in the Dog and Cat. Edited by S.F. Swaim. Philadelphia, W.B. Saunders, 1980.
2. Horne, R.D., and Henderson, R.A.: The pinna. *In* Textbook of Small Animal Surgery. Edited by D.H. Slatter. Philadelphia, W.B. Saunders, 1985.
3. Swaim, S.F., Henderson, R.A., and Sutton, H.H.: Correction of triangular and wedge-shaped skin defects in dogs and cats. J. Am. Anim. Hosp. Assoc. *16*:225, 1980.

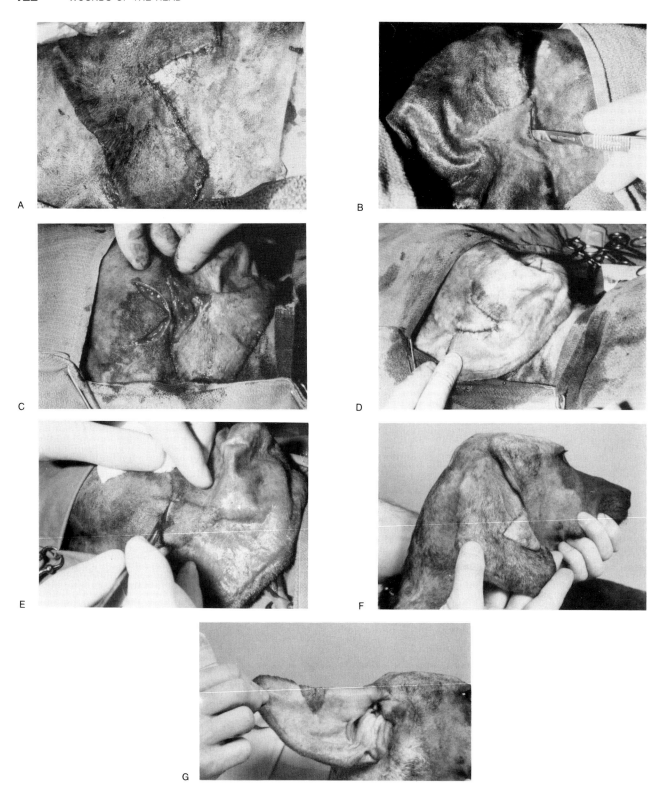

FIG. 6-9. Three-stage correction of margin defect of pinna. A, Stage I. Cheek/neck flap sutured into pinna defect. B, Stage II, Part 1. Cervical pedicle incised to form new margin. C, Stage II, Part 2. Cranial pedicle incised to cover raw undersurface of cervical flap. D, Stage II, Part 2 continued. Cranial flap sutured into place. E, Stage III. Part 1. Incising base of cranial pedicle. F, Postoperative result of concave surface. G, Postoperative result of convex surface. (A–G from Swaim, S.F., Henderson, R.A., and Sutton, H.H., Correction of triangular and wedge shaped skin defects in dogs and cats. J. Amer. Anim. Hosp. Assoc. *16*:225, 1980).

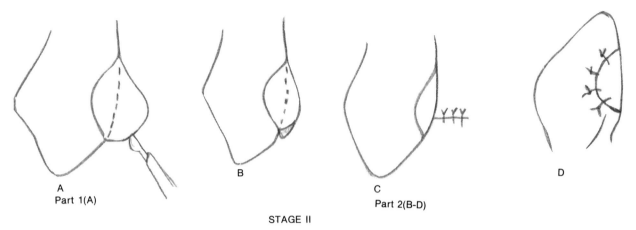

A
Part 1(A)

B

C
Part 2(B-D)

D

STAGE II

FIG. 6-10. Correction of marginal defect with two-stage flap. A, Stage II, Part 1. Incision of flap pedicle as mirror image of defect (Stage I flap) with intended fold (broken line). B, Stage II, Part 2. Folding flap pedicle loosely to cover undersurface of flap. C, Stage II, Part 2. continued. Flap folded, donor site sutured. D, Stage II, Part 2 continued. Flap sutured in place on the concave surface of ear.

DEFECTS OF THE CENTER OF THE PINNA

RECONSTRUCTION WITH FLAPS

Definition and Indications. Excision of, or trauma to, the skin and cartilage of the center of the pinna may result in defects that cannot be closed cosmetically by moving local skin (see Lacerations and Excisions of the Pinna, Suturing the Ear Flap, this chapter). The cartilage of the ear flap makes an excellent deep margin to combine with excision of a tumor because cartilage is seldom invaded by neoplastic cells. In addition, wounds and excisions of the medial (concave) aspect of the pinna involve the skin and the underlying, intimately associated cartilage. Here, defects wider than 1 cm are preferably treated by skin transfer using a graft or flap. On the lateral surface, subcutaneous tissue and typical subcutaneous blood vessels allow the skin to be advanced to close larger wounds, but here too, limited skin exists and a graft or flap may be required to fill a large defect or excision.

Technique. The ear and the side of the head and neck are surgically prepared. Flaps for central defects are prepared on the cheek/neck area if the defect is on the medial (concave) surface, and on the top of the head/neck if the defect is on the lateral (haired) surface. The pedicle flap is created on the cheek in the first stage (Fig. 6-11A). The ear defect is laid over the raw surface of the flap and their edges are sutured together (Fig. 6-11B). The ear is protected by a bandage for approximately 2 weeks, with periodic bandage changes as needed. The flap is supported under the bandage by a roll of gauze sutured to the cheek to prevent kinking

of the blood supply (Fig. 6-11B). After 2 weeks, the base of the flap is severed, shaped, and sutured to the remaining defect edge (Fig. 6-11C). Full-thickness defects may be reconstructed in three stages in a technique similar to that described for margin defects (see Defects of the Margin of the Pinna, Reconstruction with Flaps, Figs. 6-8 and 6-9, this chapter).

Aftercare. See Defects of the Margin of the Pinna, Reconstruction with Flaps, this chapter.

Advantages and Disadvantages. See Defects of the Margin of the Pinna, Reconstruction using Flaps, this chapter.

REFERENCES AND SUGGESTED READING

1. Henderson, R.A.: Reconstructive ear surgery. *In* Surgery of Traumatized Skin: Management and Reconstruction in the Dog and Cat. Edited by S.F. Swaim. Philadelphia, W.B. Saunders, 1980.
2. Horne, R.D., and Henderson, R.A.: The pinna. *In* Textbook of Small Animal Surgery. Edited by D.H. Slatter. Philadelphia, W.B. Saunders, 1985.

OBSTRUCTION OF THE VERTICAL EAR CANAL

LATERAL CANAL WALL RESECTION WITH VENTRAL PEDICLE FLAP

Definition and Indications. Hyperplasia of the auricular epithelium is a response to inflammation. Histopathologically, this lesion is characterized by increased

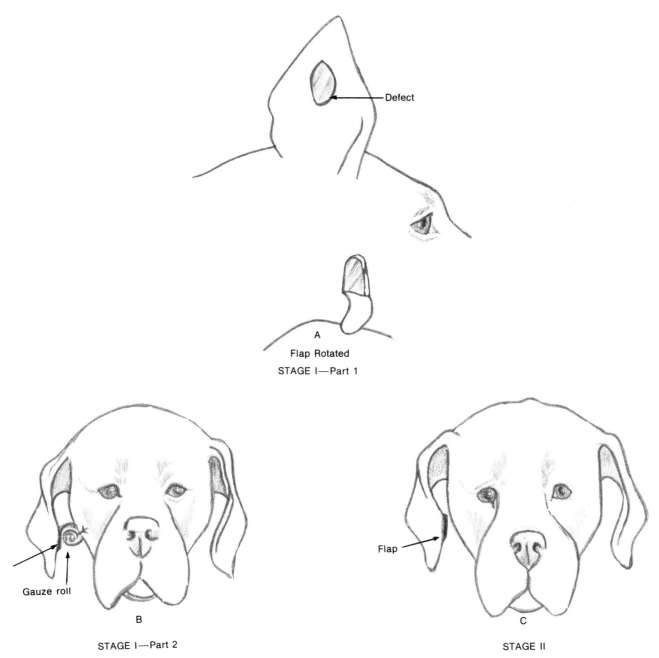

FIG. 6-11. Correction of central defect with two-stage flap. A, Stage I, Part 1. Defect in pinna, flap incised and rotated laterally. B, Stage I, Part 2. Flap sutured into distal and lateral aspects of defect with a roll of gauze sutured under base of flap. C, Stage II. Flap transferred and sutured into dorsal aspect of defect.

thickness of the epidermis and dermis with hypervascularity, epithelial ulceration, invasion of the epithelium and dermis with leukocytes, dermal fibroplasia, and glandular atrophy. This pathologic condition may cause partial obstruction of the horizontal canal and verrucous, exophytic epithelial masses that resemble granulomas on the inside of the pinna (Fig. 6-13A). The clefts and ulcerations on their surface and the deep crevices be-

tween the masses provide an environment for microbial colonization and intertriginous infection.

Straight converging incisions to remove the lateral ear canal wall with suture apposition of the ear canal epithelium to the facial skin became known as the "Lacroix procedure" (Fig. 6-12A). When it was modified by Zepp, who used the lateral canal wall as a ventral pedicle flap, it was called the "Lacroix-Zepp procedure," shortened through usage to "Zepp procedure." It is indicated as an adjunct to medical management of chronic otitis by providing access for application of medication and drainage, and for relief of obstruction of the vertical canal. A patent horizontal canal is normally considered necessary to justify the use of the Zepp procedure. The latter and the original Lacroix procedure are useful to explore the ear canal, excise neoplastic lesions or perform surgery in the horizontal canal and middle ear.

The Zepp procedure should not be performed for otitis externa without investigating the causes of the otitis and the hyperplastic skin obstructing the canal. Commonly overlooked causes of chronic otitis are atopy (inhalant dermatitis), food allergy, and hypothyroidism. Appropriate intradermal sensitivity testing, food trials,

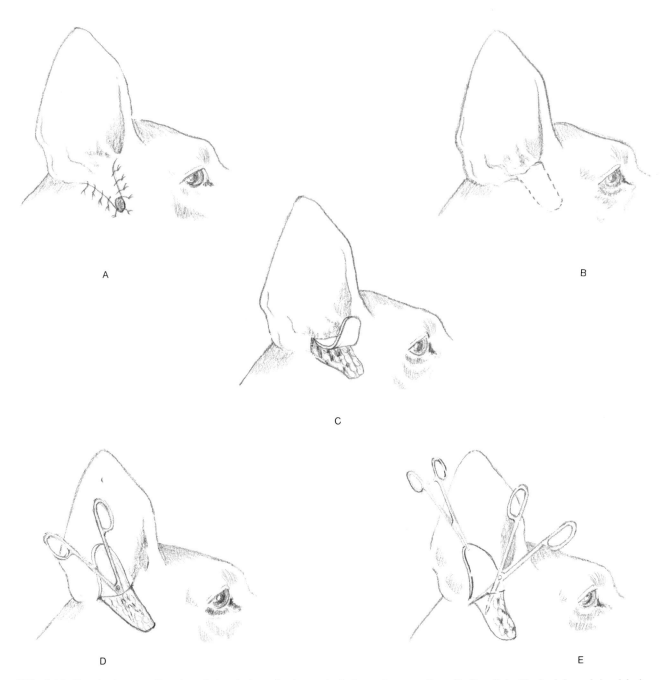

FIG. 6-12. Surgical correction for obstructed vertical canal. A, Lacroix operation. B, Parallel skin incisions joined below level of horizontal canal. C, Skin elevated dorsally. D, Vertical canal freed from parotid salivary gland and subcutis. E, Caudodorsal support of parotid salivary gland incised.

same time, masses near the orifice are excised in conjunction with the canal epithelium. The canal is spread open with large forceps rostrocaudally. The ventral horizontal canal epithelium is incised with two parallel incisions, connected as far medially as possible in the horizontal canal to create a strip of dermis and epidermis. This strip is excised to at least the level of the horizontal canal opening. This creates a defect resembling a rectangle (Fig. 6-13B). This defect is left to heal by contraction and epithelialization. If a mass is present adjacent to the canal orifice, it is removed as a wedge excision (described in the following paragraph) and may be sutured. The sutures must remain outside the horizontal canal, and the canal defect must not be sutured or the canal size would be diminished (Fig. 6-13C).

Additional masses of the inner surface of the pinna and medial canal are excised as wedges if they are narrow (Fig. 6-13D). Broad masses may be removed with a No. 11 scalpel blade creating complex triangles. Five separate incisions are required to create the complex triangle (Fig. 6-13E). Both the simple wedge and complex triangle excisions are sutured in vertical mattress or simple interrupted pattern using 5-0 or 4-0 suture.

When excess epithelium is removed from the horizontal canal, per se, the excision should involve no more than 90 degrees of the canal at any operation. Additional excisions may be indicated after 6 to 12 weeks of healing and medical care. The etiology of the hyperplastic otitis should be sought while the ear is treated.

Aftercare. The ears are protected by a bandage covering both head and ears. The ears are folded over the head or neck. The head is wrapped and the bandage is "cut out" to expose the ear canals and surgical wound for dressing changes. For the first 3 days, topical wet dressings of 0.05% chlorhexidine diacetate are applied. The "cut out" dressings are changed and debris gently wiped from the ear daily. Because these wounds produce much serum and the dressings used are wet, the head bandage usually becomes soiled and must be removed on the third or fourth postoperative day. If, when the bandage is removed, the wound remains relatively dry and the dog does not attempt to scratch the ear, the bandage is left off and a petrolatum base antibiotic ointment is applied. Topical medication is used to reduce the accumulation of dried blood, which irritates suture lines and is a source of local infection. If the wounds continue to ooze blood after bandage removal, the head bandage with cut-outs for treating the ears is reapplied for another 3 to 4 days. Sutures are removed in 7 days.

Advantages and Disadvantages. Simple excision or electrosection of these masses leaves exposed cartilage, which heals slowly by contraction and epithelialization,

and the authors prefer partial excision and suturing for faster healing. If monofilament suture is used, the ends should be left long in this instance because the sharp ends of monofilament suture cause discomfort. The horizontal canal defect must not be sutured because the lumen would be compromised. Pinpoint electrocoagulation is used to control bleeding from the cartilage because ligatures cannot be applied.

REFERENCES

1. Bojrab, M.J., and Renegar, W.R.: The ear. *In* Pathophysiology in Small Animal Surgery. Edited by M.J. Bojrab. Philadelphia, Lea & Febiger, 1981.
2. Henderson, R.A.: Reconstructive ear surgery. *In* Surgery of Traumatized Skin: Management and Reconstruction in the Dog and Cat. Edited by S.F. Swaim. Philadelphia, W.B. Saunders, 1980.

CHRONIC OTITIS WITH OBSTRUCTION OF THE HORIZONTAL CANAL

ABLATION OF THE EAR CANAL AND LATERAL BULLA OSTECTOMY

Definitions and Indication. Ablation of the ear canal is the removal of all of the vertical and horizontal ear canal cartilages, the epithelium lining these cartilages, and the osseous meatus of the temporal bone. Lateral bulla ostectomy is excision of the lateral wall of the tympanic bulla. The purpose of the bulla ostectomy is to allow obliteration of a potential space by the ingrowth of fibrous tissue. Ablation and lateral bulla ostectomy are indicated for end-stage otitis, which is defined as obstruction of the horizontal canal and chronic otitis media and/or interna. They are also used when the ear canal is heavily ossified, as is commonly seen in cocker spaniels.

Technique. *Ablation.* The skin is incised along the edge of the conca cavum laterally and across the medial wall of the vertical canal (Fig. 6-14A). Alternate sharp and blunt dissection is used to separate the cartilage from the surrounding tissue. The facial nerve is frequently incorporated in the fibro-osseous reaction. It must be gently dissected free and retracted ventrally. The dissection is continued to the horizontal canal, with dissection remaining close to the cartilage. The dissection continues to the temporal bone (Fig. 6-14B). Deeply placed Army-Navy retractors assist exposure. With care to avoid the facial nerve and internal maxillary artery and vein at the ventral edge of the dissection, the canal is severed from the temporal bone. The epithelium is curetted from the auditory canal of the temporal bone (Fig. 6-14C).

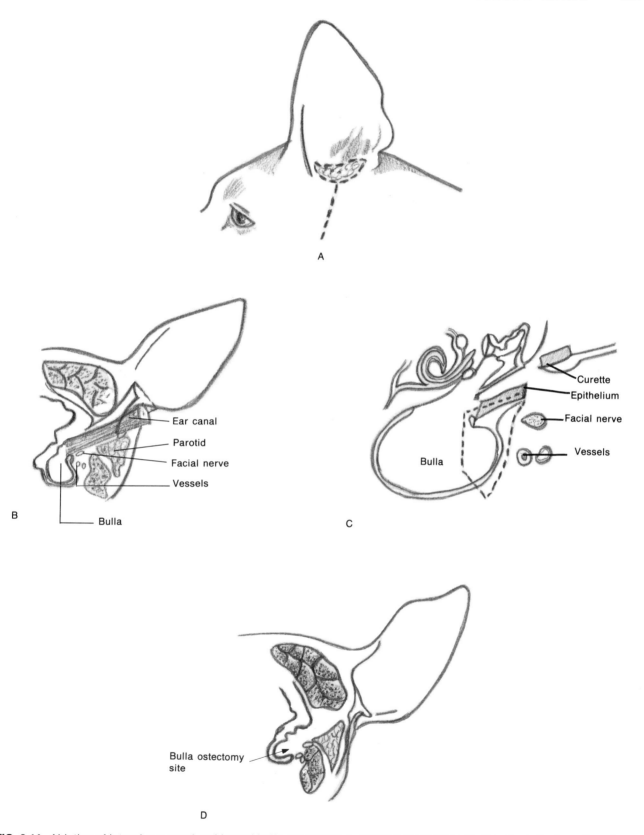

FIG. 6-14. Ablation of lateral ear canal and lateral bulla ostectomy. A, Incision for ablation (broken line). B, dissection of ear canal with anatomical relations to other structures. C, Curette removal of epithelium in osseous canal and ostectomy site (broken line). D, Incision and completed bulla ostectomy (compare to 14B).

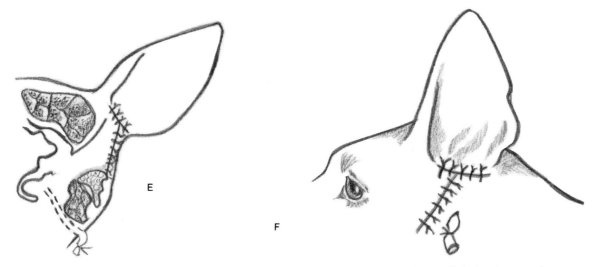

FIG. 6-14 continued. E, Drain placement and suturing of ablation. F, Sutured ablation and drain placement.

Lateral bulla ostectomy. After the ear canal has been removed, as much of the lateral and ventral wall of the bulla is removed by rongeurs as possible (Fig. 6-14C and D). Care must be taken to avoid vessels and nerves already mentioned. The remaining bulla wall is lightly curetted, avoiding the middle ear ossicles and the round and oval window.

The bulla is then irrigated. A Penrose drain is placed in the bulla cavity and the subcutis is closed with 3-0 absorbable suture. The drain exits through a separate skin incision. The skin is closed with nonabsorbable suture. The final closure is in the shape of a T (Fig. 6-14E and F). If the facial nerve was manipulated, a horizontal mattress temporary tarsorrhaphy is placed to help protect the eye until blink reflex returns.

Aftercare. Antibiotics begun just before surgery are continued for 72 hours, at which time the Penrose drain is removed The ears are protected from self-mutilation by bandaging for 3 to 5 days.

Advantages and Disadvantages. Canal ablation obviates the need of medicating the ear canal. The dissection is comparatively difficult. The inflammatory tissue may weaken or incorporate the major vessels and nerve. Injury to the facial nerve may result in temporary or permanent facial paralysis. Lethal hemorrhage may result from injuries to the major arteries. If the canal epithelium is incompletely removed, persistent ceruminous secretion and abscess will occur. Injury of the middle ear ossicles and round and oval windows may result in severe persistent head tilt or other inner ear problem signs.

REFERENCES AND SUGGESTED READING

1. Henderson, R.A.: Reconstructive ear surgery. *In* Surgery of Traumatized Skin: Management and Reconstruction in the Dog and Cat. Edited by S.F. Swaim. Philadelphia, W.B. Saunders, 1980.
2. Smeak, D.D., and DeHoff, W.D.: Total ear canal ablation: Clinical results in the dog and cat. Vet. Surg. *15*:161, 1986.

VARIOUS-SHAPED WOUNDS

7

FUSIFORM

Closure

Definition and Indications. Fusiform wounds have a lenticular shape like that of a biconvex lens. Regardless of size, most skin lesions requiring excision can be excised by creating a fusiform-shaped wound. This shape lends itself to cosmetic closure because it adapts readily to a straight line.

Techniques. In the design of a fusiform excision, the length:width ratio should approach 4:1 to help avoid the bunching of skin at the end of the excision (Fig. 7-1A). The shorter this ratio becomes, the ends of the wound bunch more and there is a greater chance of creating "dog ears" (Fig. 7-1B). Likewise, if one side of a fusiform excision is made longer than its corresponding side, a "dog ear" will form at the time of wound closure (Fig. 7-1C); therefore it is important to design the fusiform excision with equal sides.

In some instances it is impossible to achieve a 4:1 ratio, or wound edges must be of unequal length and "dog ears" occur. These may be removed in several ways. In preparation, the wound is usually sutured until it is nearly closed and the elevations of the "dog ear(s)" become(s) pronounced, and then it is corrected. In one method, the original incision is extended through the "dog ear," and the two resulting skin triangles are excised to produce a flat incision line (Fig. 7-2A through D). Another technique entails incising the "dog ear" along one side of its base, forming a large triangle of skin attached by the other side of the "dog ear" base.

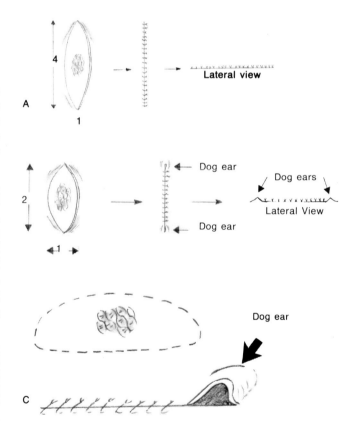

FIG. 7-1. Fusiform excision. A, Excision with 4:1 length:width ratio results in smooth closure. B, Excision with 2:1 length:width ratio may result in "dog ear" formation. C, With one side longer than the other, result is "dog ear" formation. (After Swaim, S.F.: Management and reconstruction of traumatized skin. Vet. Audio Review. Pacific Palisades, CA, Vol. 7, 1978.)

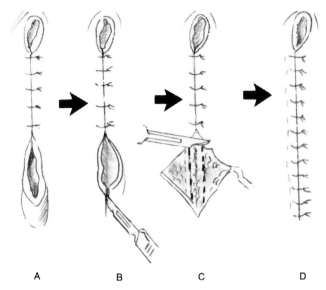

A   B   C   D

FIG. 7-2. "Dog ear" removal. A, "Dog ears" on a wound closure. B, Extending incision through "dog ear." C, Excising the two resulting skin triangles. D, Smooth closure after "dog ear" removal. (After Swaim, S.F.: Management and reconstruction of traumatized skin. Vet. Audio Review. Pacific Palisades, CA, Vol. 7, 1978.)

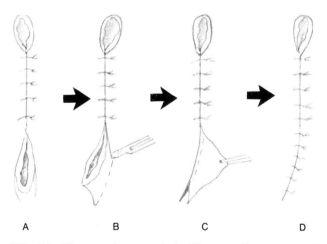

A   B   C   D

FIG. 7-3. "Dog ear" removal. A, "Dog ears" on a wound closure. B, Incising a "dog ear" along one side of its base. C, Defining and excising one large skin triangle. D, Smooth closure after "dog ear" removal. (After McGregor, I.A.: Fundamental Techniques of Plastic Surgery. 7th ed. Edinburgh, Churchill Livingstone, 1980, p. 25.)

The remaining base is incised and the result is a flat closure with a slight curve (Fig. 7-3A through D). Other methods of correcting a "dog ear" include extending the fusiform defect and closing in a straight line (Fig. 7-4A through C), or removing an arrowhead-shaped skin section in the area of the "dog ear" and closing the defect in the shape of a Y (Fig. 7-5A through C).

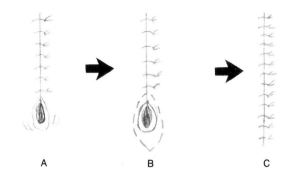

A   B   C

FIG. 7-4. "Dog ear" removal. A, "Dog ear" on a wound closure. B, Extending the fusiform to remove "dog ear." C, Smooth closure after "dog ear" removal. (After Grabb, W.C.: Basic techniques of plastic surgery. In Plastic Surgery. 3rd ed. Edited by W.C. Grabb, and J.W. Smith. Boston, Little, Brown and Co., 1979, p. 6.)

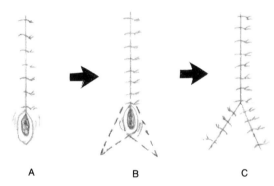

A   B   C

FIG. 7-5. "Dog ear" removal. A, "Dog ear" on a wound closure. B, Removing the "dog ear" in an arrowhead-shaped skin section. C, Y-shaped closure of resulting defect. (After Grabb, W.C.: Basic techniques of plastic surgery. In Plastic Surgery. 3rd ed. Edited by W.C. Grabb, and J.W. Smith. Boston, Little, Brown and Co., 1979, p. 6.)

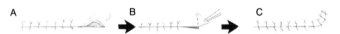

A   B   C

FIG. 7-6. "Dog ear" removal. A, "Dog ear" resulting from one side of wound being longer than the other. B, Short right angle incision made at base of "dog ear" and skin to be excised, defined. C, L-shaped closure of resulting defect. (From Grabb, W.C.: Basic techniques of plastic surgery. In Plastic Surgery. 3rd ed. Edited by W.C. Grabb, and J.W. Smith. Boston, Little, Brown and Co., 1979, p. 6.)

With a fusiform defect in which a "dog ear" results from one side of the excision being longer than the other, the "dog ear" can be corrected by making a short right angle incision at the base of the "dog ear." The excess skin that overlaps the wound edge is trimmed away to permit wound closure in the shape of an L (Fig. 7-6A through C).

with curved sides from opposite sides of the circular defect so that the long axis of the resultant fusiform is in the direction of skin tension (Fig. 7-7A through C). Skin closure is usually with simple interrupted 3-0 nonabsorbable sutures.

Aftercare. Fusiform skin closures require no special aftercare.

Advantages and Disadvantages. Fusiform excisions provide a smooth, straight wound closure. When creating a fusiform with a 4:1 length:width ratio, however, considerable normal adjacent skin must be removed to provide this ratio.

REFERENCES AND SUGGESTED READING

1. Grabb, W.C.: Basic techniques of plastic surgery. *In* Plastic Surgery. 3rd. ed. Edited by W.C. Grabb, and J.W. Smith. Boston, Little, Brown and Co., 1979.
2. McGregor, I.A.: Fundamental Techniques of Plastic Surgery. 7th ed. Edinburgh, Churchill Livingstone, 1980.
3. Stashak, T.S.: Reconstructive surgery in the horse. J. Am. Vet. Med. Assoc. *170*:143, 1977.
4. Swaim, S.F.: Principles of plastic and reconstructive surgery. *In* Textbook of Small Animal Surgery. Edited by D.H. Slatter. Philadelphia, W.B. Saunders, 1985.

TRIANGULAR

CENTRIPETAL CLOSURE

Definition and Indications. Triangular skin defects have three sides and three angles. The sides may be of any length and the angles may be of any size. Both sides and angles are usually curved because of skin elasticity and tension lines. The defects may result from traumatic injuries or excisions. One type of triangular defect has skin for wound closure available on all three sides of the defect. When this is the case, centripetal suturing is indicated to close the defect, resulting in a Y-shaped scar (Fig. 7-8A and B).

Technique. When skin is available for closure on all three sides of a triangular defect and the sides of the defect are relatively equal in length, suturing begins at the angles of the defect and progresses toward the center. Closure is done with 3-0 simple interrupted nonabsorbable sutures, begun at one of the angles of the defect and performed centripetally around the defect (Fig. 7-9A and B). If the defect is large, the skin may be undermined for a distance equal to the distance from the center of the defect to the wound edge on all three sides. In addition, some 3-0 absorbable "walking" sutures may be placed to advance the skin edges closer together and eliminate suture line tension. At the juncture of the

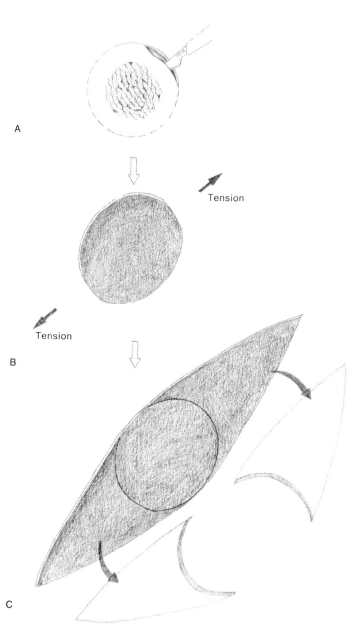

FIG. 7-7. Creating a fusiform defect after circular excision. A, Circular excision of a lesion. B, Noting direction in which tension lines tend to pull defect. C, Converting defect into a fusiform by removing two triangles of skin on sides of defect corresponding to tension line pull.

In planning a fusiform excision, it is best if the long axis of the fusiform runs parallel to skin tension lines. Because the direction of tension lines in the area may be unknown, it is best when possible to use a circular excision. By noting the long axis of the defect that is created by the adjacent tension lines, the long axis of the fusiform excision can be determined and the wound can be remodeled to create the desired fusiform shape. This is done by removing triangular-shaped segments of skin

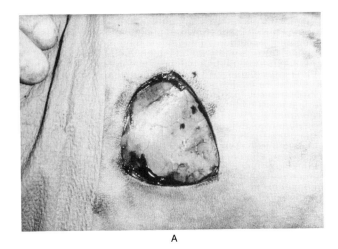

A

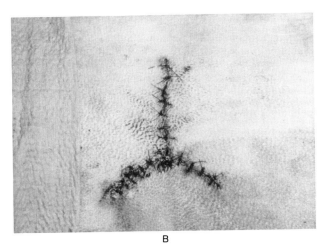

B

FIG. 7-8 Centripetal closure of a triangular defect. A, Triangular defect. B, Y-shaped closure pattern.

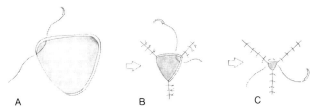

FIG. 7-9. Centripetal closure of an equal-sided triangular defect. A, closure beginning at an angle of defect. B, Closure progressing centripetally around defect. C, A half-buried horizontal mattress suture placed at juncture of three suture lines.

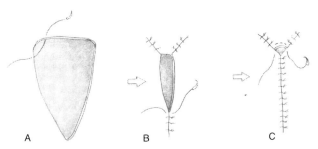

FIG. 7-10. Centripetal closure of an unequal-sided triangular defect. A, Closure beginning at an angle of defect. B, Closure progressing centripetally until two suture lines almost meet. C, Remaining defect closed and a half-buried horizontal mattress suture placed at the juncture of three suture lines.

three suture lines, a half-buried horizontal suture is placed to help preserve the blood supply to the tips of the skin segments that join (Fig. 7-9C). When the edges of the triangular defect are not of equal length, centripetal suturing should be performed until two of the suture lines come close to joining. The remaining suture line is completed to finish the closure. A half-buried horizontal mattress suture is used at the juncture of the three suture lines (Fig. 7-10A through C).

To help prevent slight elevations from forming at the ends of the suture lines, the suture material may be placed so that it takes a *small* bite into the tissue underlying the skin to help pull the skin down as the suture is tied (Fig. 7-11A and B). If, in the surgeon's judgment, the elevation is well enough defined to be considered a "dog ear," it should be removed.

Aftercare. Centripetally closed triangular defects require no special aftercare.

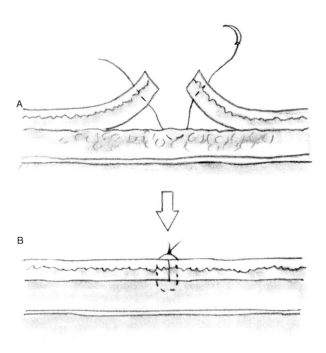

FIG. 7-11. Helping prevent elevations at ends of suture lines. A, Skin suture taking a *small* bite into underlying tissue. B, When tied, suture helps flatten skin edges.

Advantages and Disadvantages. Centripetal closure of a triangular defect is the simplest technique for wound closure. Slight elevations, not defined enough to be called "dog ears," may develop at the ends of the suture lines as closure progresses, however. In some instances, "dog ears," which require removal, may form at the angles of the closure.

REFERENCES AND SUGGESTED READING

1. Braden, T.D.: Plastic and reconstructive surgery of the canine torso. Vet. Clin. N. Am. *9*:285, 1979.
2. Johnston D.E.: Wound healing and reconstructive surgery. Am. Anim. Hosp. Assoc. Sci. Proc. *2*:383, 1975.
3. Swaim, S.F., Henderson, R.A., and Sutton, H.H.: Correction of triangular and wedge-shaped skin defects in dogs and cats. J. Am. Anim. Hosp. Assoc. *16*:225, 1980.
4. Swaim, S.F.: Principles of plastic and reconstructive surgery. *In* Textbook of Small Animal Surgery. Edited by D.H. Slatter. Philadelphia, W.B. Saunders, 1985.

UNILATERAL ROTATION FLAP

Definition and Indications. A rotation flap is a semicircular or three-fourths circular flap of skin and subcutaneous tissue that rotates about a pivot point into the defect to be closed. Triangular skin defects may only have skin available for closure on one side of the defect, or closure of such defects could result in distortion of a nearby body structure (such as the eyes, anus, or prepuce). In such instances, a rotation flap may be indicated for closure of these defects (Figs. 7-12A through C and 7-13A through C).

Technique. After evaluation of the location of a triangular defect and manipulation of the skin around the defect, it may be determined that a rotation flap is indicated to close the defect without tension. The proposed incision to create a rotation flap should be drawn on the skin with methylene blue on a cotton-tipped applicator. The incision should be long enough to make a flap that will be large enough to rotate into position without causing tension across the flap when it is sutured in place. A flap that is too small or that is less than one half of a circle depends more on stretching (tension) than rotation to be moved into place (Fig. 7-14A). If a flap has a line of tension across it as it is moved into place, this can be relieved by a small stab incision perpendicular to the line of greatest tension (Fig. 7-14B). Another technique for creating a rotation flap is to incise the curve in a progressive fashion, undermining the flap as it is cut until it covers the wound without excessive tension. Tension on a flap may also be avoided by extending the length of the side of the flap adjacent to the defect (Fig. 7-14C), allowing some shortening of the flap as it is rotated into position.

The flap should be undermined, retaining as much subcutaneous tissue or panniculus muscle with the flap as possible. Damage to any identifiable underlying direct

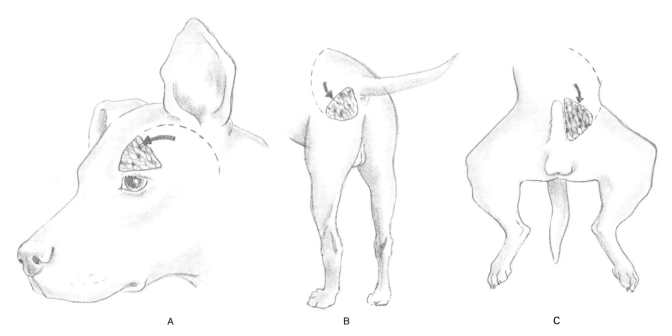

| A | B | C |

FIG. 7-12. Examples of areas where unilateral rotation flaps could be used for triangular defect closure. Skin for closure is available on only one side of the defect and in a different plane than the defect. A, Near eye. B, Near anus. C, Near prepuce.

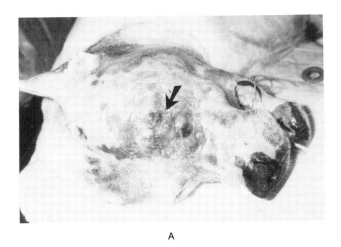

A

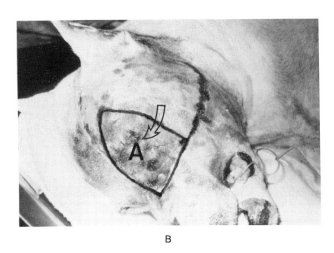

B

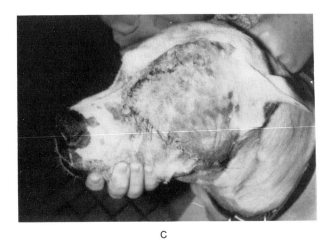

C

FIG. 7-13. Unilateral rotation flap. A, Fibrosarcoma in area of previous eye enucleation (arrow). B, Area to be excised—A is direction of rotation flap movement for reconstruction after tumor removal (arrow). C, Flap sutured in place. (Courtesy of Dr. W.W. Miller.)

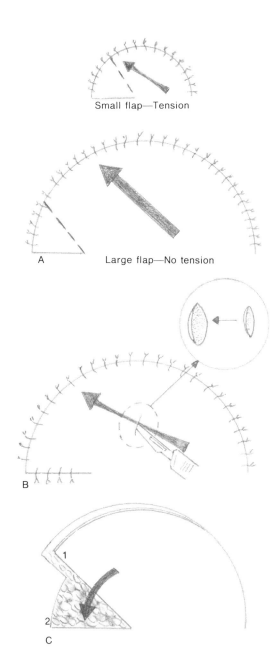

FIG. 7-14. Rotation flap tension. A, Small rotation flap has tension on closure; large flap has no tension. B, A stab incision along tension line of a flap helps relieve tension. C, Extending side of flap adjacent to defect helps relieve tension with flap rotation. Corner 1 will be sutured to angle 2.

cutaneous vessels should be avoided. This helps preserve blood supply to the flap.

As the flap is rotated and sutured into position, redundant skin appears along the outer side of the suture line. Eventually, a "dog ear" develops and must be removed for the two skin edges to be of equal length (Fig. 7-15A and B). To eliminate this "dog ear" before it occurs, a small triangle of skin (Bürow's triangle) may be

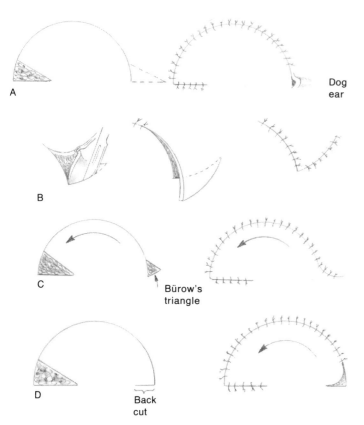

FIG. 7-15. Rotation flap "dog ears" and back cuts. A, Rotation of a flap may result in "dog ear" formation. B, "Dog ear" removal: incising along its base, defining excess skin for removal, and closure. C, Bürow's triangle of skin removed outside semicircle and tangent to it at base of flap prevents "dog ear" formation with flap rotation. D, A small back cut along diameter line of semicircle allows flap to move into position more easily. (A and B after McGregor, I.A.: Fundamental Techniques of Plastic Surgery. 7th ed. Edinburgh, Churchill Livingstone, 1980, p. 143. C, after Grabb, W.C.: Basic techniques of plastic surgery. *In* Plastic Surgery. 3rd ed. Edited by W.C. Grabb, and J.W. Smith. Boston, Little, Brown and Co., 1979, p. 47.)

removed outside the semicircle and tangent to it at the end of the incision opposite the defect (Fig. 7-15C). Removal of only the necessary amount of skin to correct the "dog ear" is preferred, however.

To allow a rotation flap to move into position easier, a short back cut may be made to help relieve tension. This back cut is made along the diameter line of the circle at the end of the incision opposite the lesion, allowing the flap to move by a combination of rotation and transposition (Fig. 7-15D). The surgeon should be aware that the back cut also reduces the vascular area at the base of the flap. In some instances it is possible to cut only the tissue responsible for the tension (skin)

without cutting the blood supply to the flap (panniculus muscle or subcutaneous tissue).

"Walking" sutures of 3-0 absorbable suture material may be used to rotate a flap into place. These should be used sparingly, however, to avoid damage to the flap's blood supply as they are tied. The skin edges are apposed using 3-0 simple interrupted nonabsorbable sutures or skin staples. If there is dead space under the flap, a one-quarter-inch diameter Penrose drain may be placed under the flap to avoid hematoma or seroma formation.

Aftercare. If a drain has been placed under a rotation flap, it is best to bandage the area to help avoid wound molestation and assess the amount and nature of any drainage that occurs. The drain should be removed when drainage has decreased to a small amount, generally after 3 to 4 days.

Advantages and Disadvantages. The use of a rotation flap to close a defect with skin available on only one side or where closure would result in distortion of a body part provides tension relief if the flap is made large enough, but requires creating a wound to correct a wound.

REFERENCES AND SUGGESTED READING

1. Braden, T.D.: Plastic and reconstructive surgery of the canine torso. Vet. Clin. N. Am. *9*:285, 1979.
2. Grabb, W.C.: Classification of skin flaps. *In* Skin Flaps. Edited by W.C. Grabb, and M.B. Myers. Boston, Little, Brown and Co., 1975.
3. Grabb, W.C., and Smith, J.W.: Basic techniques of plastic surgery. *In* Plastic Surgery. 3rd ed. Edited by W.C., Grabb, and J.W. Smith. Boston, Little, Brown and Co., 1979.
4. McGregor, I.A.: Fundamental Techniques of Plastic Surgery. 7th ed. Edinburgh, Churchill Livingstone, 1980.
5. Pavletic, M.M.: Pedicle grafts. *In* Textbook of Small Animal Surgery. Edited by D.H. Slatter. Philadelphia, W.B. Saunders, 1985.
6. Pope, E.R., and Swaim, S.F.: Shifting tissue and using flaps. Vet. Med. *81*:512, 1986.
7. Swaim, S.F.: The repair of skin: Techniques for plastic and reconstructive surgery. *In* Atlas of Canine Surgical Techniques. Edited by P.G.C. Bedford. Oxford, Blackwell Scientific Publications, 1984.
8. Swaim, S.F., Henderson, R.A., and Sutton, H.H.: Correction of triangular and wedge-shaped skin defects in dogs and cats. J. Am. Anim. Hosp. Assoc. *16*:225, 1980.

BILATERAL ROTATION FLAPS

Definition and Indications. Bilateral rotation flaps are rotation flaps designed on two sides of a triangular defect. Triangular skin defects may have skin available for closure on only two sides of the defect. In such instances, bilateral rotation flaps may be indicated for closure of such defects.

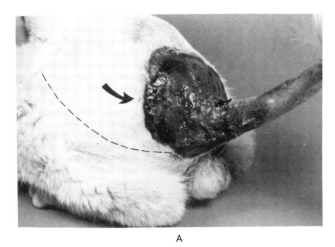
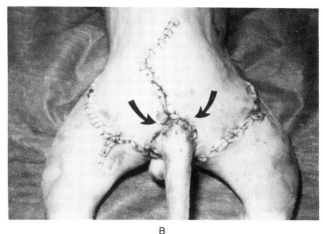

A   B

FIG. 7-16. Bilateral rotation flaps. A, Large skin defect at base of a cat's tail. Proposed incision for rotation flap (broken line). Direction of flap rotation (arrow). B, Bilateral rotation flaps rotated together to close defect (arrows). (From Pope, E.R., and Swaim, S.F.: Shifting tissues and using flaps. Vet. Med. *81*:512, 1986.)

Technique. When a triangular defect has skin available for closure on only two sides of the defect because of its location, the surgeon should manipulate the skin around the defect to ascertain whether centripetal suturing might allow wound closure. If possible, this technique should be used for closure. If centripetal closure is not possible, bilateral rotation flaps should be considered.

The technique for creating bilateral rotation flaps is as described for creating single rotation flaps; however, each flap is designed so that it rotates halfway across the defect. The leading edges of the two flaps are sutured together (Fig. 7-16A and B).

Aftercare. See Unilateral Rotation Flap, this chapter.

Advantages and Disadvantages. This technique, used when centripetal closure cannot be used, requires two smaller rotation flaps for closure to distribute skin tension on two sides of the wound rather than on just one side. In some instances, sufficient skin may not be available on one side of the defect to allow closure with one flap, but there is sufficient skin on either side of the defect to allow closure of half of the defect. The technique requires making two additional wounds to close the one already present.

REFERENCES AND SUGGESTED READING

See Unilateral Rotation Flap, this chapter.

SQUARE AND RECTANGULAR

CENTRIPETAL CLOSURE

Definition and Indications. Square skin defects have four equal sides and four right angles. Rectangular defects also have four right angles with two short and two long parallel equal sides. The sides and angles of these defects are usually curved because of skin elasticity and tension lines. These defects may result from traumatic injuries or excisions. When skin is available on all four sides of such defects, centripetal suturing is indicated to close the defect.

Techniques. With skin available for closure on all four sides of the square or rectangular defect, centripetal suturing is indicated to close the defect. Suturing a square defect begins at one of the corners of the defect and is performed centripetally around the defect using 3-0 simple interrupted nonabsorbable sutures (Fig. 7-17A and B). If the defect is large, some 3-0 absorbable "walking" sutures may be placed to advance the skin edges closer together to eliminate suture line tension. At the junction of the four suture lines that result from closure of a square defect, an intradermal purse-string-type suture may be placed to help preserve the blood supply to the tips of the skin segments that are thus joined (Fig. 7-17C).

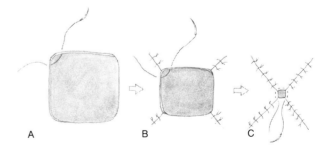

A   B   C

FIG. 7-17. Centripetal closure of a square defect. A, Closure beginning at an angle of defect. B, Closure progressing centripetally around defect. C, An intradermal purse-string-type suture is placed at junction of the four suture lines.

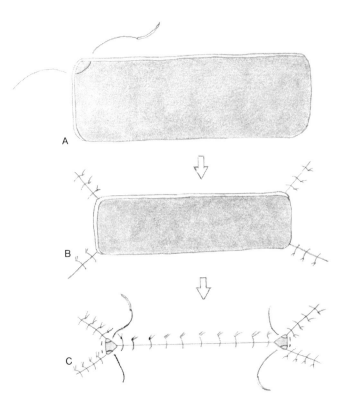

FIG. 7-18. Centripetal closure of a rectangular defect. A, Closure beginning at an angle of defect. B, Closure progressing centripetally. C, Half-buried horizontal mattress sutures placed at the junctions of three suture lines.

Rectangular defects may be closed in the same way. The result is a double Y-shaped suture line. A half-buried horizontal mattress suture is used at the junction of the three suture lines at each end of the closure (Figs. 7-18A, B, and C and 7-19A and B).

As with the centripetal closure of triangular defects,

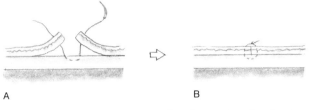

FIG. 7-20. Helping to prevent elevations at ends of suture lines. A, Skin suture taking a *small* bite into the underlying tissue. B, When tied, suture helps flatten skin edges.

slight elevations at the ends of the suture lines may be prevented by passing the suture material into underlying tissues as each simple interrupted suture is placed (Fig. 7-20A and B). If, in the surgeon's judgment, the elevation is well enough defined to be considered a "dog ear," it should be removed.

Aftercare.   Centripetally closed square or rectangular defects require no special aftercare.

Advantages and Disadvantages.   Centripetal closure of square or rectangular defects is the simplest technique for closure of such wounds. Slight elevations, which are not true "dog ears," may develop at the ends of the suture lines as closure progresses. In some instances, "dog ears," which require removal, may form at the angles of the closure.

REFERENCES AND SUGGESTED READING

1. Johnston, D.E.: Wound healing and reconstructive surgery. Am. Anim. Hosp. Assoc. Sci. Proc. *2*:383, 1975.
2. Swaim, S.F.: Principles of plastic and reconstructive surgery. *In* Textbook of Small Animal Surgery. Edited by D.H. Slatter. Philadelphia, W.B. Saunders, 1985.

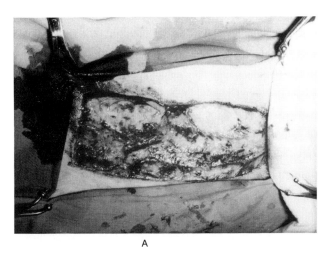
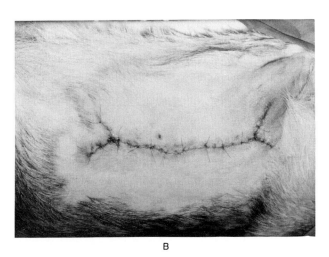

FIG. 7-19. Centripetal closure of a rectangular defect. A, Rectangular defect. B, Defect closed.

SINGLE PEDICLE ADVANCEMENT FLAP

Definition and indications.   A single pedicle advancement flap is a flap of skin that is mobilized by undermining and advanced into a defect without altering the plane of the pedicle. Square or rectangular skin defects may have skin available for closure on only one side of the defect with that skin being in the same plane as the defect. In such instances, a single pedicle advancement flap (French flap) may be indicated for closure of these defects (Figs. 7-21A through C and 7-22A and B). *These flaps can also be used to correct defects of other shapes (such as circular and oval) because the elasticity of the skin allows it to conform to other lesion shapes.*

Techniques.   The location of the square or rectangular defect should be evaluated and the skin surrounding it should be manipulated to determine if sufficient lax skin is present to use for a single pedicle advancement flap. The abundance and elasticity of skin are used to move the flap into position.

To help ensure survival of a large flap, its circulation can be enhanced by the delay phenomenon so that it can better withstand any tension placed on it during its advancement. After the flap is designed, it is incised and undermined, retaining as much subcutaneous tissue or panniculus muscle as possible and avoiding damage to any direct cutaneous vessels in the area. The flap is sutured back into its original site. The optimal time to advance the flap is 3 weeks after this initial procedure, when its blood supply has increased to a maximal level.

To create the flap, parallel incisions are made from two corners of the defect, using one edge of the defect as the leading edge of the flap. The incisons should be made at least as long as the width of the defect to allow it to be advanced into position. The flap should be undermined, retaining as much subcutaneous tissue or panniculus muscle with it as possible. Damage to any identifiable underlying direct cutaneous vessels should be avoided. This helps preserve blood supply to the flap (Fig. 7-23A). If this does not supply sufficient skin to close the defect without tension, the incision can be lengthened progressively with undermining until the flap covers the defect without tension. Depending on the laxity of the skin, it is usually necessary to make these incisions longer to ensure advancement of the flap without excess tension. When suturing the flap into place, the surgeon is faced with the problem of suturing the margins of the flap, which are stretched and shorter, to the relaxed lateral margins of the wound, which are longer. The result is "dog ear" formation at the base of the flap (Fig. 7-23B). To help equalize the length between the sides of the flap and the adjacent wound margins and avert "dog ears," a Bürow's triangle may be excised lateral to the base of the flap. The base of the triangle should be equal to the width of the defect being corrected (Fig. 7-24A and B). The authors prefer to advance the flap into place and correct any "dog ears"

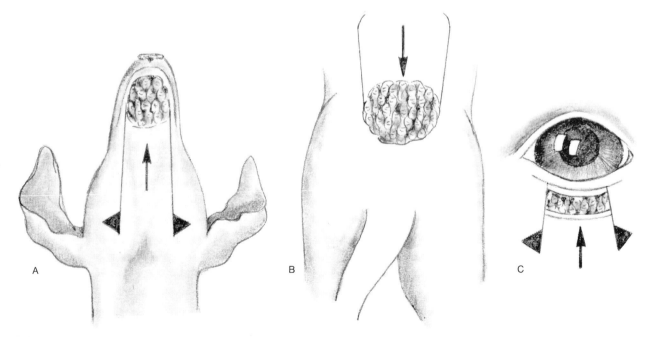

FIG. 7-21. Examples of areas where single pedicle advancement flaps could be used for defect closure. Skin for closure is available on only one side of defect and in same plane as defect. A, Cranial intermandibular area. B, Lumbosacral area. C, Palpebra.

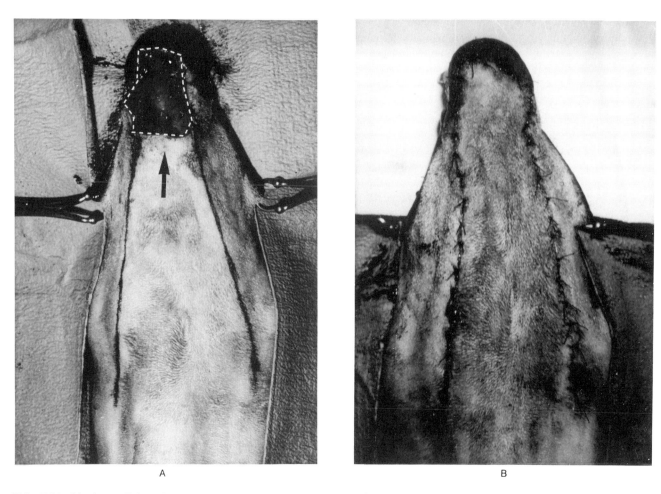

FIG. 7-22. Single pedicle advancement flap. A, Skin defect in cranial intermandibular area (broken line). Direction of advancement flap movement for closure of defect (arrow). B, Flap sutured in place.

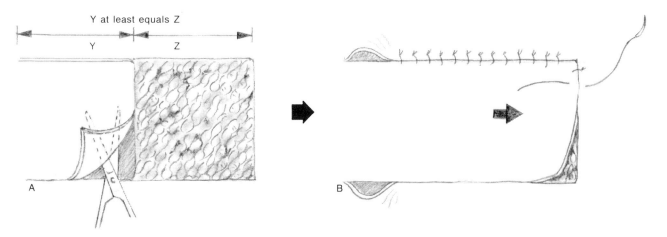

FIG. 7-23. Principles of a single pedicle advancement flap. A, Incisions to create flap should be at least equal to width of defect. Y at least equals Z. Flap is undermined. B, Flap advanced to cover defect. "Dog ears" usually form at flap base.

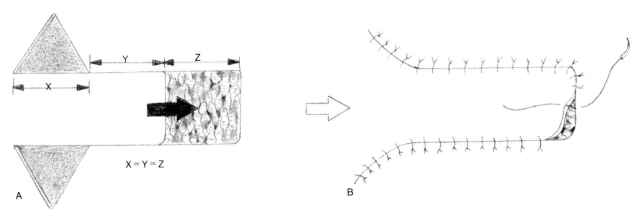

FIG. 7-24. Equalizing lengths of skin edges. A, Bürow's triangles removed lateral to flap's base. Base of triangle should be equal to width of defect. X = Y = Z. B, Flap is advanced and sutured.

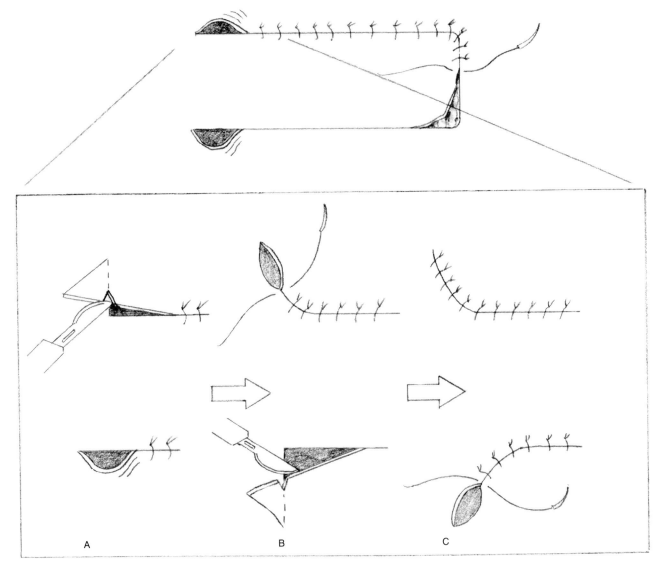

FIG. 7-25. "Dog ear" removal from base of single pedicle advancement flap. A, Incision made perpendicular to edge of flap at base of one "dog ear"; excess skin identified for removal and excised. B, Defect closed; same procedure performed on other "dog ear." C, Resulting defect from second "dog ear" removal being closed.

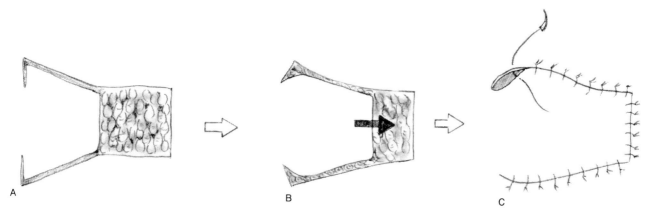

FIG. 7-26. Pantographic expansion of a single pedicle advancement flap. A, Sides of flap made divergent with slight back cuts into flap's base. B, As flap advances, back cuts open to approach a straight line. C, Flap sutured in place.

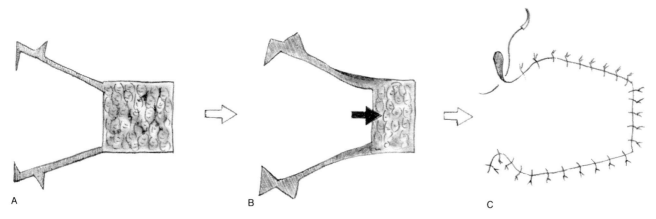

FIG. 7-27. Modified Z-plasties at flap base. A, Back cuts and lateral incisions create modified Z-plasties. B, As flap advances, Z-plasties expand. C, Flap sutured in place.

that form at the base of the flap only if they are large and unsightly. Only the amount of skin necessary to provide a smooth closure is removed (Fig. 7-25A through C).

Pantographic expansion can be used to help overcome the problem of tension on these flaps. The sides of the flap are made slightly divergent to widen the base, ensuring that the flap pedicle is not narrowed as it is developed. Small back cuts made into the base of the flap from either side open and approach being a straight line as the flap is advanced into position, making advancement easier (Fig. 7-26A through C). These back cuts also reduce the vascular area at the base of the flap. It may be possible to incise only the tissue responsible for tension (skin) without incising the blood supply to the flap (panniculus muscle or subcutaneous tissue). The addition of small incisions perpendicular to the flap incision in the tissue lateral to the flap creates modified Z-plasties when the flap is advanced

into place, thus helping relieve flap tension (Fig 7-27A through C).

Other modifications in design of single pedicle advancement flaps include curving the sides of the flap outward or angling the sides of the flap outward. These modifications have basically the same effect as pantographic expansion (Fig. 7-28A and B). "Walking" sutures of 3-0 absorbable suture material may be used to advance a flap into position, thereby gradually elongating the flap and distributing tension along it. When used, "walking" sutures should be placed sparingly and carefully to avoid damage to the flap's blood supply as they are tied. The skin edges are apposed with 3-0 simple interrupted nonabsorbable sutures or skin staples. If there is dead space under the flap, a one-quarter-inch diameter Penrose drain may be placed under the flap to avoid hematoma or seroma formation.

Aftercare. If a drain has been placed under a single pedicle advancement flap, it is best to bandage the area

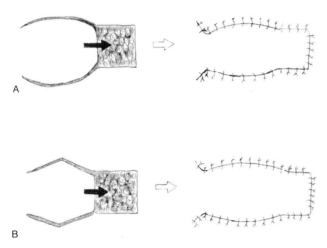

FIG. 7-28. Other designs of single pedicle advancement flaps to enhance advancement. A, Outward curvature of flap edges. B, Outward angulation of flap edges.

to help avoid wound molestation and assess the amount and nature of any drainage that occurs. The drain should be removed when drainage has decreased to a small amount, generally after 3 to 4 days.

Advantages and Disadvantages. Single pedicle advancement flaps provide an effective means of closing square, rectangular, or other shaped defects when skin is available on only one side of the defect for closure, with that skin in the same plane as the defect. This technique, however, requires creating wounds to correct a wound. If two Bürow's triangles are removed adjacent to the base of the flap with the base of each triangle as wide as the defect, relatively large wounds are created to correct a smaller wound.

REFERENCES AND SUGGESTED READING

1. Braden, T.D.: Plastic and reconstructive surgery of the canine torso. Vet. Clin. N. Am. *9*:285, 1979.
2. Grabb, W.C.: Classification of flaps. *In* Skin Flaps. Edited by W.C. Grabb, and M.B. Myers. Boston, Little, Brown and Co., 1975.
3. Grabb, W.C., and Smith, J.W.: Basic techniques of plastic surgery. *In* Plastic Surgery. 3rd ed. Edited by W.C. Grabb, and J.W. Smith. Boston, Little, Brown and Co., 1979.
4. Pavletic, M.M.: Pedicle grafts. *In* Textbook of Small Animal Surgery. Edited by D.H. Slatter. Philadelphia, W.B. Saunders, 1985.
5. Pope, E.R., Swaim, S.F.: Shifting tissue and using flaps. Vet. Med. *81*:512, 1986.
6. Stashak, T.S.: Reconstructive surgery in the horse. J. Am. Vet. Med. Assoc. *170*:143, 1977.
7. Swaim, S.F.: The repair of skin: Techniques for plastic and reconstructive surgery. *In* Atlas of Canine Surgical Techniques. Edited by P.G.C. Bedford. Oxford, Blackwell Scientific Publications, 1984.

H-PLASTY

Definition and Indications. An H-plasty is made up of two apposing single pedicle advancement flaps. Large square and rectangular defects may be closed more effectively with an H-plasty than with one such flap, provided that skin is available for closure on two sides of the wound.

Technique. Parallel incisions are made on apposing sides of the defect to create the two flaps. For each flap, the incisions are made from two corners of the defect, using one edge of the defect as the leading edge of each flap. The incisions for each flap should be made as long as the width of the defect to ensure closure of the defect without tension (Fig. 7-29A). Each flap is undermined and advanced to cover half the wound. If this does not supply sufficient skin to close the defect without tension, the incisions can be lengthened progressively with undermining of the flap until it covers the defect without tension. "Dog ears" that form are removed after the flaps are sutured in place (Fig. 7-29B). If Bürow's triangles are removed adjacent to the base of each flap to help equalize the length of the sides of the flaps and the sides of the wound, the length of the base of each triangle should be half the width of the defect being closed (Fig. 7-30A). It is advisable, however, to advance the flaps into place and remove only the skin necessary to correct "dog ears" at the bases of the flaps. Vertical mattress tension sutures may be used to help appose the edges of the two flaps, and 3-0 simple interrupted nonabsorbable sutures are used for final skin closure (Fig. 7-30B). An alternative is the use of 3-0 absorbable "walking" sutures to advance the flaps together. As with all flaps, when "walking" sutures are used, care should be taken to place as few sutures as necessary to advance the flap and to place them carefully to avoid damage to the blood vessels in the subcutaneous tissue supplying the flap. If there is dead space under the flaps, a quarter-inch diameter Penrose drain may be placed under the flaps to avoid seroma or hematoma formation.

Aftercare. See Single Pedicle Advancement Flap, this chapter.

Advantages and Disadvantages. H-plasty provides an effective method of closing square or rectangular wounds when skin is available on two sides of a defect, with that skin being in the same plane as the defect. As with other flaps, use of apposing single pedicle advancement flaps requires creating wounds to correct a wound, especially if two Bürow's triangles are removed from the base of each flap.

REFERENCES AND SUGGESTED READING

See Single Pedicle Advancement Flap, this chapter.

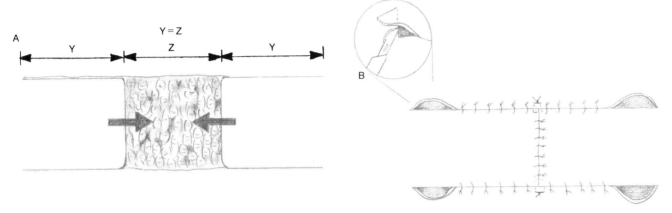

FIG. 7-29. H-plasty. A, Each flap is equal in length to width of defect. Y = Z. B, "Dog ears" removed after flaps are sutured.

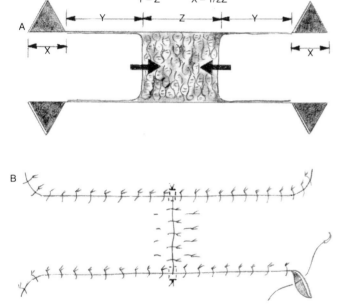

FIG. 7-30. H-plasty with Bürow's triangles removed. A, Base of each triangle is one-half the width of the defect being closed and length of each flap equals width of defect. X = 1/2 Z, Y = Z. B, Flaps sutured. Vertical mattress tension sutures help to appose flap edges.

TRANSPOSITION FLAP

Definition and Indications. A transposition flap is a piece of skin and subcutaneous tissue that is generally rectangular in shape. It turns on a pivot point to reach the adjacent defect to be covered. The defect is usually, but not always, at a right angle from the axis of the flap. Basically, square or rectangular skin defects may have skin available on only one side of the defect, and closure of such defects could cause distortion of a nearby body structure (such as the eye, ear, or anus). When the skin for closure of such defects is in a different plane from the defect, a transposition flap may be indicated for closure of these defects (Fig. 7-31A through C). Defects on the proximal portion of the thoracic and pelvic limb may be closed using transposition flaps from the craniolateral thoracic area or caudolateral abdominal area, respectively (Fig. 7-32A through D). *These flaps can be used to reconstruct defects of other shapes also (circular, oval, etc.) because the elasticity of the skin allows it to conform to other defect shapes.*

Technique. The area around the defect should be evaluated by manipulation of the skin to determine if a transposition flap is feasible. When designing a transposition flap, it should be remembered that the flap becomes shorter in effective length the farther it is rotated (Fig. 7-33). The proper design of a transposition flap will prevent undue tension. If a flap is to close a defect without tension, the diagonal distance from the pivot point of the flap (point at the base of the flap farthest from the defect) to the far point of the defect must equal the diagonal distance of the flap as measured from the pivot point. Thus the flap must be longer than the defect to be effective (Fig. 7-34A). This helps to compensate for loss of effective length as the flap is rotated. A flap designed with a diagonal shorter than the diagonal from the pivot point to the far point of the defect will have tension across it when it is transposed (Fig. 7-34B).

To design a flap that will transpose at a 90° angle with no tension, one edge of the defect should be incorporated into one edge of the flap. The width of the base of the flap should be at least equal to the width of the defect, and the diagonal from the pivot point of the flap to the farthest corner of the defect should be equal to the diagonal from the flap's pivot point across the flap (Fig. 7-35A and B). A flap designed in this manner will have no tension across it, but will have a sizeable "dog-ear" opposite the pivot point (Fig. 7-36A and B). If

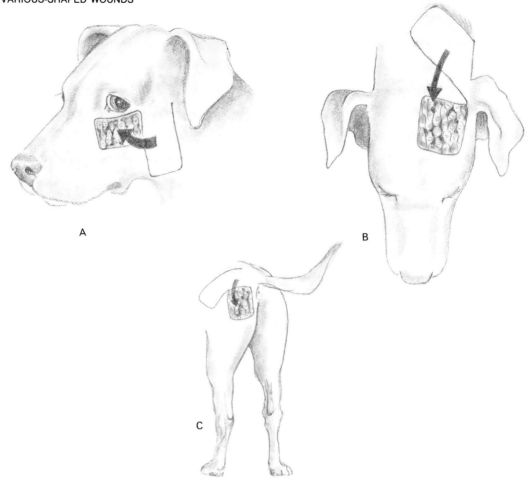

FIG. 7-31. Examples of areas where transposition flaps could be used for defect closure. Skin for closure is available on only one side of defect and in a different plane than the defect. A, Periocular area. B, Dorsal cranial area. C, Perianal area.

excision of the "dog ear" could damage the blood supply entering the base of the flap, the "dog ear" should not be removed at the time of flap transposition. The edges of the "dog ear" should be sutured, and 14 to 21 days postoperatively, after the flap has developed a blood supply from the recipient site, the "dog ear" may be removed if desired.

A transposition flap that is designed with the flap diagonal shorter than the diagonal from the pivot point to the far corner of the defect will have a diagonal tension line across it after it is transposed into position (Fig. 7-37A through C). Because the skin of the dog and cat is relatively elastic and mobile, the veterinary surgeon may be able to get by without strict adherence to the rules of flap length. It is best, however, to keep the principles in mind when designing any flap, especially when there is a potential for tension on the flap. If a flap has a tension line across it as it is moved into place, it can be relieved by a small stab incision perpendicular to

the line of greatest tension (Fig. 7-37C). The stab incision should incise only the skin and not the underlying panniculus muscle or subcutaneous tissue.

In addition to measurements for a transposition flap, a piece of sterile towel should be used to plan the flap. The towel is cut to the shape and size of the proposed flap. This flap pattern is laid over the proposed donor site and the edges of the pattern and the underlying skin are pinched together to be certain that the donor site can be closed after the flap is rotated into place (Fig. 7-38A and B). The base of the pattern is then held firmly in place while the distal end of the pattern is rotated to cover the defect to ascertain if the proposed flap can be used for closure (Fig. 7-38C).

To help ensure the survival of a large flap, its circulation can be enhanced by the delay phenomenon so that it can better withstand the torsion placed on it during its transposition. After the flap is designed, it is incised and undermined, retaining as much subcutaneous

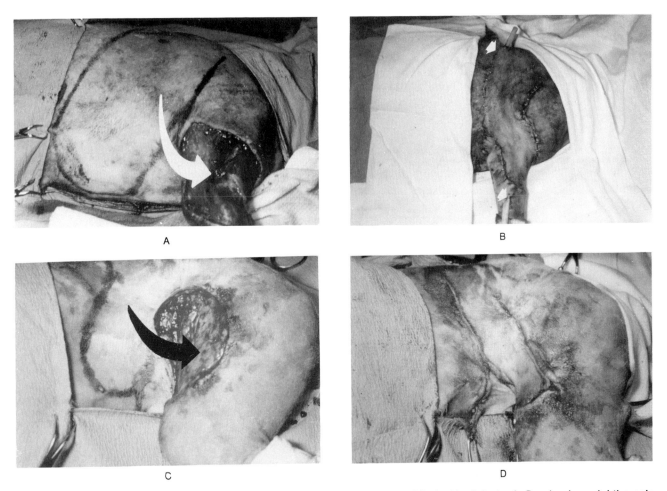

A

B

C

D

FIG. 7-32. Transpositon flaps from thoracoabdominal area to correct proximal limb skin defects. A, Proximal cranial thoracic limb defect; thoracic transposition flap designed for transposition (arrow). B, Flap transposed to correct defect. Penrose drain under flap (arrows). C, Proximal cranial pelvic limb defect with abdominal transpostion flap designed for transposition (arrow). D, Flap transposed to correct defect. (Courtesy of I. Sanchez.)

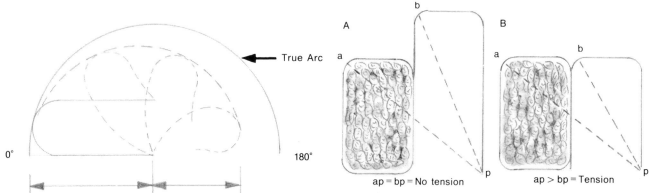

FIG. 7-33. Transposition flaps lose effective length the farther they are rotated. (After Grabb, W.C.: Classification of skin flaps. *In* Skin Flaps. Edited by W.C. Grabb, and J.W. Smith. Boston, Little, Brown and Co., 1975, p. 149.)

FIG. 7-34. No tension versus tension across a transposition flap. A, Diagonal from flap's pivot point to far point of defect (ap) equals diagonal of flap measured from pivot point (bp). Result: no tension. B, Diagonal from flap's pivot point to far point of defect (ap) is longer than diagonal of flap measured from pivot point (bp). Result: tension.

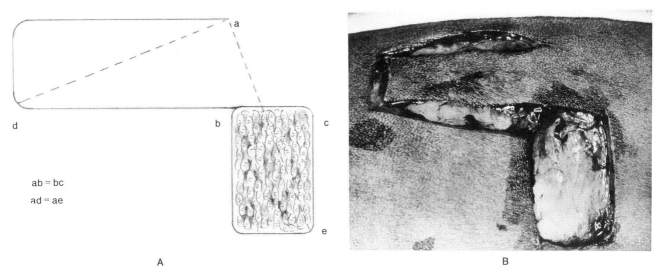

FIG. 7-35. Properly designed transposition flap that will rotate 90 degrees. A, One edge of defect incorporates one edge of flap. Width of flap base equals width of defect (ab = bc). Diagonal from flap's pivot point to farthest corner of defect equals diagonal across flap from its pivot point (ad = ae). B, Flap in vivo.

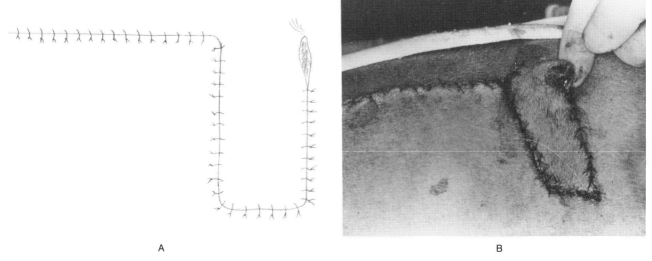

FIG. 7-36. Properly designed transposition flap rotated 90 degrees. A, Flap rotated into position with no tension on flap. Donor site closed. A "dog ear" forms at base of flap opposite pivot point. B, Flap in vivo.

tissue or panniculus muscle as possible with it. The flap is sutured back into its original site. The optimal time to transpose the flap is 3 weeks after this initial procedure, when its blood supply has increased to a maximal level.

If it is determined by the measurements and towel pattern that a transposition flap can be used for closure, the towel pattern is traced with sterile methylene blue to delineate the flap (Fig. 7-38D). The flap is incised and undermined, retaining as much subcutaneous tissue or panniculus muscle with the flap as possible (Fig. 7-38E),

then transposed into the freshened defect. Simple interrupted sutures of 3-0 absorbable suture material may be used to join the deep surface of the flap to the recipient bed tissue. This helps to eliminate dead space in which blood and tissue fluid can accumulate to interfere with vascularization of the flap. If employed, these sutures should be used sparingly and placed carefully to avoid damaging the blood supply to the flap. The edges of the flap are then sutured to the edges of the recipient area using 3-0 simple interrupted nonabsorbable sutures or

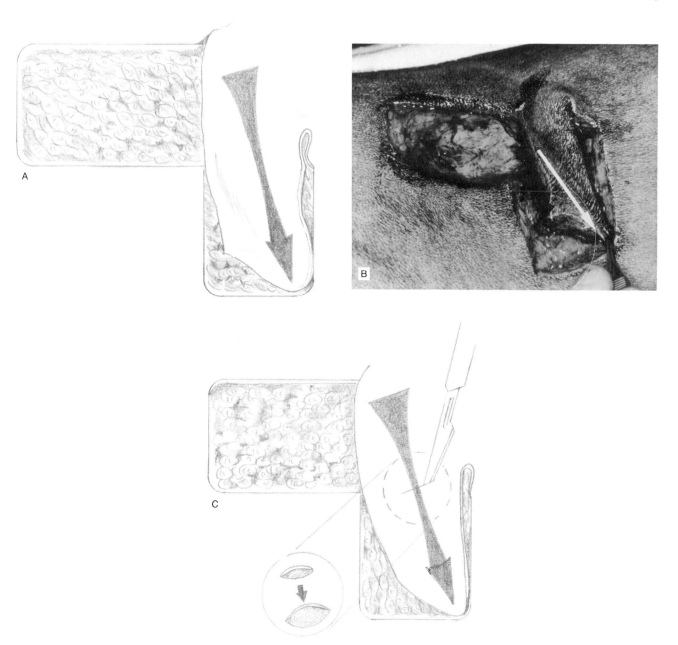

FIG. 7-37. Improperly designed transposition flap rotated 90 degrees. A, Flap rotated into position with tension across flap. B, Flap in vivo. C, Stab incision made in center of line of tension for tension release.

skin staples. If there is dead space under the flap, a one-quarter-inch diameter Penrose drain may be placed under the flap to avoid hematoma or seroma formation (Fig. 7-38F).

The donor site of the flap is closed using "walking" sutures to advance the skin edges together. A simple continuous subcuticular suture of 3-0 absorbable suture material may be used to help join the wound edges. Final skin apposition is with simple interrupted 3-0 nonabsorbable sutures or staples (Fig. 7-38G). Axial

pattern flaps can be designed containing direct cutaneous vessels that ensure a good blood supply to the flap (see Proximal Pelvic Limb, Axial Pattern Flap—references, Chapter 9).

Aftercare. If a drain has been used under a transposition flap, it is best to bandage the area to help avoid wound molestation and to assess the amount and nature of any drainage that occurs. The drain should be removed when drainage has decreased to a small amount, generally 3 to 4 days postoperatively.

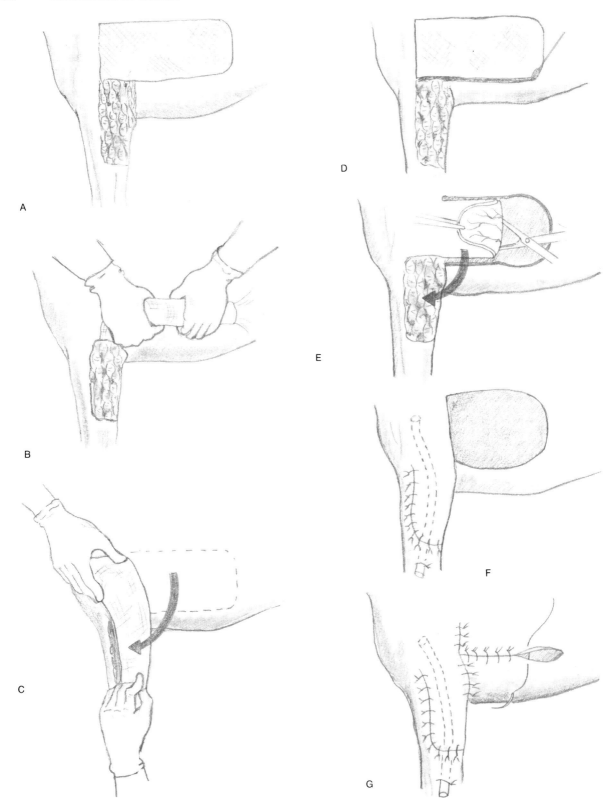

FIG. 7-38. Designing and rotating a transposition flap. A, Pattern of sterile towel cut to proper length and width laid along proposed donor site. B, Edges of pattern and underlying skin pinched together to ascertain if donor site can be closed after flap removal. C, Base of pattern held firmly in place while its distal end is rotated to cover defect. D, If manipulations reveal the pattern to be the proper size, it is traced on the donor site. E, Flap incised and undermined. F, Flap rotated into position and a Penrose drain placed under it. G, Donor site closed.

Advantages and Disadvantages. Transposition flaps provide tension relief when used to close a defect where skin is available on only one side of the defect or where closure could result in distortion of a body part, but require creating a wound to correct a wound.

REFERENCES AND SUGGESTED READING

1. Grabb, W.C., and Smith, J.W.: Basic techniques of plastic surgery. *In* Plastic Surgery. 3rd ed. Edited by W.C. Grabb, and J.W. Smith. Boston, Little, Brown and Co., 1979.
2. Grabb, W.C.: Classification of skin flaps. *In* Skin Flaps. Edited by W.C. Grabb, and M.B. Myers. Boston, Little, Brown and Co., 1979.
3. Johnston, D.E.: Wound healing and reconstructive surgery. Am Anim. Hosp. Assoc. Sci. Pro. *2*:383, 1975.
4. McGregor, I.A.: Fundamental Techniques of Plastic Surgery. 7th ed. Edinburgh, Churchill Livingstone, 1980.
5. Pavletic, M.M.: Pedicle grafts. *In* Textbook of Small Animal Surgery. Edited by D.H. Slatter. Philadelphia, W.B. Saunders, 1985.
6. Pope, E.R., Swaim, S.F.: Shifting tissue and using flaps. Vet. Med. *81*:512, 1986.

CIRCULAR

LINEAR CLOSURE

Definition and Indications. A circular defect has all points at the edges of the defect equidistant from the center of the defect. Because of tension lines in the skin, circular defects are not perfectly round. They may result from traumatic injuries or lesion excision.

Linear closure entails suturing one side of the circular defect to the opposite side with "dog ear" removal as required. The technique should be used to close circular wounds where edge-to-edge skin apposition results in little or no "dog ear" formation.

Technique. The skin around a circular defect should be manipulated to determine the amount available for closure and the potential for "dog ear" formation with closure. After determining the direction in which the tension lines tend to pull the circle, the sides parallel to the direction of pull are sutured together at their midportion with a simple interrupted 3-0 nonabsorbable suture. The two remaining smaller defects are sutured. "Dog ears" that form are removed and the resulting defects are sutured (Figs. 7-39A through D and 7-40A through C).

Aftercare. No special aftercare is needed with linear wound closure.

Advantages and Disadvantages. Linear closure is the simplest and least time-consuming technique for closing circular defects. It may require the removal of extra normal skin when "dog ears" are excised.

REFERENCES AND SUGGESTED READING

1. Swaim, S.F., Lee, A.H., and McGuire, J.A.: Techniques for reconstructing circular skin defects in dogs. Vet. Surg. *13*:18, 1984.
2. Swaim, S.F.: Principles of plastic and reconstructive surgery. *In* Textbook of Small Animal Surgery. Edited by D.H. Slatter. Philadelphia, W.B. Saunders, 1985.

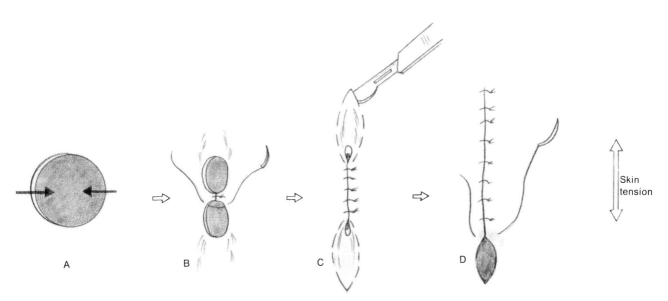

FIG. 7-39. Linear closure of a circular defect. A, Circular defect. B, Suturing center of defect and closing 2 smaller defects. C, Removing "dog ears." D, Smooth closure of resulting defects. (From Swaim, S.F., Lee, A.H., McGuire, J.A.: Techniques for reconstructing circular skin defects in dogs. Vet. Surg. *13*:20, 1984.)

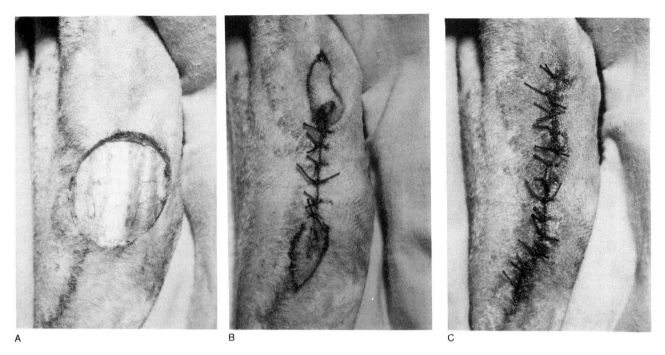

FIG. 7-40. Linear closure of a circular defect in vivo. A, Circular defect. B, Center of defect closed. "Dog ears" at ends. C, smooth closure after "dog ear" removal.

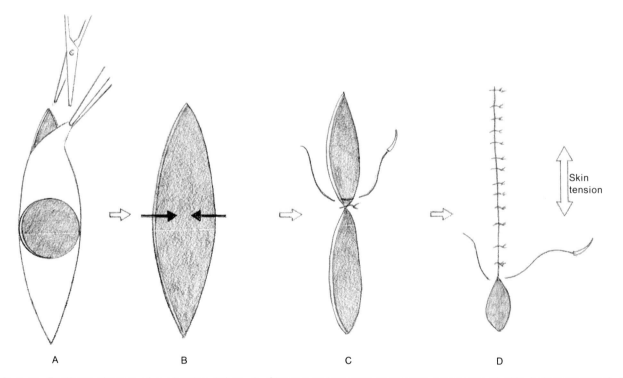

FIG. 7-41. Fusiform closure of a circular defect. A, Circular defect with triangular segments of skin being removed. B, Resultant fusiform. C, Central suture placed, creating two smaller fusiforms. D, Final straight suture line. (From Swaim, S.F., Lee, A.H., and McGuire, J.A.: Techniques for reconstructing circular skin defects in dogs. Vet. Surg. *13*:20, 1984.)

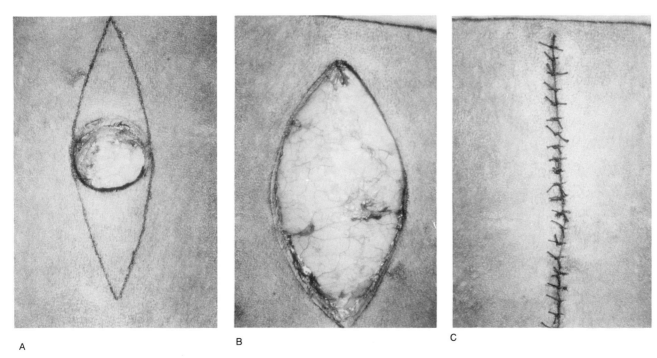

FIG. 7-42. Fusiform closure of a circular defect in vivo. A, Skin to be removed to create fusiform defect. B, Resultant fusiform defect. C, Final straight suture line.

FUSIFORM CLOSURE

Definition and Indications. Fusiform closure of circular defects entails converting the circular defect to a fusiform shape. Because the ideal length:width ratio of a fusiform defect is 4:1 to prevent "dog ear" formation, this technique should be used in areas where there is abundant skin to allow conversion to a fusiform.

Technique. After determining the direction in which skin tension lines pull the circular defect, two triangular-shaped segments of skin with curved sides are excised from opposite sides of the circular defect so that the long axis of the resultant fusiform defect is in the direction of skin tension. The widest part of the defect is closed with a simple interrupted 3-0 nonabsorbable suture, followed by closure of the two smaller defects. If the defect is large, "walking" sutures of 3-0 absorbable suture material may be used to advance the skin edges closer together before placing the skin sutures (Figs. 7-41A through D and 7-42A through C).

Aftercare. No special aftercare is needed with fusiform closure of circular defects.

Advantages and Disadvantages. Fusiform excisions provide a smooth straight wound closure. When creating a fusiform with a 4:1 length:width ratio, however, considerable normal adjacent skin must be removed to provide this ratio.

REFERENCES AND SUGGESTED READING

See Linear Closure, this chapter.

THREE-POINT OR FOUR-POINT CLOSURES

Definition and Indications. Three- or four-point closure of circular defects entails converting the defect to a three- or four-armed defect. If this type of closure is to be used, it should be on defects in areas with sufficient skin to allow removal of the "dog ears" that form.

Techniques. Three or four equidistant points are selected around the circumference of the circle. A suture of 3-0 nonabsorbable suture material is passed through one point and taken to each remaining point around the circle, where it is passed horizontally as an intradermal suture. It is then passed back out through the skin next to the first point. As the suture is tied, the three or four points are pulled together, forming three or four fusiform-like defects, which will have "dog ears" associated with them. These "dog ears" are removed with a fusiform excision and the remaining defects are sutured with simple interrupted 3-0 nonabsorbable sutures (Figs. 7-43A through D, 7-44A through C, 7-45A through D, and 7-46A through C).

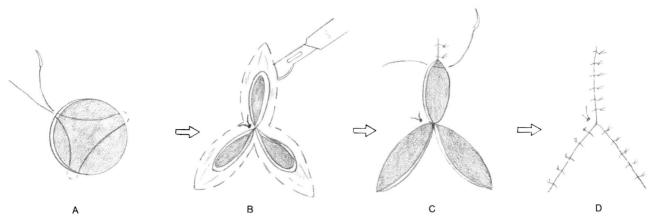

FIG. 7-43. Three-point closure of a circular defect. A, Preplacement of suture to create a three-armed defect. B, Tying suture creates a three-armed defect with "dog ears." "Dog ears" being removed. C, Closing three-armed defect. D, Completed three-armed suture line. (From Swaim, S.F., Lee, A.H., and McGuire, J.A.: Techniques for reconstructing circular skin defects in dogs. Vet. Surg. *13*:21, 1984.)

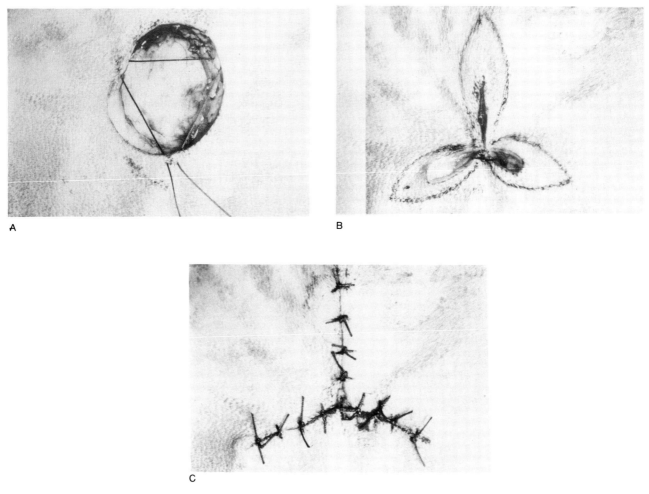

FIG. 7-44. Three-point closure of a circular defect in vivo. A, Preplaced suture to create a three-armed defect. B, Three-armed defect with "dog ears" outlined. C, "Dog ears" removed and three arms sutured.

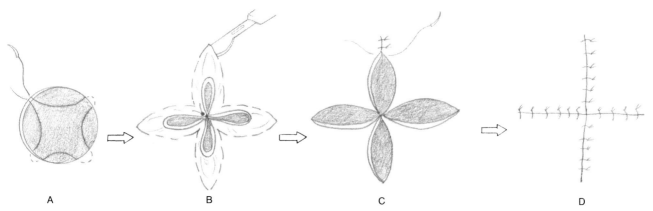

FIG. 7-45. Four-point closure of a circular defect. A, Preplacement of suture to create a four-armed defect. B, Tying suture creates a four-armed defect with "dog ears." "Dog ears" are removed. C, Closing four-armed defect. D, Completed four-armed suture line. (From Swaim, S.F., Lee, A.H., and McGuire, J.A.: Techniques for reconstructing circular skin defects in dogs. Vet. Surg. *13*:21, 1984.)

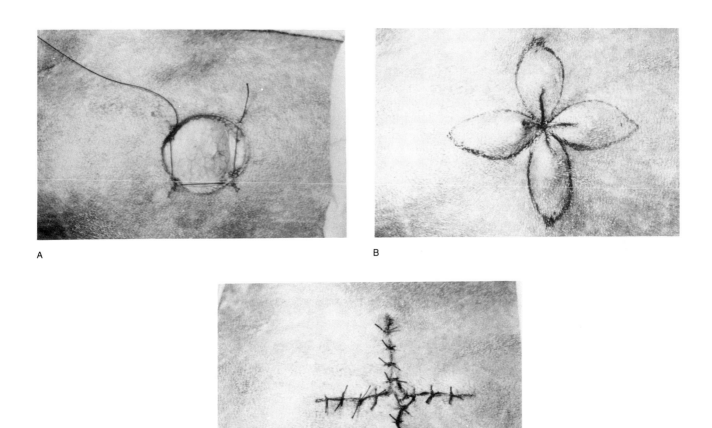

FIG. 7-46. Four-point closure of a circular defect in vivo. A, Preplaced suture to create a four-armed defect. Suture will be passed back through skin near first bite. B, Four-armed defect with "dog ears" outlined. C, "Dog ears" removed and four arms sutured.

Aftercare.   No special aftercare is needed with three-point or four-point closure of circular defects.

Advantages and Disadvantages.   The disadvantage of this technique is that a large amount of normal skin must be removed in the form of "dog ears" to obtain a smooth closure.

REFERENCES AND SUGGESTED READING

See Linear Closure, this chapter.

BOW-TIE CLOSURE

Definition and Indications.   Bow-tie closure of a circular defect requires the conversion of the circular defect to a bow-tie shape ("knot" and two "bows"). This technique should be considered when edge-to-edge apposition of the wound edges results in relatively large "dog ears" and skin around the circular defect is sufficient to allow removal of some of it to provide a smooth closure.

Technique.   Two equilateral triangles are removed from opposite sides of the circular defect. The central axis of the triangles is 30 degrees from the long axis of the skin tension lines. The apex of each triangle points toward the center of the circle, with each triangle as high as the radius of the circle. After the triangles of skin are removed, the resulting skin flaps are undermined, moved, and sutured into their new positions. These maneuvers divide the circular defect into a series of smaller fusiform defects to be closed. Suturing is with 3-0 simple interrupted nonabsorbable sutures. The angular tips of the flaps may be sutured with half-buried horizontal mattress sutures to preserve the blood supply to the flap tips. In essence, removal of the triangles of skin and transposition of the resultant flaps prevents "dog ears" before they occur (Figs. 7-47A through E, 7-48A through D).

Aftercare.   No special aftercare is needed with bow-tie closure of circular defects.

Advantages and Disadvantages.   The bow-tie technique provides a smooth closure of circular defects by removing "dog ears" before they occur, and less normal skin is removed in preventing "dog ears" than is removed with other techniques (for example, fusiform, three-point, or four-point). The disadvantage of the technique is that wounds are created to correct another wound.

REFERENCES AND SUGGGESTED READING

See Linear Closure, this chapter.

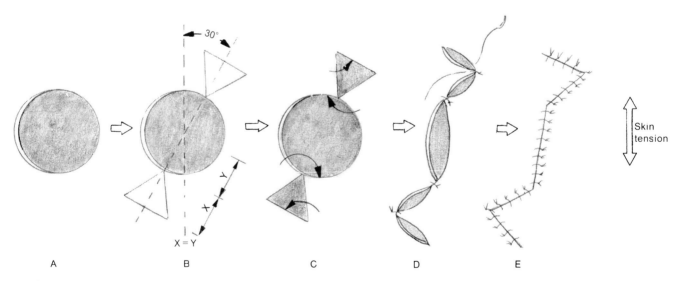

FIG. 7-47. Bow-tie closure of a circular defect. A, Circular defect. B, Equilateral triangles designed for removal. Triangles are 30 degrees off greatest tension line pull. Triangles are as high as circle's radius (x = y). C, After triangle removal, flaps will be transposed into new positons (arrows). D, Transposition of flaps breaks defect into several small fusiforms. E, Completed suture line. (From Swaim, S.F., Lee, A.H., and McGuire, J.A.: Techniques for reconstructing circular skin defects in dogs. Vet. Surg. *13*:22, 1984.)

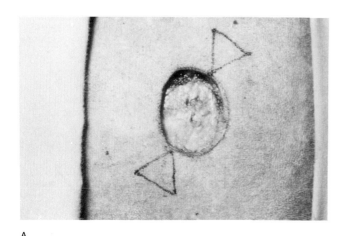

A

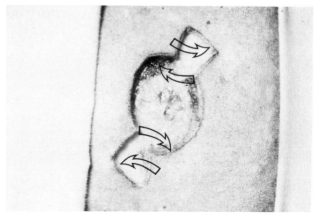

B

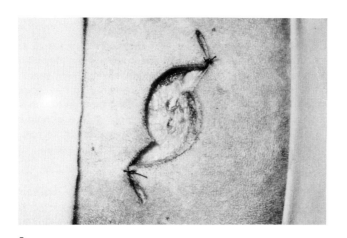

C

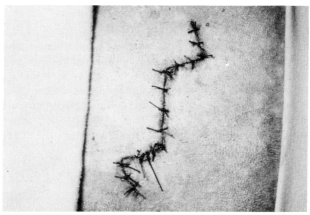

D

FIG. 7-48. Bow-tie closure of a circular defect in vivo. A, Circular defect with equilateral triangles designed for removal. B, Defect after triangles removed, and proposed flap transposition (arrows). C, One set of flaps transposed. D, Completed suture line.

COMBINED-V CLOSURE

Definition and Indications. Combined-V closure of a circular defect requires creating two V-shaped flaps on opposite sides of the circle to close the circle. The technique is indicated to close circular defects when there is a sparsity of skin surrounding the defect and all of the skin must be used to close the defect rather than any being removed as "dog ears" (as in closure of circular defects on the limbs).

Technique. Two V-shaped flaps on opposite sides of the circular defect are designed as two equilateral triangles as described for the bow-tie technique. The central axis of each triangle, however, is 45 degrees from the long axis of the defect as produced by the skin tension lines. To make the V-shaped flaps, only two sides of each triangle are incised, with the vertex of the V pointing to the long axis of the defect. After the flaps

are incised and undermined, they are moved and sutured into their new position. The angular tips of the flaps may be sutured with half-buried horizontal mattress sutures to preserve the blood supply to the flap tips. When the tip of the V-shaped flap is sutured to the side of the circular defect, this should be done so that a small fusiform defect is formed with sides of equal length.

This converts the original circular defect into smaller, irregular fusiform defects. The skin of each of the flaps is used to close half of the larger central fusiform defect. When distributing the skin of each flap to close its half of the defect, a central suture technique may be used, whereby a suture is placed between the center of each flap and its corresponding concave side of the wound. A suture is then placed in the center of each of the resulting defects. This central suturing of defects is continued until closure is complete. A "fudging" technique may also be used if necessary to provide smooth

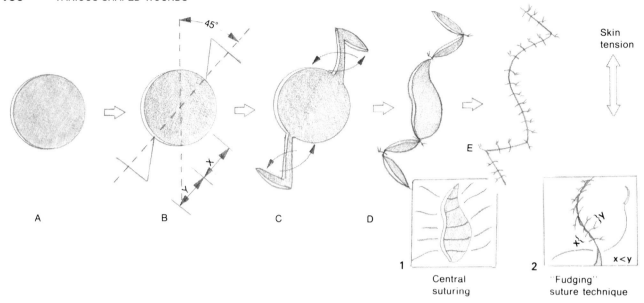

FIG. 7-49. Combined-V closure of a circular defect. A, Circular defect. B, V-shaped flaps designed like two sides of an equilateral triangle. Flaps are 45 degrees off greatest tension line pull; flap points directed toward tension line. Flaps are as wide as circle's radius (x = y). C, Flaps will be transposed into new positions (arrows). D, Transposition of flaps breaks defect into several small fusiforms. E, Skin of each V-shaped flap closes half of circle. Inset 1: Central suturing by placing sutures between center of flap and its corresponding concave side of wound (1, 1), followed by placing sutures in center of resulting 3 defects (2, 2, 2). Central suture placement continues until wound is closed. Inset 2: "Fudging" suture technique distributes flap skin to prevent "dog-ears". "Fudging" sutures are close together on convex side of wound and farther apart on concave side of wound (X < Y). (From Swaim, S.F., Lee, A.H., McGuire, J.A.: Techniques for reconstructing circular skin defects in dogs. Vet. Surg. *13*:22, 1984.)

closure. With this technique, simple interrupted sutures are placed so that they are closer together on the flap and farther apart on the concave side of the wound. This distributes any "dog ear" that might form all along the suture line (Figs. 7-49A through E and 7-50A through D). Suturing is with 3-0 simple interrupted nonabsorbable sutures.

Aftercare. No special aftercare is needed with combined-V closure of circular defects.

Advantages and Disadvantages. The combined-V technique allows closure of circular defects without removal of normal skin. The skin of the flaps is used to close the defect. This type of closure is advantageous on the limbs, where skin is not as abundant for "dog ear" removal as on the trunk. The disadvantage of the technique is that wounds are created to correct another wound.

REFERENCES AND SUGGESTED READING

See Linear Closure, this chapter.

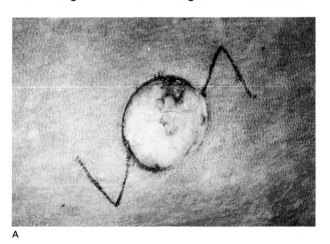

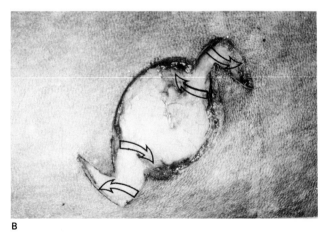

FIG. 7-50. Combined-V closure of a circular defect in vivo. A, Circular defect with V-shaped flaps designed. B, Incision of flaps and proposed transposition (arrows).

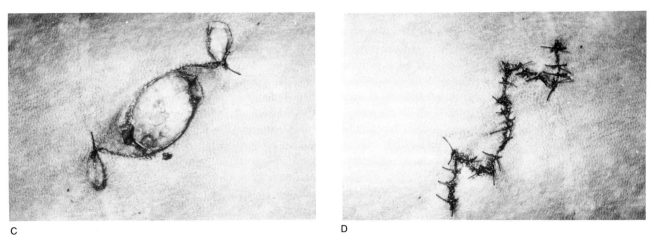

C

D

FIG. 7-50 continued. C, One set of flaps transposed. D, Completed suture line.

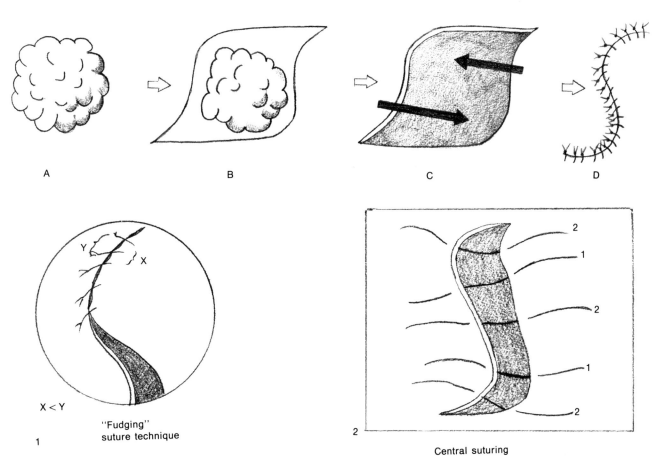

A B C D

X < Y

"Fudging"
suture technique

1

2

Central suturing

FIG. 7-51. S-plasty for removal of a circular lesion. A, Circular lesion. B, Curvilinear S-shaped lines around lesion. C, Resulting defect after excision. Curvilinear sides will be sutured together (arrows) using "fudging" suture technique. D, Completed suture line. Inset 1: "Fudging" suture technique with sutures placed close together on convex side of wound and farther apart on concave side of wound (X < Y). (From Swaim, S.F., Burkhalter, J.E., and Bell, P.J.: A tissue conserving technique for skin excision. Aub. Vet. *37*:20, 1980.) Inset 2: Central suturing by placing sutures between most convex parts of defect and their corresponding concave part(s) (1, 1), followed by placing sutures in centers of remaining 3 defects (2, 2, 2). Central suture placement continues until wound is closed.

S-PLASTY CLOSURE

Definition and Indications. S-plasty refers to the shape of the suture line after completion of the technique. The technique is indicated as a tissue-conserving method for removing one or two adjacent skin lesions.

Techniques. A curvilinear S-shaped line is drawn on either side of the one or two adjacent lesions to enclose the lesion(s). After lesion removal, the two remaining convex segments of skin are moved across the defect in opposite directions to close the defect. If necessary, the "fudging" technique may be used to place the simple interrupted 3-0 nonabsorbable sutures. Sutures are placed closer together on the convex edge of the wound than they are on the concave side. This distributes any "dog ear" that might form all along the suture line. Another technique to distribute "dog ears" all along the suture line is the central suturing technique. A suture is placed between the most convex parts of the wound and their corresponding concave portions. A suture is then placed in the center of each of the three remaining defects. This central suturing of defects is continued until closure is complete (Figs. 7-51A through D, 7-52A through D, and 7-53A and B.

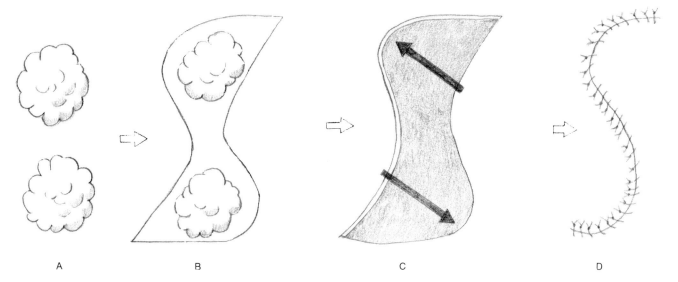

A   B   C   D

FIG. 7-52. S-plasty for removal of two adjacent circular lesions. A, Two adjacent lesions. B, Curvilinear S-shaped lines drawn around lesions. C, Resulting defect after excision. Curvilinear sides will be sutured together (arrows) using "fudging" suture technique. D, Completed suture line. (From Swaim, S.F., Burkhalter, J.E., and Bell, P.J.: A tissue conserving technique for skin excision. Aub, Vet. *37*:20, 1980.)

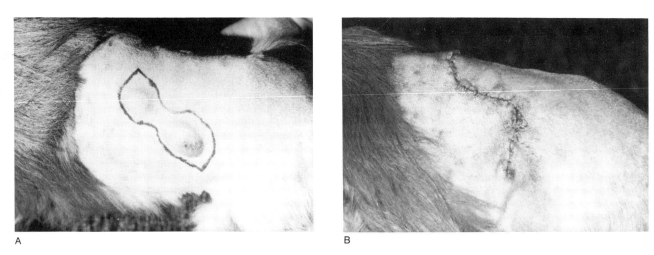

A   B

FIG. 7-53. S-plasty for removal of 2 adjacent circular inclusion cysts in vivo. A, S-plasty designed around lesions. B, Defect closure after cyst removal.

Aftercare. No special aftercare is needed with S-plasty closure of circular defects.

Advantages and Disadvantages. The S-plasty technique allows removal of one or two adjacent circular skin lesions in such a way that tissue is conserved. Much less normal skin is removed with the technique than would be removed with a fusiform excision. Careful placement of the sutures is necessary to ensure that any "dog ear" skin is evenly distributed along the suture line.

REFERENCE AND SUGGESTED READING

1. Swaim, S.F., Burkhalter, J.E., and Bell, P.J.: A tissue-conserving technique for skin excision. Aub. Vet. *37*:20, 1980.

CRESCENT-SHAPED

"FUDGING" SUTURE AND CENTRAL SUTURING CLOSURE

Definition and Indications. Crescent-shaped wounds have one side longer than the other. Closure entails removal of "dog ears" at some point in the closure process. The "fudging" and central suturing techniques distribute skin that would result in a "dog ear" all along the suture line. These techniques should be used on crescent-shaped defects where the length of the defect is relatively long and there is little discrepancy between the length of the wound edges.

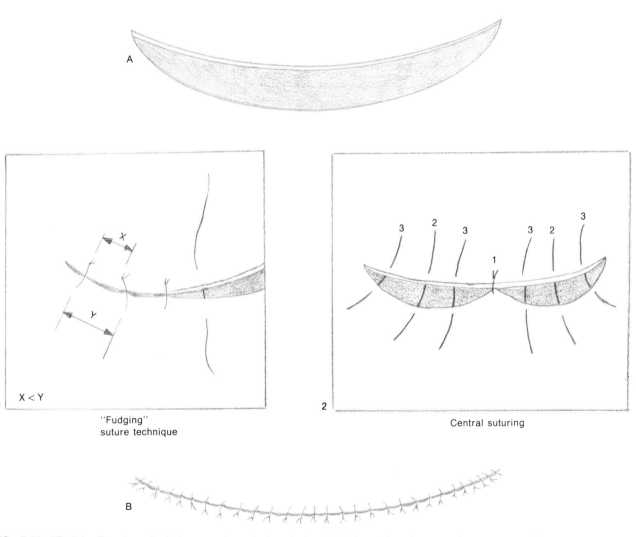

FIG. 7-54. "Fudging" suture technique and central suturing technique for closure of a crescent-shaped defect. A, Crescent-shaped defect with little discrepancy between lengths of wound edges. Inset 1: "Fudging" suture technique. Sutures are placed close together on short side of defect and farther apart on long side of defect (X < Y). Inset 2: Central suturing by placing a suture in the center of wound (1), followed by placing sutures in the center of the 2 remaining defects (2, 2). Central suture placement is contunued (3, 3, 3, 3, etc.). B, Completed suture line.

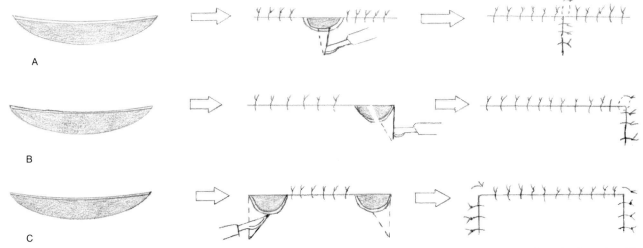

FIG. 7-55. Linear closure with "dog ear" removal for closure of crescent-shaped defects. A, Closure from both ends with central "dog ear" removal. B, Closure from one end with "dog ear" removal at opposite end. C, Closure from center toward ends with "dog ear" removal at ends. (From Swaim, S.F.: Principles of plastic and reconstructive surgery. *In* Textbook of Small Animal Surgery. Edited by D.H. Slatter. Philadelphia W.B. Saunders, 1985, p. 448.)

Techniques. With the "fudging" technique, simple interrupted 3-0 nonabsorbable sutures are placed so that they are slightly closer together on the short side of the wound and farther apart on the long side of the wound. With the central suture technique, a suture is placed in the center of the wound, followed by central placement of a suture in the two remaining defects. The central placement of sutures in defects is continued until closure is complete (Fig. 7-54A and B).

Aftercare. No special aftercare is needed with the "fudging" or central suturing techniques for closure of crescent-shaped defects.

Advantages and Disadvantages. The "fudging" and central suturing techniques allow closure of crescent-shaped wounds without removing extra normal skin as "dog ears." Careful suture placement may be necessary to distribute "dog ear" skin evenly along the suture line with either technique.

REFERENCES AND SUGGESTED READING

1. Gorney, M.: Tissue dynamics and surgical geometry. *In* Biological Aspects of Reconstructive Surgery. Edited by D.A. Kernahan, and L.M. Vistnes. Boston, Little, Brown and Co., 1977.
2. Swaim, S.F.: Principles of plastic and reconstructive surgery. *In* Textbook of Small Animal Surgery. Edited by D.H. Slatter. Philadelphia, W.B. Saunders, 1985.

LINEAR CLOSURES WITH "DOG EAR" REMOVAL

Definition and Indications. Crescent-shaped defects may be closed by various linear closure techniques with the removal of "dog ears" as they develop. This type of closure is indicated when there is little discrepancy between the length of the wound edges.

Techniques. Simple interrupted 3-0 nonabsorbable sutures may be placed from either end of the defect toward its center. As a "dog ear" forms in the center of the suture line, it is removed and the defect is closed (Fig. 7-55A). Alternately, suturing may be started at one end of the defect, progressing to the other end of the defect with "dog ear" removal at the other end of the defect (Fig. 7-55B). Suturing may also be started in the center of the defect and progress toward either end with the removal of "dog ears" at the ends of the suture line (Fig. 7-55C).

Aftercare. No special aftercare is needed with linear closure and "dog ear" removal on crescent-shaped defects.

Advantages and Disadvantages. This type of closure results in a smooth closure of the skin; however, extra normal skin must be removed in the form of "dog ears."

REFERENCES AND SUGGESTED READING

1. Borges, A.F.: Dog ear repair. Plast. Reconst. Surg. *69*:707, 1982.
2. Grabb, W.C.: Basic techniques of plastic surgery. *In* Plastic Surgery. 3rd ed. Edited by W.C. Grabb, and J.W. Smith. Boston, Little, Brown and Co., 1979.
3. Swaim, S.F.: Principles of plastic and reconstructive surgery. *In* Textbook of Small Animal Surgery. Edited by D.H. Slatter. Philadelphia, W.B. Saunders, 1985.

ONE-HALF BOW-TIE CLOSURE

Definition and Indications.   One-half bow-tie technique entails removing only one triangle of skin (one bow) from the edge of a crescent-shaped skin defect. This technique is indicated where there is a large discrepancy between the lengths of the sides of a defect. Removal of the triangle of skin from the long side of the defect will help to equalize the length of the sides of the defect to make closure easier. In other words, a large "dog ear" is removed before it occurs.

Technique.   An equilateral triangle of skin is de-signed on the skin on the long side of the defect. One angle of the triangle is in contact with the wound edge and points toward the center of the defect. The triangle is as high as the distance from the center of the defect to the long edge of the defect at the point where the triangle is designed.

After the triangle of skin is removed, the skin on either side of the triangle is undermined and the angles of skin are moved into their new positions and sutured with simple interrupted 3-0 nonabsorbable sutures. These maneuvers shorten and straighten the long side of the defect so that it more nearly matches the length of

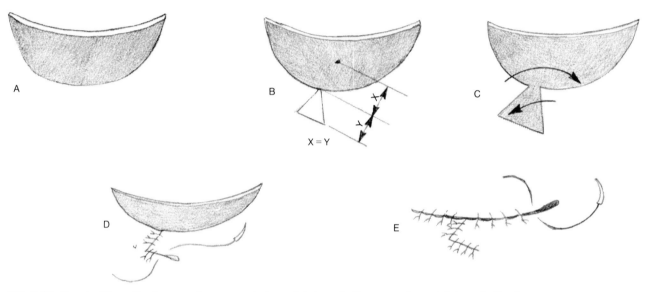

FIG. 7-56. One-half bow-tie closure of a crescent-shaped defect. A, Crescent-shaped defect. B, Equilateral triangle designed on skin adjacent to long side of defect. Height of triangle equal to distance from center of defect to long edge of defect at point where triangle is designed (x = y). C, After triangle is removed, flaps are transposed into new positions (arrows). D, Flaps sutured in place. Long side of defect is shortened. E, Remaining defect is closed using "fudging" suture technique.

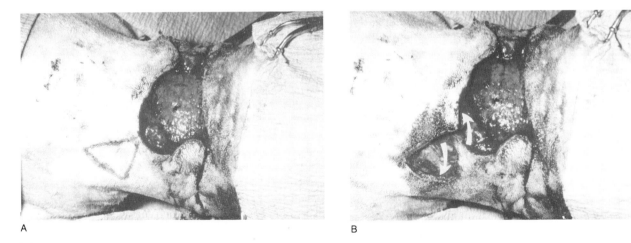

FIG. 7-57. One-half bow-tie closure of a defect with large discrepancy of wound edge lengths in vivo. A, Equilateral triangle designed adjacent to long side of defect. B, Triangle of skin has been removed. Flaps will be transposed to shorten wound edge (arrows).

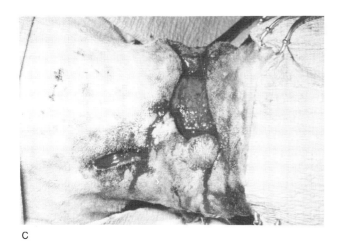

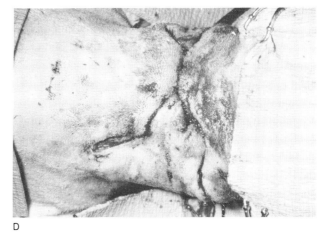

C

D

FIG. 7-57 continued. C, Flaps sutured in position. Long side of defect has been shortened. D, Final closure. (From Swaim, S.F., Lee, A.H., and McGuire, J.A.: Techniques for reconstructing circular skin defects in dogs. Vet. Surg. *13*:24, 1984.)

the short side of the defect. The remaining defect is sutured using the "fudging" suture technique, whereby sutures are placed closer together on the short side of the wound and farther apart on the long side of the wound. Alternately, the central suture technique could be used to produce a smooth closure by placing sutures to divide resulting defects continuously in half until the wound is closed (Figs. 7-56A through E, and 7-57A through D).

Aftercare. No special aftercare is needed with the one-half bow-tie closure of crescent-shaped defects.

Advantages and Disadvantages. The one-half bow-tie technique provides a smooth closure of crescent-shaped defects with considerable discrepancy between the length of the edges. The technique, however, requires creating a wound to correct a wound, but this is necessary to prevent "dog ears."

REFERENCES AND SUGGESTED READING

See Linear Closure, this chapter.

CHEVRON-SHAPED

Y CLOSURE

Definition and Indications. Chevron-shaped wounds are basically in the shape of a V, with an associated angular flap. In some of these wounds, part of the flap may have been lost or has to be debrided as a result of necrosis. The resulting chevron-shaped defect may be closed in the shape of a Y. The flap is usually free and

does not require any undermining. When dealing with a loose flap of skin, the size and position of the flap as well as the length of time since injury may be important factors with regard to the flap's blood supply. A large ventrally based flap that has folded back on itself as the result of gravity may have more impaired circulation, owing to the kinking of blood vessels at its base, than a dorsally based flap. This is especially true if the flap has been present for a long time (Fig. 7-58A and B).

Technique. The surgeon should evaluate a chevron-shaped flap carefully before deciding on the technique for reconstruction. It may be necessary to progressively cut the edges of the flap away until fresh bleeding is

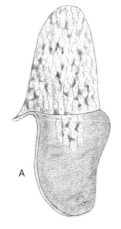
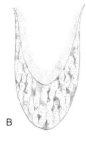

A   B

FIG. 7-58. Skin flap survival. A, A large ventrally based flap folded at base may have impaired blood supply and loss of tissue viability (shaded area). B, A dorsally based flap may have a better blood supply with less nonviable tissue (shaded area).

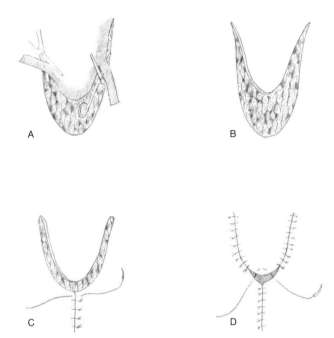

FIG. 7-59. Y-shaped closure of a chevron-shaped defect. A, Edges of a flap are progressively trimmed until fresh hemorrhage is seen at wound edge. B, Viable tissue of skin flap. C, Suturing begun at point of chevron and continued until tension develops. D, Arms of Y closed and a half-buried horizontal mattress suture placed at juncture of three suture lines.

seen at the skin edges before suturing the flap back in place (Fig. 7-59A and B). A small, dorsally based flap of short duration may have a better blood supply than the previously described flap.

The skin on each side of the chevron should be undermined. "Walking" sutures of 3-0 absorbable suture material may be used to advance the skin on either side of the defect closer together if the defect is large. Starting at the point of the chevron, the two sides are drawn together to form the stem of the Y, using simple interrupted 3-0 nonabsorbable sutures (Fig. 7-59C). Suturing is continued as far as possible without causing too much tension. As tension starts to develop on this suture line, the remainder of the defect is closed to form the arms of the Y. The suture at the junction of the three lines should be a half-buried horizontal mattress suture (Fig. 7-59D).

When a flap associated with a chevron-shaped wound has been amputated because of avascular necrosis or because of its long, narrow shape, a triangular defect is formed, and centripetal closure of the defect should be considered.

Aftercare. Y-shaped closure of chevron-shaped wounds requires no special aftercare.

Advantages and Disadvantages. Y-shaped closure provides a simple means of closing chevron-shaped wounds or wounds in which the flap has been amputated. When flaps have been amputated, however, slight elevations that are not true "dog ears" may develop at the ends of the suture line as closure progresses.

REFERENCE AND SUGGESTED READING

1. Swaim, S.F., Henderson, R.A., and Sutton, H.H.: Correction of triangular and wedge-shaped skin defects in dogs and cats. J. Am. Anim. Hosp. Assoc. *16:*225, 1980.

Advantages and Disadvantages. Chemical cauterization is less costly and time-consuming than surgery. Open excision provides no real advantage or disadvantage in comparison to the principal alternative technique, closed excision, in which the sac is packed with string or plastic before dissection.

The surgical positioning of the animal may pose disadvantages. Failure to adequately pad the end of the table beneath the hind limbs (Fig. 8-1A) may cause femoral nerve paresis. Animals with compromised cardiopulmonary function should not be placed in such a steep incline that respiration might be impaired.

REFERENCE AND SUGGESTED READING

1. Walshaw, R.: Anal sac disease. *In* Current Techniques in Small Animal Surgery II. Edited by M. J. Bojrab. Philadelphia, Lea & Febiger, 1983.

PERIANAL SINUSES

SAUCERIZATION

Definition and Indications. Perianal sinus is a common name for a pyogranulomatous inflammation of the perianal tissues. A unifying description of the etiopathology of this condition does not exist. Current theory has been established by case reports, retrospective case analysis, empirical evidence, and anecdotal reports. Pyodermatitis is the only consistent histopathologic finding. Presently, it appears that superficial contamination of the perianal region leads to abscess and ulceration of cutaneous glands and hair follicles. The inflammatory sinuses formed may extend into the anal sphincter muscle, subcutaneous tissues, pelvic canal, and peritoneal cavity. Distant infections such as peritonitis and bacterial endocarditis may be sequelea. The presenting lesion may be: (1) one or more large sinuses, (2) a matrix of interlinking sinus tracts, or (3) in rare instances, true fistulas that extend from the anal canal to the skin (Fig. 8-3A). Approximately 75% of affected dogs are German sheperd, with equal male/female ratio. Synonyms for this condition are perianal fistula, fissure, and anal furunculosis.

Saucerization is the conversion of a confined or draining inflammatory process to a broad, shallow, shelfless open wound. Without saucerization, the wound will not heal. Saucerization may be used to treat the larger cutaneo-subcutaneous perianal sinuses that are isolated in occurrence (Fig. 8-3B) as contrasted with the multiple, small or densely communicating sinuses described in the next section.

Technique. Food is withheld and mild cathartics are administered 24 hours before surgery. Cleansing enemas are given the evening before surgery. The rectum is packed 4″ × 4″ povidone-iodine-soaked cotton sponges. The dog is prepared and positioned for perineal surgery (see Open Anal Sac Excision and Fig. 8-2A, this chapter).

Each sinus is probed with curved hemostatic forceps or a catheter (Fig. 8-3B). The sinus is incised along its complete length (Fig. 8-3C). The overlying skin flaps are excised (Fig. 8-3D) at their respective bases so that no cutaneous shelf remains (Fig. 8-3E). The depth of the wound is superficially debrided or electrofulgurated to remove chronic granulation tissue and promote renewed wound contraction. Deep tracts are excised. Hemostasis is obtained by pressure, pinpoint electro-coagulation, or clamping and twisting of small vessels. If possible, no ligatures should remain in the surgical wound. The wound is left open to heal by contraction and epithelialization. The cotton sponges used to pack the rectum are removed immediately after surgery.

Because hypothyroidism and/or autoimmune proctitis have been associated with perianal sinuses, the prudent surgeon will investigate these possibilities with T3 and T4 analysis and rectal mucosal biopsy concurrent with other surgical therapy, especially in severe or recurrent disease.

Aftercare. Because mixed bacterial populations are always present, a broad spectrum systemic antibiotic such as amoxicillin is used until healing is complete. A tail brace may be constructed of heavy aluminum splint rods to support the tail and facilitate cleansing (Fig. 8-3F). Warm water sprays or "Sitz" type antiseptic baths with sponge and bowl are used 2 to 3 times daily. After cleansing, the authors prefer a topical spray emollient and enzymatic debriding agent.* Continued withholding of food for an additional 3 to 5 days or feeding a low-residue food reduces fecal contamination. Water is provided free-choice and daily water-soluble vitamins are administered. The perineum is inspected for recurrence every 2 weeks during healing and then monthly for 6 months.

Advantages and Disadvantages. No single treatment for perianal sinuses produces consistently good results; therefore surgical combinations are frequently necessary to manage the diverse presentations of this disease. Saucerization spares the anal sphincter and nerves because it is a superficial treatment. It is increasingly ineffective as the number and depth of the sinuses increase. Postoperative nursing is required for 6 to 8 weeks, and inadequate owner compliance with nursing may make the procedure less effective. The surgeon has the option of closing a saucerized defect, which reduces the time of healing (see Perianal Sinuses, Debridement

---

*Granulex, Beecham Laboratories, Bristol TN 37620.

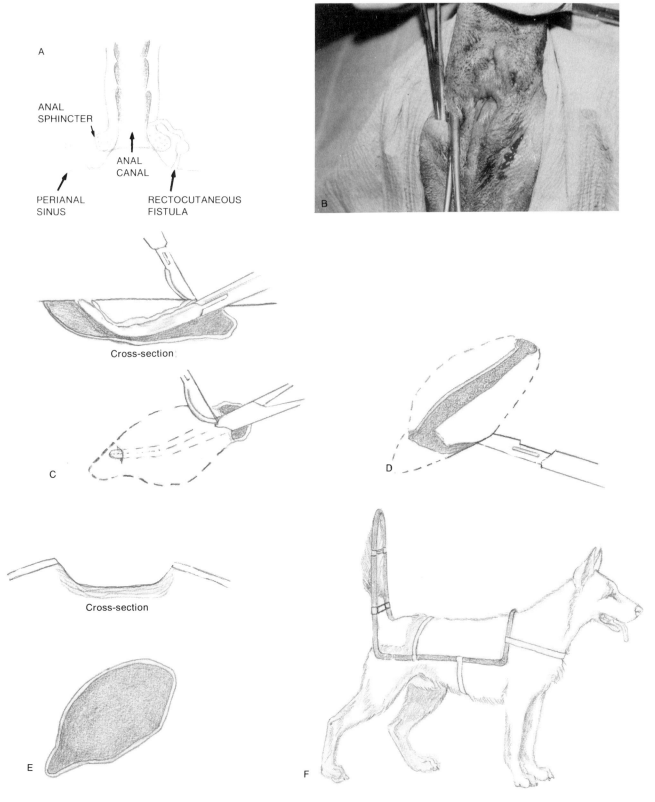

FIG. 8-3. Saucerization of perianal sinus. A, Perianal sinus and rectocutaneous fistula. B, Probing a large perianal sinus. C, Cross-section of large solitary sinus with forceps inserted and incision being made in overlying skin. D, Excision of overlying flaps of skin. E, Broad, open, shelfless, saucerized wound viewed in cross-section and from above. F, Optional tail brace secured with adhesive tape.

and Epluchage, this chapter). When closure is chosen, the surgeon should obliterate all recesses of dead space by using a monofilament, absorbable suture.

REFERENCES AND SUGGESTED READING

1. Goring, R.L., and Bright, R.M.: Perianal fistulas in the dog: Retrospective evaluation of surgical treatment by deroofing and fulgration. Vet. Surg. *15*:392, 1986.
2. Houlton J.E.F.: Anal furunculosis: A review of seventy cases. J. Small Anim. Pract. *21*:575, 1980.
3. Houlton J.E.F.: Canine anal furunculosis: A modified approach. J. Small Anim. Pract. *21*:585, 1980.
4. Vasseur, P.: Perianal fistula in the dog: A retrospective analysis of surgical techniques. J. Amer. Anim. Hosp. Assoc. *17*:188, 1981.
5. Vasseur, P.: Results of surgical excision of perianal fistulas in dogs. J. Am. Vet. Med. Assoc. *185*:60, 1984.
6. Walshaw, R.: Perianal fistula in the dog. *In* Current Techniques in Small Animal Surgery II. Edited by M.J. Bojrab. Philadelphia, Lea & Febiger, 1983.

SURGICAL DEBRIDEMENT AND EPLUCHAGE

Definition and Indications. Perianal sinus is a common name for a pyogranulomatous inflammatory process (see Perianal Sinuses, Saucerization, this chapter). One form of the disease is characterized by draining tracts and malodorous sanguinopurulent discharge. Pain causes licking, crying, and sporadic aggression. Although the inflammatory tracts usually do not penetrate the rectal mucosa, submucosa, or anal sacs, chronic and extensive involvement may allow infiltration of the anal sphincter with the same pyogranulomatous inflammation and fibrosis that, in advanced cases, may cause tenesmus or partial continence.

Debridement is the general removal of foreign matter and devitalized tissue from the affected tissue. The forceps elevation and scissor removal of any devitalized or contaminated tissue remaining after debridement is termed epluchage. Debridement and epluchage are primarily indicated for clusters of interlinking sinuses that cannot be treated by saucerization (Fig. 8-4A).

Technique. Solid food is withheld and a mild cathartic is administered 24 hours before surgery. Cleansing enemas are given the evening before surgery. The rectum is packed with 4" × 4" povidone-iodine-soaked cotton sponges following anesthesia. The dog is prepared and positioned for perineal surgery (see Open Anal Sac Excision and Fig. 8-2A, this chapter). Before beginning debridement, each sinus is probed to examine for true rectocutaneous fistulas, which are managed by incision, debridement, and suture obliteration. Then, the

anal sacs are excised (see Open Anal Sac Excision, this chapter) regardless of their degree of involvement, and the wound remaining after removing the anal sac is sutured or incorporated into the sinus excision.

The involved tissue is circumscribed with a scalpel to the anocutaneous junction (Fig. 8-4B). Debridement commences at the anocutaneous junction, dissecting the skin free from the underlying anal sphincter, and the dissection is continued centrifugally from the anus (Fig. 8-4C). No subcutaneous tissue lies between the skin and the anal sphincter to facilitate dissection (see Fig. 8-1A). If dissection is commenced distant to the anus and continued centripetally, the subcutaneous tissue plane directs dissection cranial to the external anal sphincter which may be excised or impaired. After initial debridement, epluchage of residual diseased tissue is continued until, ideally, none remains (Fig. 8-4D). Portions of the thickness of the anal sphincter may be excised; however, if the sphincter is extensively involved, it should be spared. In this instance, antibiotics, perineal washes, and open drainage are used to try to resolve the inflammation and salvage as much anal sphincter as possible.

The final shape of the excision depends on the area of tissue involved. Hemostasis is accomplished by pressure, pinpoint electrocoagulation, or clamping and twisting, of small vessels. The wound is vigorously irrigated before closing. Monofilament absorbable ligatures are used if needed, but braided ligatures are avoided. The wound may be left open to contract and epithelialize or closure may be delayed. If the debridement and epluchage appear particularly effective in removing diseased tissue, immediate closure may be chosen. If immediate closure is chosen, dead space must be obliterated and any area that would form a dependent cavity, if sutured, should be left unsutured and allowed to contract and epithelialize. The authors prefer to suture the wound whenever possible. The skin is sutured to the anorectal mucosa. Walking sutures of 4-0 monofilament absorbable material are effective in obliterating dead space and supporting the skin sutures, which are usually under moderate tension. The skin is sutured with monofilament suture using a vertical mattress pattern, tying knots on the wound edge away from the anus (Fig. 8-4E).

It is usually not possible to shift local skin to close large 360-degree defects, and in this instance partial suturing is used (Fig. 8-4F). Although flaps are effective in this area, shifting local skin is preferred because flaps are at increased risk in the presence of infection. Because perianal adenoma/carcinoma and squamous cell carcinoma may present as chronic ulcerated lesions, excised tissues should be submitted for histopathologic analysis. The cotton sponges that were placed in the rectum are removed immediately following surgery.

Aftercare. A tail brace is constructed to reduce fecal contamination caused by the tightly carried, broad German sheperd tail (see Fig. 8-3F). Multiple daily perineal irrigations and systemic amoxicillin are used until the wound is healed. The perineum is inspected for recurrence every 2 weeks during healing and then monthly for 6 months.

Advantages and Disadvantages. All diseased tissue is removed and primary closure is possible. Because the source wound is classified as infected or dirty, the resulting debrided wound is considered dirty as well, and special precautions are necessary, including reducing the amount of suture remaining in the wound and the use of systemic antibiotics to reduce the chance of postoperative infection. Depending on the degree of involvement, the anus may stricture as a result of the disease or surgery, requiring an anoplasty (see Anal Stricture, Anoplasty, this chapter).

REFERENCES AND SUGGESTED READING

1. Goring, R.L., and Bright, R.M.: Perianal fistulas in the dog: Retrospective evaluation of surgical treatment by deroofing and fulgration. Vet. Surg. *15*:392, 1986.
2. Houlton, J.E.F.: Canine anal furunculosis: A modified approach. J. Small Anim. Pract. *21*:585, 1980.
3. Houlton, J.E.F.: Anal furunculosis: A review of seventy cases. J. Small Anim. Pract. *21*:575, 1980.
4. Vasseur, P.: Perianal fistula in the dog: A retrospective analysis of surgical techniques. J. Am. Anim. Hosp. Assoc. *17*:188, 1981.
5. Walshaw, R.: Perianal fistula in the dog. *In* Current Techniques in Small Animal Surgery II. Edited by M. J. Bojrab. Philadelphia, Lea & Febiger, 1983.

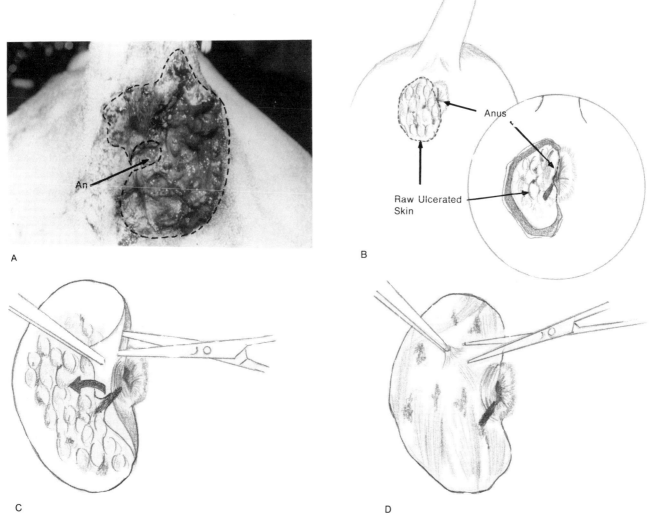

FIG. 8-4. Debridement and epluchage of perianal sinuses. A, Multiple small perianal sinus tracts to right of anus, and excision area (inside broken lines). B, Incision circumscribes sinuses on left of anus (inset); anal sac has been excised. C, Debridement at the anocutaneous junction continued centrifugally. D, Epluchage of remaining abnormal tissue until healthy tissue remains.

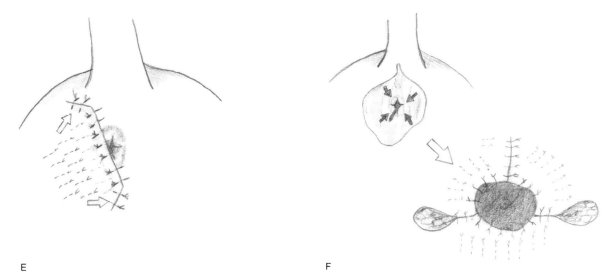

E   F

FIG. 8-4 continued. Debridement and epluchage of perianal sinuses. E, "Walking" suture closure and areas of "dog ear" removal (arrows). F, Centripetal closure for 360-degree excision with two partially sutured lateral areas.

ANAL STRICTURE

ANOPLASTY

Definition and Indications. The fibrous contracture that results from chronic perianal sinus infection, extensive excisions or cryodestruction of perianal sinuses, and rectal pull-through causes strictures of the anus (Fig. 8-5A). If 270 degrees of the anus are involved, clinical signs of tenesmus or obstruction may be present. The surgical interruption of these fibrous bands is termed anoplasty.

Neoplasia of the anal canal or surrounding skin must not be mistaken for anal stricture. Abnormal tissues should be submitted for histopathologic examination. If this technique is not successful, partial or total rectal pull-through may be indicated.

Technique. The contents of the rectal canal are manually removed, the hair removed from the surgical site, and the anus scrubbed and prepared for surgery. Povidone-iodine-soaked sponges are placed into the rectum to prevent gross soilage.

The fibrous scar is incised perpendicular to the anocutaneous junction extending 1 cm deep into normal anal sphincter or subcutaneous tissue (Fig. 8-5B). Both the skin and rectal mucosa should be incised for the same distance.

The incision is sutured in the opposite direction to create a new anocutaneous junction using 5-0 absorbable suture (Fig. 8-5C). Small interrupted sutures should be used to create a perfect mucocutaneous junction (Fig. 8-5D). This procedure may be repeated in up to three additional quadrants during the same procedure to adequately open the anal canal. The gauze sponge is removed after the procedure.

Aftercare. The authors use no special aftercare. If a stool softener is to be used, it must be started 2 days before surgery to modify the initial bowel movement and discontinued within 3 days after surgery, because distension of the anal orifice by the stool may help prevent recurrent stricture.

Advantages and Disadvantages. The advantage of this technique is its technical simplicity. The principal disadvantage is that it is possible to create incontinence if multiple individual anoplasties are created and made too large, or if too many are created. The stricture may recur if the anoplasties are too small or too traumatic, or if the mucocutaneous anastomosis is not accurate.

REFERENCES

1. Bojrab, M.J.: Editor's Note (on Anoplasty). *In* Current Techniques in Small Animal Surgery II. Edited by M.J. Bojrab. Philadelphia, Lea & Febiger, 1983.
2. Walshaw, R.: Anoplasty. *In* Current Techniques in Small Animal Surgery II. Edited by M.J. Bojrab. Philadelphia, Lea & Febiger, 1983.

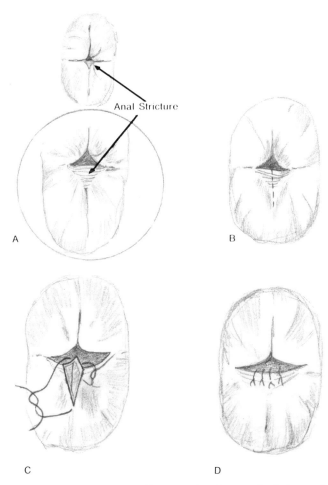

surgery, the term is applied to reconstruction of the perineum after excision of the redundant perivulvar folds.

Episioplasty is not a commonly indicated surgical procedure. Even though perivulvar folds are common, pyoderma of these folds is not. Atopy is commonly manifested as perivulvar inflammation and should be ruled out or managed before surgical intervention. Improved pet health care, antiseptic baths, and antibiotic therapy have reduced the incidence of "filth-type" infections in all but certain predisposed individuals.

Technique. The inflammation of the skin of the vulva and fold should be controlled before scheduling surgery. The perivulvar region is clipped and prepared for sterile surgery. The recesses of the folds should be scrubbed well because of greater potential of bacterial inhabitation. A purse-string suture is placed in the anus and, depending on the surgeon's preference, the dog is placed in dorsal recumbent lithotomy position with the hind limbs tied cranially (Fig. 8-6B) or in perineal position (see Fig. 8-2A).

Heavy sharp scissors or a scalpel may be used to excise the redundant skin folds (Fig. 8-6C). Excision of these folds alone may not solve the problem; the subcutaneous tissue dorsal to the vulva must also be removed to prevent recession of the vulva (Fig. 8-6D). When possible, a 1 cm margin of skin should be maintained dorsal to the vulva for suture placement, and the incision ends should taper to points to eliminate "dog ears."

Because the incision nearest the vulva will be shorter than the perineal incision, there is the potential for "dog ear" development as closure proceeds. To help prevent this, the subcutaneous tissue is approximated beginning dorsally at the midpoint of the wound using absorbable 4-0 simple interrupted sutures. After the first suture is tied, the midpoints of each half of the remaining incisions are approximated, and this is repeated until the skin edges are almost apposed (Fig. 8-6E). To further help distribute skin and prevent "dog ear" formation, the "fudging" technique can be used when placing skin sutures, with sutures closer together on the short side of the wound and farther apart on the longer-side wound edge (Fig. 8-6F).

Aftercare. Immediately after surgery, the surgical site is washed, antiseptic solution is applied again, and the purse-string suture in the anus is removed. Affected skin is treated with a topical antibacterial such as bacitracin, polymixin, neomycin ointment* until infection is controlled. Because self-mutilation is a potential complication of surgery in this area, Elizabethan collars,

FIG. 8-5. Anoplasty to relieve anal stricture. A, Strictured anus and close-up (inset). B, Area of incision of anal stricture (broken line). C, Sutures placed for creating a new elongated mucocutaneous junction. D, Completed anoplasty.

REDUNDANT PERIVULVAR FOLDS

EXCISION OF REDUNDANT PERIVULVAR FOLDS (EPISIOPLASTY)

Definition and Indications. Redundant perivulvar folds are apron-like folds of redundant perineal tissue that partially or completely cover the vulva (Fig. 8-6A). The recesses of the perivulvar fold are the sites of intertriginous irritation and chronic pyoderma. Hypoplasia of the vulva and obesity, seen mostly in mature bitches, contribute to the occurrence of this condition. Hypoplasia of the vulva may occur secondary to performance of ovariohysterectomy before the first estrous cycle.

Episioplasty is technically defined as an operation to reconstruct a deformity of the vulva, but in veterinary

*Neosporin ointment, Burroughs Wellcome Co. Research, Triangle Park, NC.

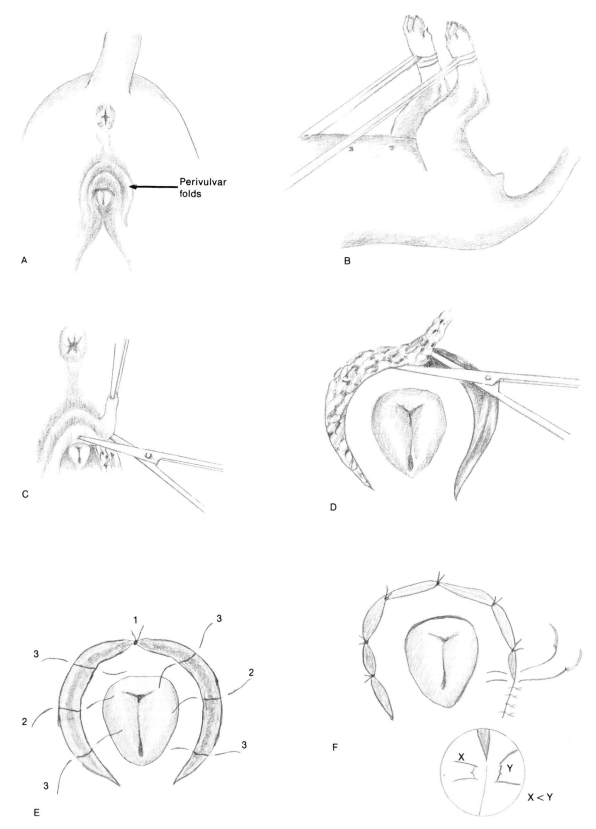

FIG. 8-6. Excision of perivulvar folds. A, Perivulvar folds. B, Lithotomy position for episioplasty. C, Cutaneous folds being removed with scissors. D, Subcutaneous fat being excised. E, Order of placement of subcuticular sutures to help prevent "dog ears." F, Placement of skin sutures using "fudging technique" (inset).

sidebars, or wire basket type muzzles may be necessary to protect the wound for the first several days after surgery.

Advantages and Disadvantages. There are no direct advantages or disadvantages to this procedure because there are no commonly applied alternatives. The lithotomy position offers a flat operating field, but sacrifices the gravitational pull on the folds of the perineal position. The surgeon must allow for this change. Allowing a bitch to have one estrus cycle before ovariohysterectomy and regulation of the animal's weight are advantageous because they may help to prevent this condition.

REFERENCES AND SUGGESTED READING

1. Krahwinkel, D.J.: Correction of specific skin diseases. *In* Surgery of Traumatized Skin: Management and Reconstruction in the Dog and Cat. Edited by S.F. Swaim. Philadelphia, W.B. Saunders, 1980.
2. Krahwinkel, D.J., and Bone, D.: Surgical management of specific skin disorders. *In* Textbook of Small Animal Surgery. Edited by D.H. Slatter. Philadelphia, W.B. Saunders, 1985.

INGROWN TAIL

VERTEBRAL EXCISION AND RECONSTRUCTION

Definition and Indications. Ingrown tail is observed primarily in the Boston terrier and English bull-dog breeds and in Manx cats. Pathologically, ventral or spiraling curvature of ankylosed coccygeal vertebrae causes skin folds, immobile tail, and/or anal obstruction (Fig. 8-7A). When this condition is combined with obesity, partial fecal obstruction, cutaneous secretions, and trauma, an intertriginous infection develops, primarily beneath the tail. These infections cannot be managed medically because the tail is immobile and prevents cleansing. Synonyms for this condition are screw tail and corkscrew tail.

Vertebral amputation and reconstruction is the removal of the osseous deformity with preservation of the tail stub. This technique is recommended when owners do not want the tail amputated and are willing to occasionally bathe the recess that remains ventral to the tail.

Technique. Because this is potentially a contaminated surgical procedure, prophylactic antibiotics may be given. The clinical presentation is variable, so a "standard procedure" must be modified for each animal. Variable configurations of ankylosis cause the problems associated with the skin folds, as well as the patterns of intertriginous infection, to differ. The specific malformation to be described in this technique is ventral curving deviation and ankylosis of the coccygeal vertebrae (Fig. 8-7A and B). In this circumstance, the tail covers the anus and cannot be elevated during defecation; thus pyodermatitis occurs in the skin on the ventrum of the tail and perianal skin ventral to the anus.

The perineum is surgically prepared by clipping,

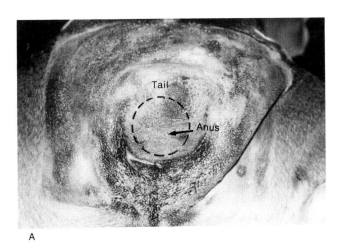

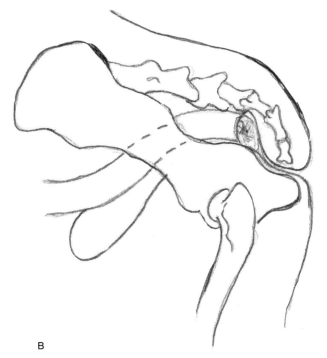

FIG. 8-7. Ingrown tail: Vertebral excision and reconstruction of tail. A, Ventral deviation of English bulldog's tail with intertriginous infection. Location of anus under tail (broken line). B, Ventral deviating ankylosed vertebrae obstructing anus.

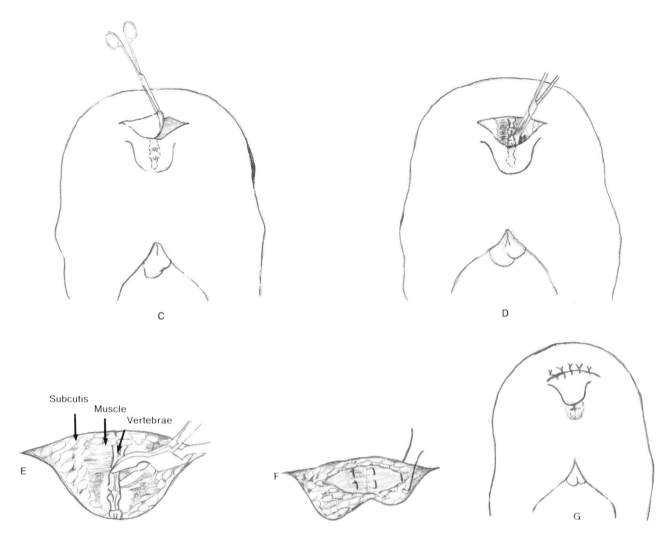

FIG. 8-7 continued. Ingrown tail: Vertebral excision and reconstruction of tail. C, Transverse fusiform skin/subcutaneous excision at the dorsal tail base. D, Coccygeal muscles and rectum being separated from the coccygeal vertebrae. E, Coccygeal vertebrae being amputated at the point where they begin to deviate ventrally. F, Apposition of coccygeal muscles and subcutaneous tissues. G, Final skin closure and appearance of perianal region.

scrubbing, and applying a surgical antiseptic. The area beneath the tail and skin folds cannot be clipped; therefore extra time should be spent in cleansing this area because of the likelihood of fecal impaction and residual pathogenic bacteria. Although no special bowel preparation is used, it is usually possible to use forceps to pack the rectum with povidone-iodine-impregnated gauze sponges even when the anus is covered by the tail stub.

With the dog in sternal recumbency, a transverse fusiform skin incision is performed at the base of the tail to allow access to the coccygeal vertebrae. The excision should be large enough that its closure will result in cosmetic reduction of tail volume, and elevation of the remaining soft tissues of the tail will open the anal canal (Fig. 8-7C). Using alternate sharp and blunt dissection, the coccygeal vertebrae are exposed. The coccygeal

muscle tendons are incised as close to the vertebrae as possible, and the soft tissues that loosely attach the rectum to the vertebrae are divided (Fig. 8-7D). Coccygeal vessels are ligated as they are encountered. Bone-cutting forceps are used to amputate through the first coccygeal vertebrae or where the ventral deviation begins (Fig. 8-7E). The vertebrae are sharply dissected from the tail stub and removed. The bone may be intimately associated with the "end" of the stub, causing a perforation as this portion is freed. A perforation at this location is sutured.

If dissection and excision of the vertebrae expose the dorsal portion of the rectum, the coccygeal muscles are sutured with 3-0 absorbable horizontal mattress sutures to support the rectum dorsally and prevent a dorsal perineal hernia. Additional skin and subcutaneous tissue are excised as necessary to reduce the volume of the tail stub, remove additional folds, and improve skin apposition. The subcutaneous tissues and skin are apposed in layers with suture patterns and materials of the surgeon's choice (Fig. 8-7F and G).

Aftercare. The rectal packing is removed. Cool compresses are applied for the first 2 days, and the surgical wound and peripheral tissues are bathed twice daily with dilute antiseptic solution in conjunction with topical antibiotic therapy to control the remaining pyoderma.

Advantages and Disadvantages. Amputation of the coccygeal vertebrae with maintenance of the tail "stub" alleviates obstruction of the anal canal and is cosmetically preferred by most owners. The intertriginous zone presists, however, and may require periodic cleansing by the owner. With dorsal approach and reconstruction of the tail, the area may be less likely to become contaminated than with procedures that invade the inflamed skin during amputation of the tail. Regardless of whether this procedure or tail amputation is used, if the coccygeal muscles are incised cranial to the anus, they must be apposed dorsal to the rectum or a rectal deviation and perineal hernia may result.

REFERENCES AND SUGGESTED READING

1. Krahwinkel, D.J., Correction of specific skin diseases. *In* Surgery of Traumatized Skin: Management and Reconstruction in the Dog and Cat. Edited by S.F. Swaim. Philadelphia, W.B. Saunders, 1980.
2. Krahwinkel, D.J., and Bone, D.: Surgical management of specific skin disorders. *In* Textbook of Small Animal Surgery. Edited by D.H. Slatter. Philadelphia, W.B. Saunders, 1985.

AMPUTATION

Definition and Indications. Another form of ingrown tail anomaly is a pathologically spiraling curvature of ankylosed coccygeal vertebrae which may cause skin folds cranial to the tail head and/or an infected recess beneath the tail with or without occlusion of the anus (Fig. 8-8A and B). This malformation of the coccygeal vertebrae, coupled with obesity, cutaneous secretions and trauma, also creates an intertriginous inflammation that cannot be managed medically. Synonyms for this condition are screw tail and corkscrew tail.

Amputation is the removal of the coccygeal vertebrae and skin. It is indicated as an alternative when the owner is unconcerned as to whether the dog has a tail stub or not.

Technique. Each animal will vary as to degree of involvement. The procedure chosen must be adapted to the individual animal. The perineum is surgically prepared by clipping, scrubbing, and applying a surgical antiseptic. The areas between the tail and skin folds are difficult to clean. Although no special bowel preparation is required, the rectum is packed with povidone-iodine-soaked gauze sponges and the anus is closed with a temporary purse-string suture to reduce the potential for soilage of the surgical site. The animal is positioned in sternal recumbency.

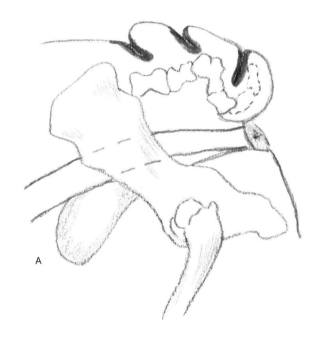

A

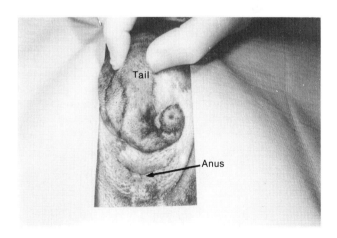

B

FIG. 8-8. Ingrown tail: Amputation. A, "Corkscrew" tail, showing skin folds which are sites of intertriginous infection (extra bold lines). B, Tail pad elevated to show ankylosed caudal vertebrae and one form of "corkscrew" tail.

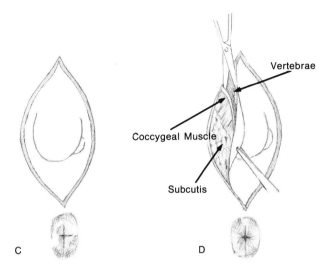

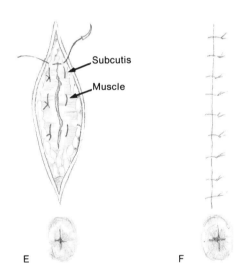

FIG. 8-8 continued. Ingrown tail: Amputation. C, Elliptical skin incision circumscribing the tail base. D, Skin and subcutis reflected, and coccygeal muscles being dissected from the vertebrae. E, Coccygeal muscles reapposed and first suture placed in subcutis. F, Completed operation with a smooth perineum.

A dorsoventral elliptical skin incision is made, incorporating the tail and its surrounding skin folds Fig. 8-8C). Blunt dissection centripetally allows access to the ankylosed coccygeal vertebrae (Fig. 8-8D). After the coccygeal vertebrae are exposed, the coccygeal muscle tendons are incised from the vertebrae, and the soft tissues that loosely attach the rectum to the vertebrae are bluntly separated. Bone-cutting forceps are used to amputate through the first coccygeal vertebrae because ankylosis frequently prevents disarticulation (see Fig. 8-7E). The circumscribed skin and vertebrae are removed. Hemorrhage from the lateral and median coccygeal vessels is controlled by ligation.

The coccygeal muscles are apposed with absorbable 3-0 interrupted horizontal mattress sutures to support the rectum dorsally if the excision of the vertebrae is cranial to the anal sphincter (Fig. 8-8E). Additional skin and subcutaneous tissue are excised if necessary to improve the appearance of the closure. The subcutaneous tissues and skin are sutured in layers, with suture patterns and materials of the surgeon's choice. The result is a smooth vertical closure dorsal to the anus (Fig. 8-8F).

Aftercare. Prophylactic antibiotics may be given perioperatively. Cool compresses are applied for the first 2 days, and the surgical wound and peripheral tissues are bathed twice daily with dilute antiseptic solution for several days.

Advantages and Disadvantages. Amputation requires less surgical time. Amputation of the coccygeal vertebrae and skin fold is not as cosmetic as maintenance of a tail stub, but excision of the tail alleviates the folds.

REFERENCES AND SUGGESTED READING

1. Krahwinkel, D.J.: Correction of specific skin diseases. *In* Surgery of Traumatized Skin: Management and Reconstruction in the Dog and Cat. Edited by S.F. Swaim. Philadelphia, W.B. Saunders, 1980.
2. Krahwinkel, D.J., and Bone D.: Surgical management of specific skin disorders. *In* Textbook of Small Animal Surgery. Edited by D.H. Slatter. Philadelphia, W.B. Saunders, 1985.

WOUNDS ON THE LIMBS

9

PROXIMAL THORACIC LIMB

ELBOW HYGROMA:

Penrose Drainage

Definition and Indications. A hygroma is a cystic cavity containing fluid that, in the dog, is usually an accumulation of serum between the skin and a bony prominence (Fig. 9-1A). Hygromas are caused by pressure and trauma, probably because early callus development is too slow or insufficient, and occur most frequently over the olecranon, greater trochanter, and ischium. Synonyms for elbow hygroma are elbow seroma and olecranon bursitis; however, the bursa of the triceps tendon is not associated with this lesion. In elbow hygroma, the serum accumulation occurs in the subcutaneous space superficial to the triceps muscle fascia over the olecranon. Some dogs are predisposed to hygromas because of their thin skin and small quantity of subcutaneous fat pad. In other dogs, concurrent hip dysplasia or pain from other orthopedic problems may render the dog less able to protect the elbow from being traumatized when attempting to lie down.

Penrose drainage is the placement of a Penrose drain through the hygroma cavity for the purpose of continuous drainage. Drainage is continued until the granulation tissue that lines the cavity walls has the opportunity to unite and obliterate the cavity.

Technique. *Aspiration.* The size and breed of the dog should be considered, and appropriate diagnostic tests conducted to rule out possible intercurrent orthopedic conditions. Small, more acute hygromas that are not infected or ulcerated may be treated by aseptic aspiration and pressure coaptation bandage. Aspiration is rarely successful for larger hygromas.

Penrose Drainage. If the hygroma recurs after aspiration or an alternate treatment is sought for a larger, more chronic hematoma, Penrose drainage is recommended. If both forelimbs are affected with small hygromas, they may be explored and drained at the same operation. Large bilateral hygromas should be staged because the postoperative bandaging requires that extension spicas be applied.

The elbow is prepared for aseptic surgery. A stab incision is made in the proximal part of the hygroma. Sterile forceps are used to probe the cavity. The most dependent portion of the cavity is determined and the skin is incised to permit digital exploration of the cavity. The cavity is palpated, fibrin septae are interrupted, fibrin remnants are removed, and the cavity is irrigated (Fig. 9-1B). One or more 1/4 inch diameter Penrose drain(s) is (are) drawn through the cavity and fixed proximally and distally. The redundant skin and volume of large hygromas may be reduced by plicating the skin with 2-0 monofilament horizontal or vertical mattress sutures. To prevent incorporation of the drain in the plication sutures, the sutures should be placed but not tied. Then the drain is placed and fixed and the plicating sutures are tied (Fig. 9-1C and inset). The cavity is then irrigated with saline or Ringer's solution a final time.

The Penrose drain is fixed by placing a loose 3-0 simple interrupted suture in the skin near the drain emergence. The drain is placed between the suture ends over the initial fixating knot and the ends are retied

181

tightly, fixing the drain. This secures the drain and prevents injury to the skin at the drain fixation point.

Aftercare. Antibiotics are not used unless the hygroma is infected. If infection is present, the antibiotic used should be chosen based on results of culture and sensitivity examination. The wound is covered with a nonadherent dressing, and the elbow is covered by a heavy cotton and absorbent gauze bandage. This bandage is changed daily. The absorbent bandage can usually be replaced with an absorbent bandage incorporated into a spica-type bandage (Fig. 9-1D) after 3 or 4 days. When the elbow is wrapped in a spica-type bandage, the majority of the padding should be placed around, rather than on, the olecranon, thus preventing pressure injury of the skin (see Pressure Sores, Chapter 4). Small (2 to 3 cm diameter) hygromas may be managed without the spica using only an absorbent padded

bandage. For larger hygromas, the spica is intended to protect the elbow by preventing pressure over it and limiting movement of the skin over the olecranon during healing. Its efficacy is re-evaluated every 5 to 7 days. The absorbent portion of the spica with its overlying padding may be changed by incising the tape over the area, but if any portion of the bandage is soiled, wet, loose, or causing irritation, the entire bandage should be replaced. The coapting spica bandage (or padded bandage for small hygromas), plicating sutures (if used), and drain remain in place concurrently for 2 to 4 weeks until the subcutaneous tissue firmly adheres to the underlying olecranon. The period of drainage is longer for larger hygromas. The wound is kept under a smaller padded bandage for 1 week after the drain is removed (Fig. 9-1D inset). The animal should be restricted from hard surfaces or provided with padding for the elbows until

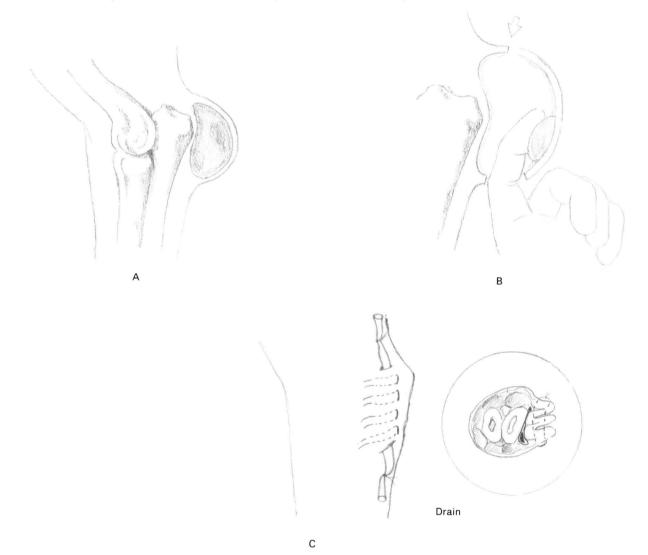

Drain

FIG. 9-1. Elbow hygroma correction with Penrose drain. A, Midsaggital section of the lesion. B, Digital exploration through ventral incision, and dorsal incision (arrow). C, Plicated hygroma with drain fixed and viewed in cross-section (inset).

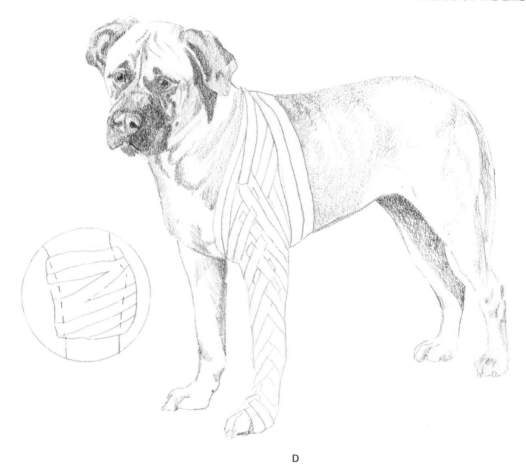

D

FIG. 9-1 continued. D, Spica-type tape bandage applied and smaller heavily padded elbow bandage (inset).

adequate protective callus has had an opportunity to form.

Advantages and Disadvantages. Complete dissection and excision of elbow hygromas was recommended at one time. Comparatively, the drainage technique is simple, inexpensive, and effective. The integrity of the skin is not compromised by incision and sutures, and pressure from lying on the elbow does not compromise a suture line. Latex drains are preferred to silastic and other materials. Chronic hygromas are lined by mature collagen, which may not heal even when apposed. Latex induces a mild inflammatory response that converts the hygroma wall from a chronic to a more acute inflammation, and healing progresses. Penrose drainage cannot be used when the hygroma has ulcerated.

REFERENCES AND SUGGESTED READING

1. Johnston, D.E.: Hygroma of the elbow in dogs. J. Am. Vet. Med. Assoc. *167*:213, 1975.

2. Krahwinkel, D.J., and Bone, D.: Surgical management of specific skin disorders. *In* Textbook of Small Animal Surgery. Edited by D.H. Slatter. Philadelphia, W.B. Saunders, 1985.

Suture Obliteration

Definition and Indications. See Elbow Hygroma, Penrose Drainage, this chapter. Suture obliteration is obliteration of the hygroma cavity by apposing the debrided walls of the hygroma with sutures.

Technique. The patient is prepared for aseptic surgery in a routine manner. The limb is draped as for orthopedic surgery on the elbow. The hygroma is incised on its lateral surface, and the incision is extended to the proximal and distal limit of the cavity (Fig. 9-2A). Fibrinous septae and blood clots are digitally disrupted from their attachments and removed by irrigation (Fig. 9-2B). The cavity of a chronic hygroma is lined by mature granulation tissue. Because this tissue is predominantly collagen, and little fibroblastic activity is present, it is necessary to superficially debride the lining.

Debridement may be accomplished by alternately scraping the cavity with a scalpel blade and rubbing with dry gauze sponges (Fig. 9-2C). Debridement is sufficient when capillaries are oozing blood and the tissue is a blushed pink color. Deep debridement that results in marked hemorrhage should be avoided. The stretching of the skin by the hygroma will have created redundant skin, which must be excised (Fig. 9-2D). Because the hygroma was incised on its lateral surface, additional skin may be excised from the edges of the incision to keep the lengths nearly equal, and the final suture line will rest on the lateral aspect of the elbow.

Wound closure is commenced by obliterating the cavity with multiple rows of 3-0 or 4-0 simple interrupted absorbable sutures that approximate the debrided granulation tissue of the skin/subcutaneous layer to the granulation layer, which covers the triceps tendon and olecranon (Fig. 9-2E). These rows of sutures are similar to "walking" sutures except that the tissue is not advanced with each row. Rather, the sutures obliterate the dead space. The final skin suture line of 3-0 monofilament suture must lie lateral to, not on, the olecranon or pressure will cause dehiscence (Fig. 9-2F).

Aftercare.   A forelimb spica-type splint, as described for Penrose drainage hygroma treatment (Fig. 9-1D) is

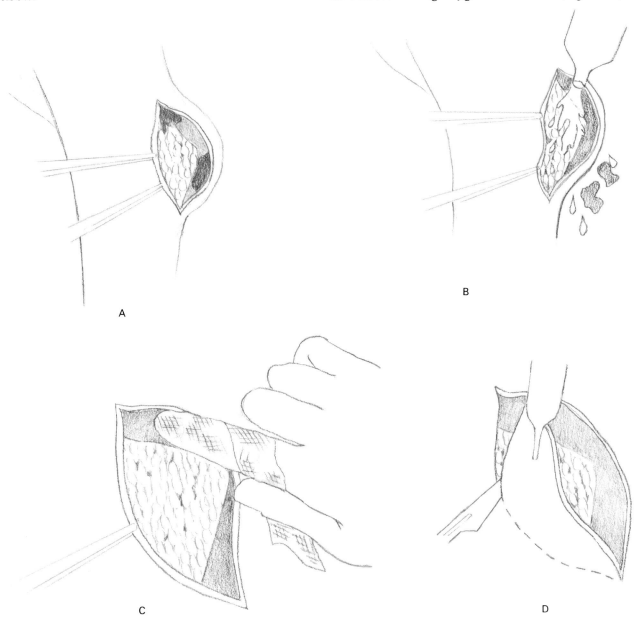

FIG. 9-2. Elbow hygroma corrected by suture obliteration. A, Incised hygroma exposing the cavity. B, Blood clots and fibrous septa removed. C, Debridement of the cavity with a gauze sponge. D, Redundant skin removed.

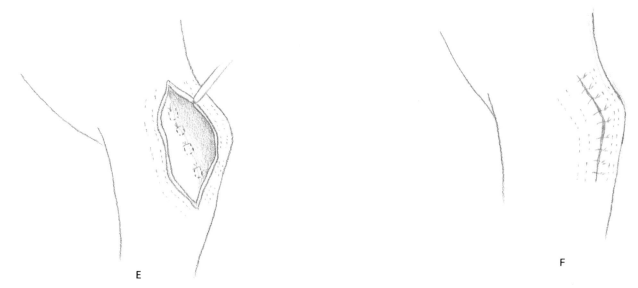

FIG. 9-2 continued. E, Sutures obliterate the cavity. F, Skin sutures positioned laterally.

applied and maintained for 10 days. The bandage that immobilizes the elbow following surgery is important for surgical success because movement disrupts the fragile capillary buds, which are necessary to lead to union of the debrided granulation surfaces. After the splint and sutures are removed, the elbow is protected with a light padded bandage until the tissues are strong enough to bear weight. The animal's bed and primary rest area should also be padded to protect the elbow.

Advantages and Disadvantages. The debridement and suture obliteration method described here results in a shorter period of bandaging, but is more difficult and has the potential of wound breakdown. The most serious complication, dehiscence, may result in chronic infection and an "ulcer" (see Elbow Ulceration, this chapter).

REFERENCE

1. Horne, R.D.: Auburn University, Personal communication, 1974.

ELBOW ULCERATION

Debridement and Closure or Advancement Flap

Definition and Indications. Chronic nonhealing ulcers of the skin over the olecranon may be caused by hygromas that become infected and dehisce after surgery or when trauma causes necrosis. Debridement and closure involve circumferential undermining and shifting of local skin to cover the ulcer. An advancement flap uses skin primarily from one side of the ulcer for coverage. If the inciting hygroma for an ulcer was small, adequate local skin is usually available to allow the wound to be debrided and closed or to advance a flap of local skin. These techniques, however, should not be used if the skin sutures must be placed under tension.

Techniques. *Debridement and Closure.* The dog is prepared for aseptic surgery, and the ulcer is thoroughly scrubbed and irrigated. Perioperative antibiotics are used because the ulcer must be considered infected, and an antibiotic-laden padded bandage may be used until the wound appears healthy. The margin of skin is excised (Fig. 9-3A) and the surface of the ulcer is debrided. Debridement may be accomplished by alternating use of scalpel, scissors, and a dry gauze sponge rubbed on the tissue (Fig. 9-3B). Particulate matter and tissue debris are flushed from the wound.

After all devitalized tissue is excised, the skin is undermined circumferentially (Fig. 9-3C). Because of the chronic inflammation, the wound margins and subcutaneous tissue are vascular. Hemorrhage should be controlled before the wound is closed. If adequate local skin is available, the wound may be sutured directly. With the elbow in extension, the skin is apposed with 3-0 monofilament vertical mattress sutures (Fig. 9-3D). "Walking" sutures of 3-0 absorbable material may be used to help move the tissues and attempt to place the suture line to one side of the olecranon.

Advancement Flap. See Single Pedicle Advancement Flap, Chapter 7. With larger ulcers, the suture line may be moved to one side of the elbow by creating an advancement flap, but if it is difficult to appose the skin without tension, a transposition flap should be used

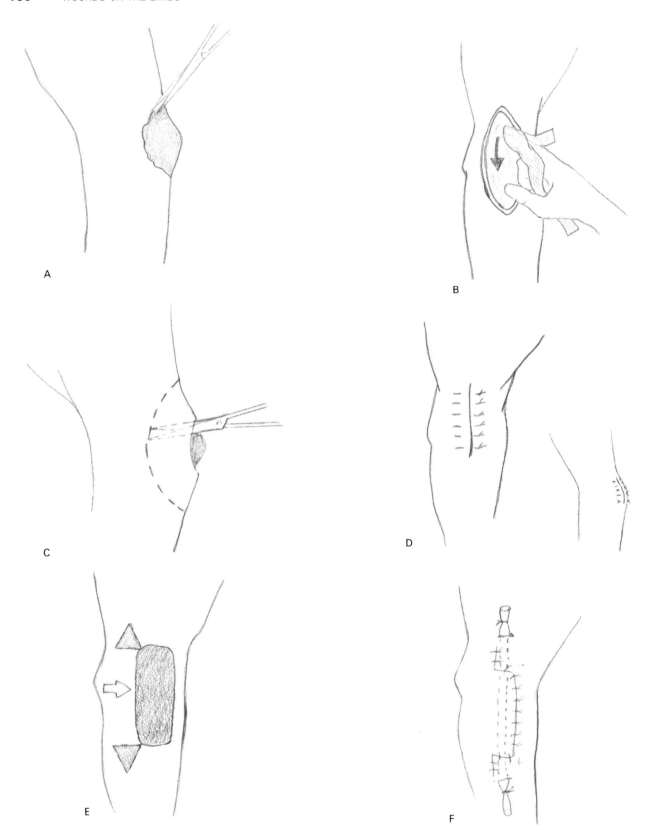

FIG. 9-3. Elbow ulceration corrected by debridement and closure or advancement flap. A, Debridement of ulcer margin. B, Debridement of ulcer surface with a sponge. C, Undermining ulcer margin. D, Direct apposition with vertical mattress sutures (caudal and side view). E, Preparation of advancement flap. F, Closure of flap over drain.

instead, see Elbow Ulceration, Transposition Flap, this chapter. To create an advancement flap, parallel incisions are made at the proximal and distal ends of the debrided ulcer, and Bürow's triangles may be removed to prevent "dog ears" (Fig. 9-3E). The flap is advanced and sutured in place, and a Penrose drain are placed if drainage is deemed necessary (Fig. 9-3F). "Walking" sutures may be used to give additional support and obliterate dead space.

Aftercare. A forelimb spica-type splint, as described for Penrose drainage hygroma treatment (see Fig. 9-1D), should be applied postoperatively. Bandage changes should follow the general guidelines for elbow hygromas that have been obliterated by suture (see Elbow Hygroma, Suture Obliteration, this chapter).

Advantages and Disadvantages. Local tissue used for reconstruction reduces the complexity of reconstruction associated with designing a flap. Direct closure should be reserved for small ulcers; however, with this technique, the final position of the suture line cannot be easily controlled and usually centers on the caudal aspect of the elbow, which predisposes it to injury and dehiscence. An advancement flap may allow better placement of the suture line, but requires making a larger wound to correct a smaller wound.

REFERENCES AND SUGGESTED READING

1. Johnston, D.E.: Hygroma of the elbow in dogs. *In* Current Techniques in Small Animal Surgery. Edited by M.J. Bojrab. Philadelphia, Lea & Febiger, 1975.
2. Krahwinkel, D.J., and Bone, D.: Surgical management of specific skin disorders. *In* Textbook of Small Animal Surgery. Edited by D.H. Slatter. Philadelphia, W.B. Saunders, 1985.
3. Krahwinkel, D.J.: Correction of specific skin diseases. *In* Surgery of Traumatized Skin: Management and Reconstruction in the Dog and Cat. Edited by S.F. Swaim. Philadelphia, W.B. Saunders, 1980.

Transposition Flap

Definition and Indications. See Elbow Ulceration Debridement and Closure or Advancement Flap, this chapter. If the resulting ulcer is large, the remaining local skin may be inadequate to allow the wound to be debrided and closed or to advance a flap. In this instance, a transposition flap is rotated from the adjacent area to cover the defect.

Technique. See Transposition Flap, Chapter 7. Perioperative antibiotics as directed by culture and sensitivity examination are used because the ulcer must be considered infected. The wound is prepared for surgery by applying a preoperative antibiotic-laden sterile dressing under a padded bandage. The dressing is used until the wound appears healthy, which may mean several

days. The dog is prepared for aseptic surgery, and the ulcer is thoroughly scrubbed and irrigated. The margin of the epithelium around the ulcer and the granulating base of the ulcer crater are debrided. Debridement may be accomplished by the alternating use of scalpel, scissors, and a dry gauze sponge rubbed on the tissue until all devitalized tissue is removed (see Fig. 9-3A and B). Particulate matter and tissue debris are flushed from the wound.

The skin is undermined circumferentially in an effort to attempt direct closure or evaluate the possibility of an advancement flap (see Fig. 9-3C). If the tension present is considered too great for direct closure or advancement flap, a transposition flap is prepared from skin on the caudomedial aspect of the humerus dorsal to the ulcer (Fig. 9-4A and B). The dimensions of the flap are made so that the width of the flap is the same as the width of the defect. Ideally, the length of the flap should be such that the diagonal from the pivot point of the flap to its far corner is equal in length to the diagonal from the pivot point to the farthest corner of the debrided ulcer. The wound created to harvest the flap may extend onto the thoracic wall if necessary for additional length or breadth. The flap is elevated with as much subcutaneous tissue as possible to provide blood supply. The recipient site may be very vascular because of the chronic inflammation; hemorrhage should be controlled before transposing the flap and closing the wound.

The flap is transposed and sutured in place with 3-0 simple interrupted monofilament sutures (Fig. 9-4C), followed by similar closure of the donor site (Fig. 9-4D). The "dog ear" that forms at the bend of the flap base is ignored because its correction may compromise the blood supply to the flap. If necessary, the "dog ear" can be corrected at a later time. If capillary hemorrhage is significant, a 1/4 inch diameter Penrose drain may be placed under the flap.

Aftercare. A forelimb spica-type splint, as described for Penrose drainage hygroma treatment, (see Fig. 9-1D) should be applied postoperatively. Bandage changes should follow the general guidelines for elbow hygromas that have been obliterated by suture (see Elbow Hygroma, Suture Obliteration, this chapter).

Advantages and Disadvantages. Designing a transposition flap is more difficult than transferring local tissue to close an ulcer. Although transposition flaps are more time-consuming in initial application and require making a wound to correct a wound, they are time-efficient if they prevent the need to repair a tension-induced dehiscence. Preparation of the wound for an attempted direct closure or advancement flap does not interfere with the use of a transposition flap as described if manipulation of the skin reveals that direct closure on an advancement flap would produce excessive tension.

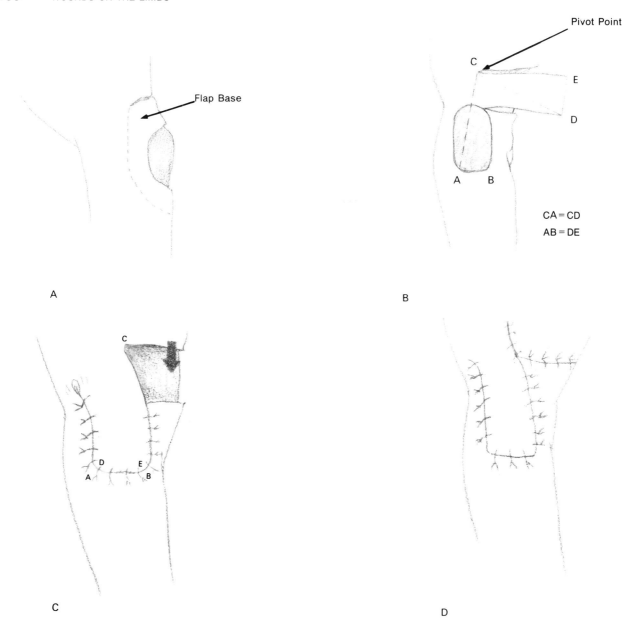

FIG. 9-4. Elbow ulceration corrected by transposition flap. A, Lateral view of debrided ulcer, undermined skin (broken line) and flap base. B, Caudal view of flap raised (CA = CD and AB = DE). C, Flap transposed and sutured, shifting of skin over donor site (arrow). D, Donor site sutured.

REFERENCE AND SUGGESTED READING

1. Leighton, R.L.: Chronic ulcer of the olecranon treated by skin graft. Vet. Med. *79*:55, 1984.

MID AND DISTAL THORACIC LIMB

POUCH FLAP

Definition and Indications.   A pouch flap is a double pedicle flap that is created on the body and used to reconstruct a defect on an extremity by moving the extremity to the flap (Fig. 9-5A through D).

Technique.   It may be wise to bandage the animal's leg along its side for 2 to 3 days before surgery to ascertain if it will tolerate the leg bandaged in this position.

The lateral thoraco-abdominal area and the limb to be reconstructed, including the paw on that limb, should be prepared for aseptic surgery. The animal is placed in lateral recumbency with the affected limb uppermost. Epithelial tissue at the wound edge is removed. The

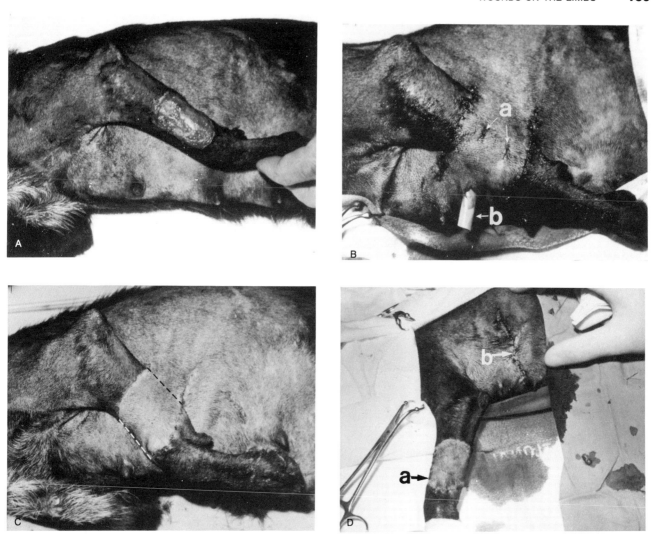

FIG. 9-5. Pouch flap to reconstruct a forelimb defect. A, Forelimb with skin defect in position for pouch flap. B, Pouch flap from thoracic area over defect. Tacking sutures hold flap against wound (a). Penrose drain placed (b). C, Healed pouch flap after 14 days' placement. Incision lines drawn to separate flap from body (broken lines). D, Pouch flap on limb (a). Donor site closed (b).

defect is covered with a surgical sponge soaked in a 1:40 dilution of chlorhexidine diacetate* while the flap is prepared. The limb is placed along the animal's side in the most comfortable position, which minimizes stress on the joints. The level of the proximal edge of the defect along the animal's side is noted and an incision is made in the thoracic or abdominal skin perpendicular to the limb's axis. Then a second incision is made parallel to the first at the level of the distal edge of the defect so that the distance between the incisions is equal to the dorso-ventral dimension of the limb defect (Fig. 9-6A).

If the wound completely encircles the limb, the flap is undermined, the limb is flexed, and the paw is passed under the flap. The limb is moved until the defect lies under the flap. Simple interrupted 3-0 nonabsorbable monofilament[†] sutures are used to suture the edges of the flap and wound together (Fig. 9-6B). If the wound involves only the lateral aspect of the limb with normal skin on the medial aspect of the leg and the defect is not too long, the flap is undermined and elevated. Skin on either side of the flap is advanced beneath the flap using "walking" sutures and the edges are sutured together with 3-0 simple interrupted monofilament nonabsorbable sutures (inset). When the limb is passed under the flap, the normal skin on the medial side of the leg is in contact with the sutured skin under the flap rather than the subcutis of the thorax. The raw undersurface of the flap is in contact with the wound on the lateral aspect of the leg.

---

*Nolvasan solution, Ft. Dodge Laboratories, Ft. Dodge, IA.

[†]Monofilament as used in this chapter excludes stainless steel.

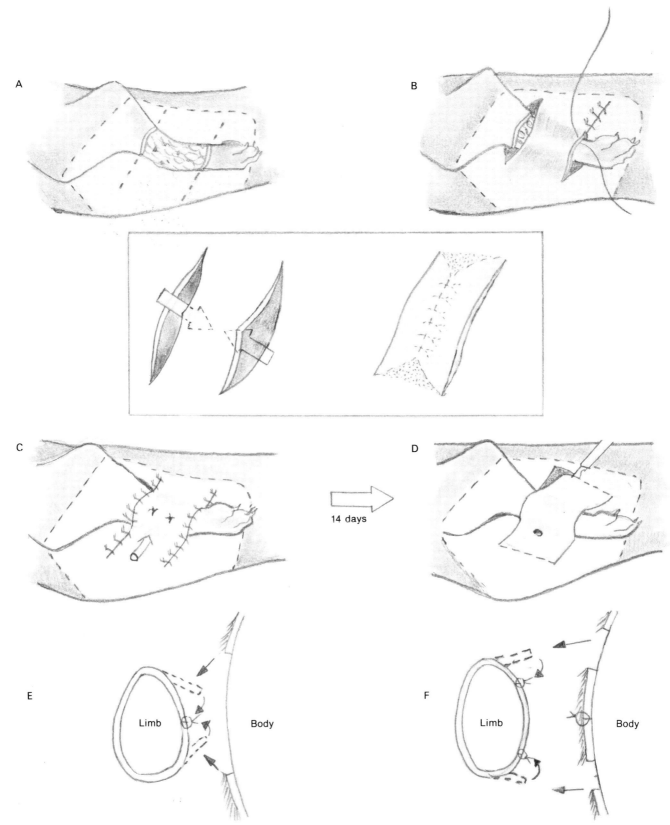

FIG. 9-6. Pouch flap to reconstruct a forelimb skin defect. A, Limb wound with proposed flap site. B, Suturing flap to the wound. Inset: Suturing adjacent skin edges together under flap. C, Placement of drain under limb/flap area. D, Cutting flap attachments. E, Final flap transfer when defect encircles limb. F, Final flap transfer when defect does not encircle limb.

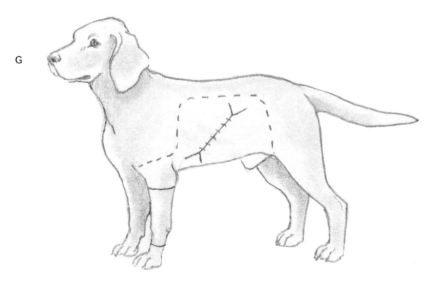

FIG. 9-6 continued. G, Flap transferred to limb, donor site sutured.

Two or three tacking sutures may be placed to immobilize the flap to the defect. A small Penrose drain should be placed in the most dependent base of the flap to allow drainage of any fluid that may accumulate in the space around the limb and flap. This is especially important if the wound completely encircles the limb and the adjacent skin edges have not been sutured together under the flap as described above (Fig. 9-6C).

After approximately 14 days, the thoraco-abdominal bases of the flap are incised, allowing sufficient skin for complete closure of the defect if the defect completely encircled the limb (Fig. 9-6D). If the medial surface of the limb has adhered to the body wall, it should be dissected free. The two edges of the flap are wrapped around the remaining defect, then trimmed and sutured together on the medial side of the limb with 3-0 simple interrupted nonabsorbable sutures (Fig. 9-6E). If the defect did not completely encircle the limb, the two edges of the flap are sutured to the remaining freshly debrided skin edges of the defect with the same type of suture material and pattern (Fig. 9-6F). The thoraco-abdominal donor site is closed by undermining and advancing the skin edges together with "walking" sutures and skin apposition sutures or skin staples (Fig. 9-6G). If the development of adequate blood supply in the flap is questionable after 14 days, the flap may be left attached to the body longer or separated from the body in stages as a surgical delaying technique (severance of one pedicle of the flap followed by severance of the second pedicle 3 to 5 days later).

Aftercare. After suturing the flap to the limb, the limb is bandaged against the body for *approximately 14 days*, with periodic bandage changes, especially if there is copious drainage. When bandaging, extra absorbent bandage material should be placed over the drain. Care should be taken to avoid pressure over the carpus and olecranon to prevent pressure sores. Donut-type pads may be placed over these areas when bandaging (see Pressure Sores, Chapter 4). After the flap has been completely transferred to the limb, it should be protected by a bandage for another 7 to 10 days.

Advantages and Disadvantages. Such flaps are cosmetic because they provide a full-thickness, fully haired piece of skin for reconstruction. The direction of hair growth is acceptable on the forelimb. Pouch flaps are functional because such skin can withstand the trauma to which it will be subjected on the distal limb. These flaps have the advantage of having two pedicles (one dorsal and one ventral) that support the limb against the body while vascular linkage develops between the flap and the defect. These flaps work best on the thoracic limbs of small dogs and cats because bandaging this limb along the animal's side is relatively comfortable for the animal. After the limb is released from its side, the animal may be lame in that limb for a few days.

REFERENCES AND SUGGESTED READING

1. Alexander, J.W., Hoffer, R.E., and MacDonald, J.M.: The use of tubular flap grafts in the treatment of traumatic wounds on the extremity of the cat. Feline Pract. *6*:29, 1976.
2. Johnston, D.E.: The repair of skin loss on the foot by means of a double-pedicle abdominal flap. J. Am. Anim. Hosp. Assoc. *12*:593, 1976.

3. Pope, E.R., and Swaim, S.F.: Shifting tissue and using flaps. Vet. Med. *81*:512, 1986.
4. Swaim, S.F.: The repair of the skin: Techniques for plastic and reconstructive surgery. *In* Atlas of Canine Surgical Techniques. Edited by P.G.C. Bedford. Oxford, Blackwell Scientific Publications, 1984.
5. Swaim, S.F.: Foot salvage techniques in dogs and cats: Options, "Do's" and Don'ts". J. Am. Anim. Hosp. Assoc. *21*:511, 1985.
6. Sykes, G.P.: Pouch graft: Resurfacing the distal extremity of a dog. Canine Pract. *7*:28, 1980.
7. Yturraspe, D.J., Creed, J.E., and Schwach, R.P.: Thoracic pedicle skin flap for repair of lower limb wounds in dogs and cats. J. Am. Anim. Hosp. Assoc. *12*:581, 1976.

STRIP GRAFTS

Definition and Indications. Strip grafts are 5 mm wide strips of full-thickness skin that are placed in 2 mm deep, parallel linear grooves, 3 to 5 mm apart, cut in a bed of healthy granulation tissue. These grafts provide skin coverage for defects where local flaps or moving local tissue cannot be used for wound closure (mid and lower limb skin defects) (Fig. 9-7A through C).

Techniques. Once a wound has formed a bed of healthy granulation tissue that is starting to epithelialize, strip grafts may be applied. The animal is placed in lateral recumbency with the affected area exposed. The wound surface is prepared by wiping it with a surgical sponge. While the wound is protected with a sterile sponge soaked in a 1:40 dilution of chlorhexidine diacetate*, the area around the wound and the lower craniolateral thoracic area are prepared for aseptic surgery.

With a No. 15 scalpel blade, parallel 2 mm deep longitudinal incisions are made about 3 to 5 mm apart in the granulation tissue (Fig. 9-8A). As the granulation tissue is incised, it should retract to form a groove wide enough to accommodate a 5-mm-wide strip graft. If not, the scalpel blade may be used to trim some of the granulation tissue off the sides of the groove.

Using a sterile splintered wooden applicator stick or sterile toothpick dipped in methylene blue, 5-mm-wide parallel lines are drawn on the lower craniolateral

---

*Nolvasan solution, Fort Dodge Laboratories, Fort Dodge, IA.

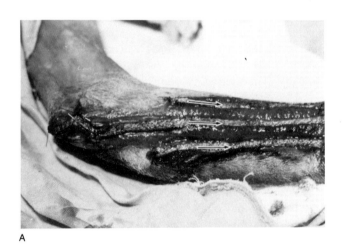

A

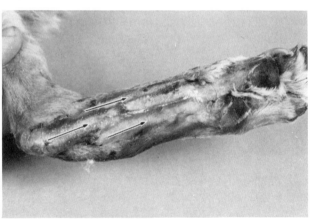

B

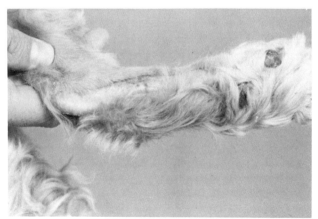

C

FIG. 9-7. Strip grafts to correct a pelvic limb skin defect. A, Three strip grafts in a bed of granulation tissue (arrows). B, Strip grafts after 14 days' placement (arrows). C, Healed strip grafted wound. (A and B from Swaim, S.F., Lee, A.H., Newton, J.C., and McGuire, J.A.: Evaluation of strip skin grafts in dogs. J. Am. Anim. Hosp. Assoc. *23*:115, 1987).

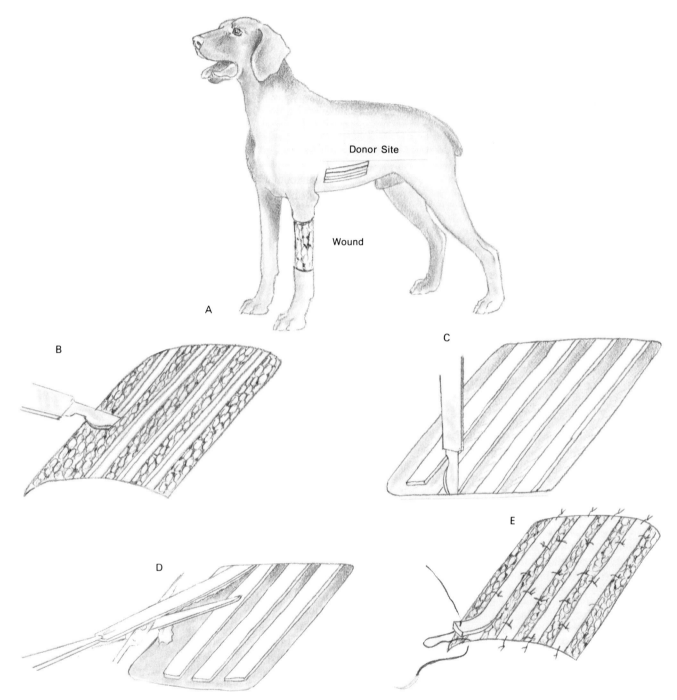

FIG. 9-8. Strip grafts to reconstruct a forelimb skin defect. A, Dog with limb wound showing donor site. B, Cutting grooves in granulation tissue. C, Cutting strip grafts free on one end. D, Removing subcutaneous tissue from strip grafts. E, Suturing strip grafts into grooves.

thoracic area. The number of strips created will be one fewer than the number of lines drawn. The strips are formed as each line and one end of the strips are incised with a No. 15 scalpel blade (Fig. 9-8B). Sequentially, each strip is elevated and tensed with thumb forceps, the subcutaneous fat is removed with scissors (Fig. 9-8C), and the other end of each strip is cut free.

The strips are laid in the previously cut grooves with the hair growth on the graft going in the same direction as the hair around the defect. A simple interrupted 3-0 monofilament nonabsorbable suture is placed at each end of each strip to anchor the grafts and at intervals as deemed necessary along the strips to further anchor each strip into its groove (Fig. 9-8D).

alternative to making the pattern of the wound is to measure the wound at its widest and longest points. These points are marked on the donor site and a basically rectangular graft is drawn within them (inset).

The pattern is removed from the donor area and the traced line is incised with a No. 15 scalpel blade. The graft is removed (Fig. 9-10D) and placed on a piece of sterile cardboard (such as the back of a writing tablet that has been autoclaved), dermal side up. Long doubled strands of 2-0 silk or sterile string are placed at intervals around the edge of the graft and pulled through slits cut in the edge of the cardboard, thus stretching the graft. Alternately, the graft may be fixed to the cardboard with sterile hypodermic needles. Scissors and thumb forceps are used to remove all subcutaneous tissue from the graft (Fig. 9-10E), and a No. 11 scalpel blade is used to cut parallel rows of staggered incisions in the graft. Incisions are approximately 1 cm long and 0.5 cm apart (Fig. 9-10F).

The graft is removed from the cardboard and placed on the wound so that the direction of hair growth on the graft matches that on the skin around the defect. Using 3-0 or 4-0 monofilament nonabsorbable suture in a simple interrupted or simple continuous pattern, one edge of the graft is sutured to its corresponding wound edge, or alternatively, skin staples may be used. Two to 3 mm of skin are trimmed from the opposite side of the graft before it is sutured in place to ensure expansion of the mesh holes (Fig. 9-10G). If a rectangular piece of skin was harvested from the donor site instead of one patterned after the wound, one edge is sutured to an edge of the defect, and the graft is trimmed to fit the defect and then sutured to the remaining wound edges.

The graft is further immobilized on the defect by placing 3-0 or 4-0 monofilament nonabsorbable simple interrupted tacking sutures between adjacent slits in the graft at points where the graft lies over concave or convex portions of the wound and at other intermittent places, but not through all adjacent slits (Fig. 9-10H).

The donor site is closed by undermining and advancing the skin edges together with "walking" sutures and skin apposition sutures or skin staples.

Aftercare. See Strip Grafts, this chapter.

Advantages and Disadvantages. Slits of a mesh graft provide flexibility so that the graft conforms better to concave and convex surfaces as well as irregular edges. The grafts are more stable because they are immobilized on the wound surface by sutures through the slits. Granulation tissue grows up into the slits of the graft to help immobilize it and provide vessels that grow into the cut edges of the dermis for revascularization. The slits allow serum, blood, and exudate to drain from under the graft, permitting it to contact the wound

for revascularization. A disadvantage of mesh grafts is their uncosmetic appearance early in the wound healing process; however, as they heal, the mesh slits become less noticeable as they get smaller and hair regrows on the graft. As a graft is expanded more, the cosmetic effect is diminished, but too little expansion may result in the accumulation of blood, serum, or exudate under the graft with a poor graft take. If an animal tends to produce excess granulation tissue, it may grow up through the mesh holes and partially overgrow the surface of the graft. Topical application of a steroid generally reduces the granulation tissue.

REFERENCES AND SUGGESTED READING

1. Swaim, S.F.: Principles of mesh grafting. Compend. Contin. Educ. 4:194, 1982.
2. Swaim, S.F., Pope, E.R., Lee A.H., and McGuire, J.A.: Evaluation of a practical skin grafting technique. J. Am. Anim. Hosp. Assoc. 20:637, 1984.
3. Swaim, S.F.: The full-thickness mesh graft. Vet. Med. 81:524, 1986.

PROXIMAL PELVIC LIMB (STIFLE AND ABOVE)

BODY FLAP

Definition and Indications. A body flap is a flap of skin created on the caudal distolateral abdominal area to cover a defect of the stifle area by moving the pelvic limb cranially to insert the stifle under the flap. After 14 days, the flap is transected from the donor site with enough skin to fold medially to cover the medial aspect of the stifle (Fig. 9-11A through E). The technique works best on cats and small female dogs.

Technique. The lateral thoraco-abdominal area and the limb to be reconstructed should be prepared for aseptic surgery. The animal is placed in lateral recumbency with the affected limb uppermost. If the wound is covered with healthy granulation tissue, the wound surface is wiped with a surgical sponge. If epithelium is present at the wound edge, it is removed. The defect is covered with a surgical sponge soaked in a 1:40 dilution of chlorhexidine diacetate* while the flap is prepared. The limb is placed along the animal's side in a position that does not place undue stress on the joints to determine the best position for the flap (Fig. 9-12A).

An incision matching the lateral aspect of the stifle defect in curvature and length is made in the skin along

---

*Nolvasan solution, Ft. Dodge Laboratories, Ft. Dodge, IA.

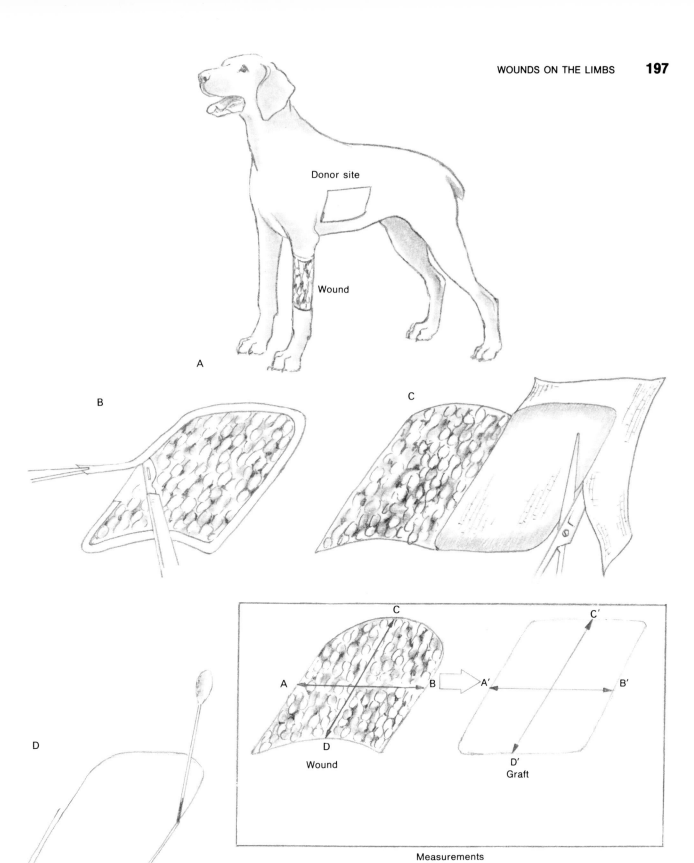

FIG. 9-10. Mesh graft to reconstruct a forelimb skin defect. A. Dog with limb wound showing donor site. B, Removing epithelium from wound edge. C, Cutting a pattern of wound from sterile cloth. D, Tracing pattern on donor site. Inset: Alternative technique for planning a graft. Take length and width measurements of wound, draw graft on donor site with same measurements.

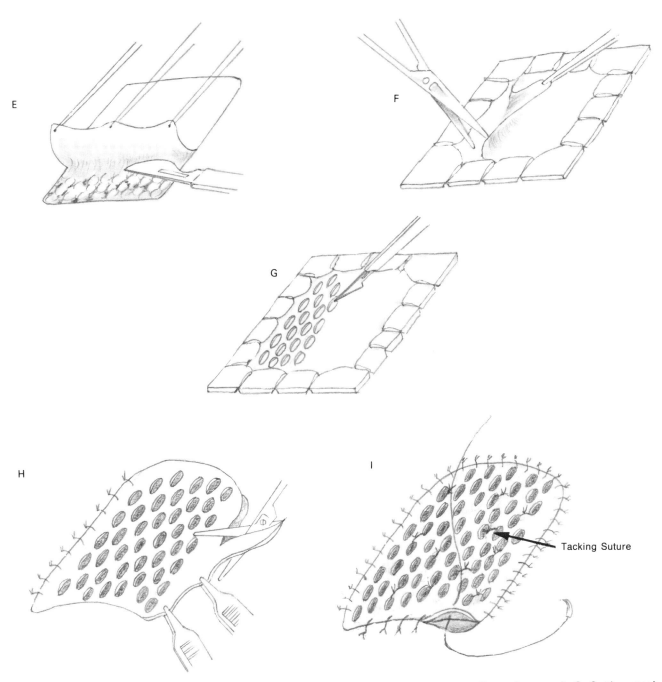

FIG. 9-10 continued. E, Removing graft from donor site. F, Removing the subcutaneous tissue from graft. G, Cutting mesh holes in graft. H, Trimming the opposite edge of the graft after first edge is sutured. I, Suturing graft in place and tacking it to wound surface.

the ventrolateral aspect of the abdomen. The skin cranial to the incision is undermined. The stifle is advanced cranially and the defect is inserted under the flap (Fig. 9-12B). The edge of the flap is sutured to the lateral aspect of the stifle defect using 3-0 nonabsorbable monofilament simple interrupted sutures (Fig. 9-12C).

After approximately 14 days, the attachment of the flap to the side of the body is cut free, cutting sufficient skin from the body to cover the medial aspect of the stifle defect. As a guideline, the calculated amount of skin to cover the lesion plus at least another centimeter of skin should be taken to allow coverage of the medial aspect of the defect (Fig. 9-12D). Pinching the abdominal skin in the area of the lesion with the thumb and fingers may give the surgeon an idea of how much skin can be removed without causing a difficult closure of the resultant defect. The edge of free skin is trimmed and sutured to the medial edge of the stifle defect with the same suture material and pattern mentioned above. The donor site defect is closed by undermining and advancing the skin edges together with "walking" sutures or tension sutures and apposition sutures or staples (Fig. 9-12E and inset).

Aftercare. After the flap is sutured to the lateral aspect of the stifle defect, the limb should be bandaged

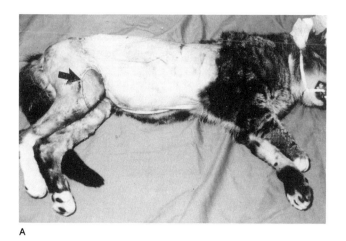

A

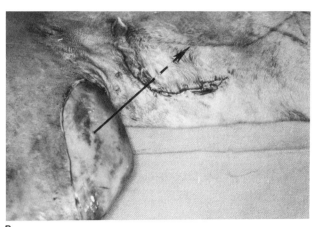

B

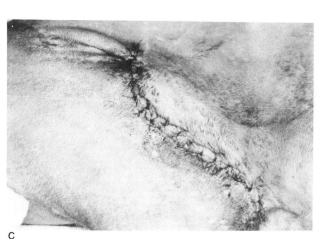

C

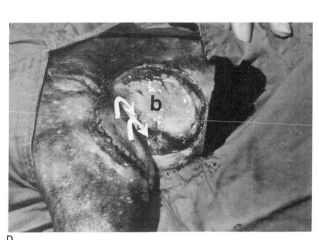

D

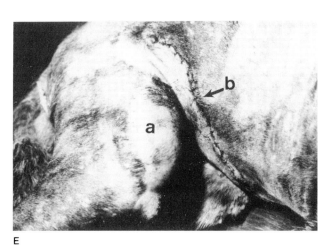

E

FIG. 9-11. Body flap to correct cranial stifle skin defect. A, Cranial stifle defect on a cat (arrow). B, Flap incised in caudo-lateral abdominal skin. Stifle will be advanced cranially to insert defect under flap (arrow). C, Edge of body flap sutured to lateral stifle skin edge. D, Fourteen days postoperatively, flap is severed from body with enough skin to fold medially to cover medial aspect of stifle (arrows). Donor site (b). E, Donor site closed (b). Flap (a) transferred to the limb. (B through E from Swaim, S.F., and Bushby, P.A.: Correction of skin defects of the stifle of dogs and cats. J. Am. Anim. Hosp. Assoc. *17*:447–448, 1981).

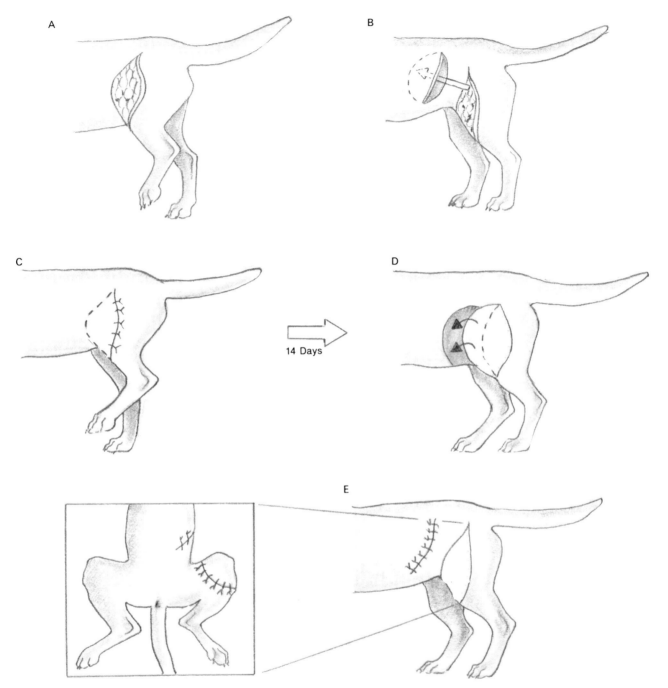

FIG. 9-12. Body flap to correct cranial stifle defect. A, Flexing stifle along caudo-lateral abdomen to determine site for flap. B, Caudo-lateral abdominal skin incised and undermined. Stifle will be advanced under flap (arrow). C, Flap edge sutured to lateral edge of stifle defect. D, Skin incised from caudo-lateral abdomen to fold over (arrows) and cover medial aspect of stifle. E, Inset: Skin sutured to medial aspect of stifle. Donor site sutured.

against the body for *approximately 14 days* with periodic bandage changes. When bandaging, extra-absorbent bandage material should be placed in the area of the remaining medial stifle defect to absorb exudate. In cats, the lateral aspect of the flap has often healed in place by 7 to 10 days, and immobilization of the leg against the body may not be necessary. If it is decided to remove the immobilizing bandage after 7 to 10 days, the cat should be observed for 12 to 24 hours for evidence of wound disruption and/or molestation. Exercise should be limited to a cage. After the flap has been completely transferred to the limb, a protective bandage may be necessary if the cat molests the suture line.

Advantages and Disadvantages. The technique provides a fully-haired, full-thickness segment of skin for closure of a large stifle defect. The technique, however, requires two surgical procedures: attachment of the flap to the lateral aspect of the defect and attachment of the flap to the medial aspect of the defect. Because a cat often rests with its stifles fully flexed, any suture lines in the area may be under tension, which may cause wound disruption and/or slowed healing. This is the reason for obtaining ample skin from the lateral abdominal area to cover the medial aspect of the stifle lesion.

REFERENCE AND SUGGESTED READING

1. Swaim, S.F. and Bushby, P.A.: Correction of skin defects of the stifle of dogs and cats. J. Am. Anim. Hosp. Assoc. *17*:445, 1981.

MESH GRAFT

Definition and Indications. See Mid and Distal Thoracic Limb, Mesh Graft, this chapter. These grafts can be used on the proximal portion of the pelvic limb to cover defects over the stifle area.

Technique. See Mid and Distal Thoracic Limb, Mesh Graft, this chapter.

Aftercare. See Mid and Distal Thoracic Limb, Mesh Graft, this chapter. Immobilization of the stifle joint while the graft takes may be accomplished with a Schroeder-Thomas splint (Fig. 9-13A). A more effective immobilization of the stifle can be accomplished with an external pin splint apparatus (Fig. 9-13C). Such joint immobilization is generally needed only during the first 10 to 14 days after grafting. Either of these immobilization techniques can be applied so that a bandage can be applied over the graft (Fig. 9-13B and D). With an external pin splint, if bandages are applied the full length of the leg to help prevent distal limb edema, the portion of the bandage over the graft may be cut out to allow for daily bandage changes without removal of the entire bandage.

Advantages and Disadvantages. See Mid and Distal Thoracic Limb, Mesh Graft, this chapter.

REFERENCES AND SUGGESTED READING

See Mid and Distal Thoracic Limb, Mesh Graft, this chapter.

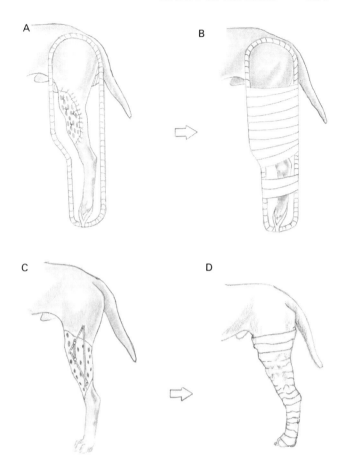

FIG. 9-13. Mesh graft immobilization and bandaging over stifle. A, Schroeder-Thomas splint on pelvic limb immobilizing stifle. B, Bandage applied over grafted area and affixed to the splint. C, Transarticular external pin splint placed in femur and tibia, immobilizing stifle. D, Bandage applied over grafted area and splint.

AXIAL PATTERN FLAP (CAUDAL SUPERFICIAL EPIGASTRIC)

Definition and Indications. An axial pattern flap is a skin flap with a single neurovascular trunk that supplies the tissue and allows it to be moved. In this case, it is based on the caudal superficial epigastric vessels and the segment of skin and underlying subcutis or mammary tissue (in females) from the second to the fifth mammae that is elevated along with the caudal superficial epigastric artery and vein. The flap may be used to reconstruct skin defects in the flank, inner thigh, and inguinal areas.

Technique. The entire ventral thoraco-abdomen, flank, groin, and pelvic limb on which the defect is located are prepared for aseptic surgery. The animal is placed in dorsal recumbency. If the wound is covered with healthy granulation tissue, it should be wiped with

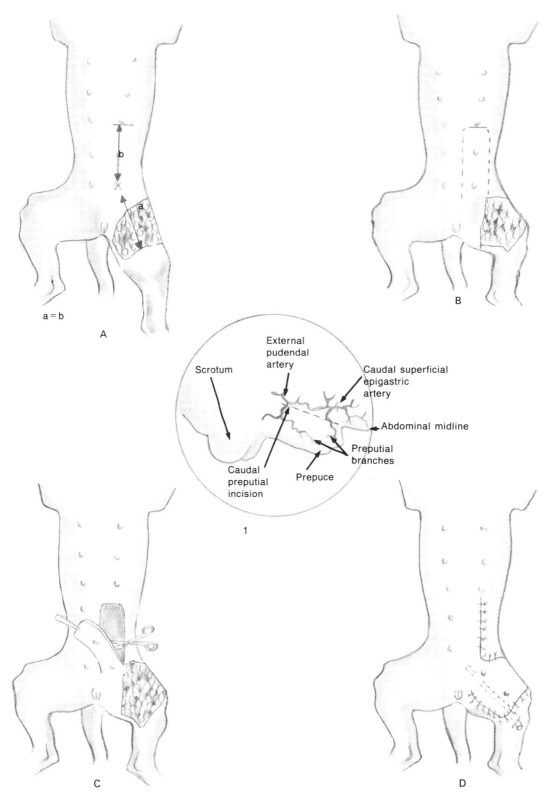

FIG. 9-14. Caudal superficial epigastric axial pattern flap to correct inner thigh defect. A, With leg extended, measurement made from origin of caudal superficial epigastric artery to distalmost edge of lesion (a). Same measurement made cranially along mammary chain and marked (b). B, An axial pattern flap based on caudal superficial epigastric vessels. Inset 1: In males, medial flap incision along dorsal base of prepuce and continued along ventral midline. C, Flap incised, undermined, and elevated. D, Flap rotated over defect and sutured, with a drain under it. Donor site closed.

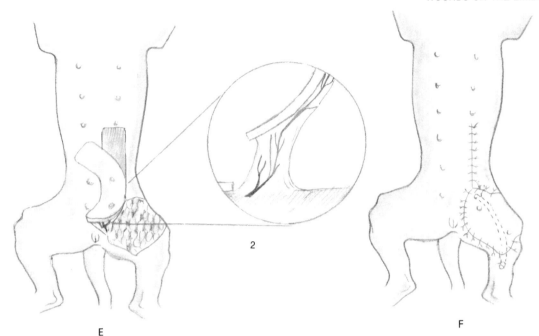

2

E   F

FIG. 9-14 continued. E, Creating an island axial pattern flap based on caudal superficial epigastric vessels. Inset 2: Skin at flap base incised, subcutaneous tissue and caudal superficial epigastric vessels left intact. F, Flap rotated over defect and sutured, with a drain under it. Donor site closed. (B, Inset 1 after Pavletic, M.M.: Pedicle grafts. *In* Textbook of Small Animal Surgery. Edited by D.H. Slatter. Philadelphia, W.B. Saunders, 1985, p. 476).

a surgical sponge and any epithelium present at the wound edge should be removed. The wound is covered with a surgical sponge soaked in a 1:40 dilution of chlorhexidine diacetate.*

A measurement is made from the emergence of the external pudendal/caudal superficial epigastric vessels, just caudal to the last mammary gland, to the farthest extent of the skin defect with the leg in extension. This length is measured cranially along the mammary chain from the origin of the vessels. The length is marked on the skin (Fig. 9-14A).

An axial pattern flap based on the caudal superficial epigastric vessels is drawn on the donor site (Fig. 9-14B). On females, a midline abdominal skin incision is made from a point 3 to 5 cm caudal to the last teat to the previously marked point on the mammary chain (Fig. 9-14B and C). On males, it is necessary to incise along the dorsal base of the prepuce and then continue the incision along the ventral midline to the desired point (inset 1). At the previously marked point, the incision is directed laterally for a distance lateral to the teats equal to the medial distance between the teats and ventral midline incision. The incision is then directed caudally and extended parallel to the ventral midline incision until it reaches the point opposite the origin of the incision (Fig. 9-14B and C). Metzenbaum scissors are used to undermine the flap of tissue deep to the cuta-

neous musculature, the musculus preputialis in males and the musculus supramammarius in females. Dissection is kept close to the aponeurosis of the external abdominal oblique muscle (Fig. 9-14C). Hemorrhage is controlled by electrocoagulation and ligation. In males, ligation of the preputial branch of the caudal superficial epigastric vessels is necessary.

After the flap is elevated, it is rotated to cover skin defects of the flank, medial thigh, or inguinal areas. Monofilament 3-0 nonabsorbable simple continuous sutures with an occasional lock stitch, simple interrupted sutures, or staples may be used to affix the flap in place at the wound edges. To prevent serum or blood accumulation under the flap, a Penrose drain is placed under the flap in such a manner that it traverses the entire length of the flap and emerges from a stab incision approximately 2 cm distal to the most dependent portion of the flap (Fig. 9-14D).

The donor site is closed by undermining the skin and advancing the edges together with "walking" sutures followed by placement of skin apposition sutures or staples (Fig. 9-14D).

To facilitate rotation of the flap to reach defects of the inner thigh, flank, or inguinal areas, the flap may be converted to an island axial pattern flap by connecting the medial and lateral flap incisions caudal to the last mammary gland. This incision is through the skin only; dissection and cutting of the underlying tissue should be avoided or done very carefully to prevent damage to the

---

*Nolvasan solution, Ft. Dodge Laboratories, Ft. Dodge, IA.

external pudendal and caudal superficial epigastric vessels that supply the flap (Fig. 9-14E and inset 2). The flap is rotated and sutured in place, and a drain is placed under it as previously described. The donor site is also closed as previously described (Fig. 9-14F).

Aftercare. Sterile absorbable surgical sponges are placed over the suture lines, with extra sponges placed over the drain tube. Absorbent bandage is wrapped around the trunk and affected limb, followed by placement of 2" adhesive tape over the wrap. The bandage should be changed daily during the first few days after surgery, when drainage is at its maximum. As the amount of drainage decreases, the bandages may be changed less often on the basis of clinical judgment. The drain should be removed when drainage is minimal, generally 5 to 7 days postoperatively.

Advantages and Disadvantages. Because this flap carries major vessels along its long axis, a relatively long flap can be made to reach defects on the pelvic limb. Compared to graft reconstruction on the limb, bandaging and immobilization of the reconstructed area are not as critical to success of the reconstruction when an axial pattern flap is used. The flap carries its blood supply with it, whereas the graft must develop a new blood supply based on strict immobilization of the grafted part while new vessels become established in the graft. Use of this flap requires making a larger skin defect to correct a smaller defect, and it places mammary tissue in an abnormal location.

REFERENCES AND SUGGESTED READING

1. Pavletic, M.M.: Caudal superficial epigastric arterial pedicle grafts in the dog. Vet. Surg. 9:103, 1980.
2. Pavletic, M.M., and Peyton, L.C.: Plastic and reconstructive surgery in the dog and cat. *In* Current Techniques in Small Animal Surgery II. Edited by M.J. Bojrab. Philadelphia, Lea & Febiger, 1983.
3. Pavletic, M.M.: Pedicle grafts. *In* Textbook of Small Animal Surgery. Edited by D.H. Slatter. Philadelphia, W.B. Saunders, 1985.

MID AND DISTAL PELVIC LIMB

POUCH FLAP

Definition and Indications. See Mid and Distal Thoracic Limb, Pouch Flap, this chapter. These flaps may be used to cover defects on the mid and distal portions of the pelvic limb. If used on the pelvic limb, these flaps work best on cats and small female dogs.

Technique. See Mid and Distal Thoracic Limb, Pouch Flap, this chapter and Figure 9-15A.

Aftercare. See Mid and Distal Thoracic Limb, Pouch Flap, this chapter.

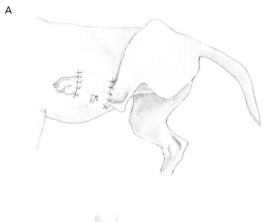

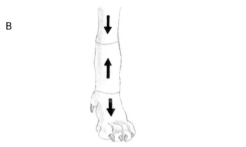

FIG. 9-15. Pouch flap to correct a distal pelvic limb defect. A, Pouch flap sutured over defect. B, Direction of hair growth on a pelvic limb pouch flap usually opposite that on surrounding areas.

Advantages and Disadvantages. See Mid and Distal Thoracic Limb, Pouch Flap, this chapter. A disadvantage of a pouch flap on the pelvic limb is that it may not be as cosmetic as when used on the front limb. The direction of hair growth on the flap is more likely to be just the opposite of that on the remainder of the limb (Fig. 9-15B). Use of a pouch flap on the pelvic limb of a large and/or a male dog is more difficult because of the size and/or the presence of genitalia that must be bandaged around.

REFERENCES AND SUGGESTED READING

See Mid and Distal Thoracic Limb, Pouch Flap, this chapter.

AXIAL PATTERN FLAP (CAUDAL SUPERFICIAL EPIGASTRIC)

Definition and Indications. See Proximal Pelvic Limb, Axial Pattern Flap (Caudal Superficial Epigastric), this chapter. This type of flap could be used to reconstruct defects on the upper medial aspect of the tibial area.

Technique. See Proximal Pelvic Limb, Axial Pattern Flap, (Caudal Superficial Epigastric), this chapter. To

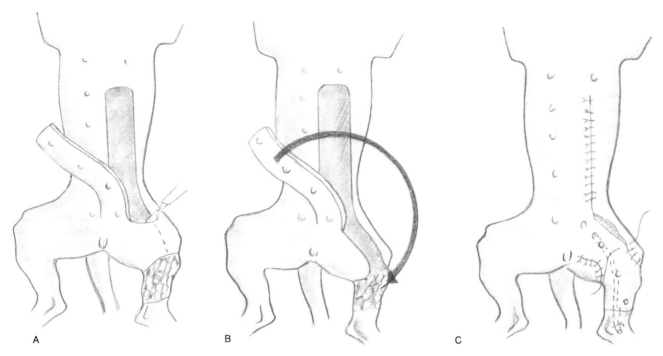

FIG. 9-16. Caudal superficial epigastric axial pattern flap to correct skin defect over tibial region. A, Flap elevated. Bridging incision being made between defect and caudolateral aspect of flap base. B, Flap rotating into place. C, Flap sutured into defect and to edges of bridging incision. (C after Pavletic, M.M.: Pedicle grafts. *In* Textbook of Small Animal Surgery. Edited by D.H. Slatter. Philadelphia, W.B. Saunders, 1985, p. 476).

reconstruct defects of the mid portion of the pelvic limb, an axial pattern flap based on the external pudendal/caudal superficial epigastric vessels can be used in combination with a bridging incision. The flap is elevated in the manner previously described, and a bridging incision is made between the caudal end of the lateralmost flap incision and the proximal aspect of the defect (Fig. 9-16A). The flap is rotated into position (Fig. 9-16B) and affixed to the edges of the defect. The remaining edges of the flap are sutured to the respective edges of the bridging incision (Fig. 9-16C). Monofilament 3-0 nonabsorbable simple continuous or simple interrupted sutures or staples are used. To help create a more cosmetic appearance, the edges of the bridging incision may be trimmed back so that the flap fits more smoothly in the defect. A Penrose drain is placed under the length of the flap, emerging 2 cm distal to the most dependent portion of the flap. The donor site is closed by undermining and advancing the skin edges together with "walking" sutures followed by placement of skin apposition sutures or staples (see Fig. 9-16C).

Aftercare. See Proximal Pelvic Limb, Axial Pattern Flap, (Caudal Superficial Epigastric), this chapter.

Advantages and Disadvantages. See Proximal Pelvic Limb, Axial Pattern Flap, (Caudal Superficial Epigastric), this chapter.

REFERENCES AND SUGGESTED READING

See Proximal Pelvic Limb, Axial Pattern Flap, (Caudal Superficial Epigastric), this chapter.

MESH GRAFT

Definition and Indications. See Mid and Distal Thoracic Limb, Mesh Graft, this chapter.

Technique. See Mid and Distal Thoracic Limb, Mesh Graft, this chapter.

Aftercare. See Mid and Distal Thoracic Limb, Mesh Graft, this chapter. Because of the shape of the pelvic limb, it may be difficult to maintain a bandage over the tibial area. Extending a dovetail type bandage above the stifle and affixing tape well to the hair over the femoral area may be beneficial in holding the bandage in place (Fig. 9-17A and B). Limiting the animal's exercise is also helpful in maintaining a bandage on the limb. If bandages are placed on the full length of the leg to help prevent distal limb edema and to help keep the bandage in place, the portion over the graft may be cut out to allow for daily bandage change without removal of the entire bandage.

If the graft is placed over the tarsal area, joint immobilization should be provided for 10 to 14 days after

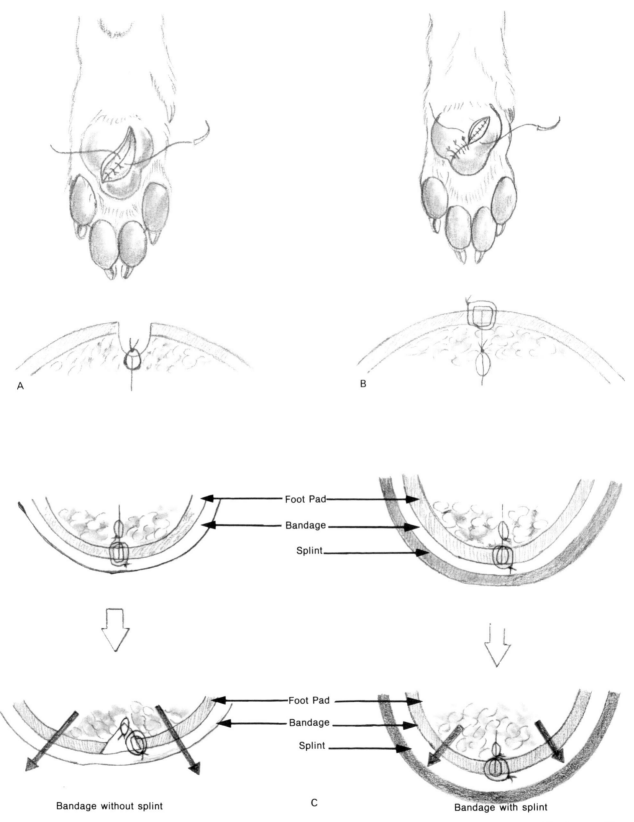

Foot Pad

Bandage

Splint

Foot Pad

Bandage

Splint

Bandage without splint

C

Bandage with splint

FIG. 9-20. Suturing and bandaging a lacerated pad. A, Simple interrupted sutures in deep tissues. B, Final apposition of wound edges with far-near-near-far sutures. C, With light bandage and no splint, weight on paw may result in sutures tearing through pad (left). Splint over bandage helps prevent sutures from tearing through pad (right).

time, it may be advisable to continue bandaging until the surgeon is convinced that healing is adequate to allow use of the paw without a bandage. The length of time for sutures to remain in place, the frequency of bandage changes, and the length of time bandages are needed are factors that vary according to wound severity and the animal's size. Clinical judgment is necessary in deciding these factors.

Advantages and Disadvantages. When pad lacerations are properly sutured, they tend to heal faster (that is, there is earlier gain of tensile strength) than lacerations that are only bandaged. They also have a better cosmetic appearance than unsutured pads. If pads are not sutured and/or bandaged properly, the wound edges may separate when weight is placed on the pad. This results in delayed healing or lack of healing.

REFERENCES AND SUGGESTED READING

1. Newman, M.E., Lee, A.H., Swaim, S.F., and Redding, R.W.: Wound healing of sutured and nonsutured canine metatarsal footpad incisions. J. Am. Anim. Hosp. Assoc. *22:*757, 1986.
2. Swaim, S.F.: Management and bandaging of soft tissue injuries of dog and cat feet. J. Am. Anim. Hosp. Assoc. *21:*329, 1985.

Abrasions and Burns: Bandaging

Definitions and Indications. Abrasion injuries of the pads may be superficial, involving only the superficial epidermal layers, or deep enough to expose the underlying connective tissue of the pad. Abrasion injuries result from prolonged walking or running, especially on a rough surface. Such injuries may also occur when an animal is accidentally dragged behind a vehicle. Pad burns may be superficial or deep and

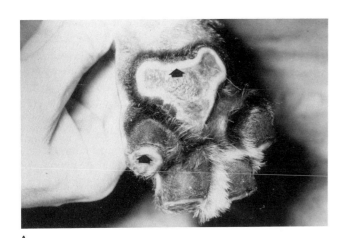
A

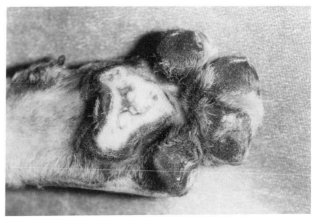
B

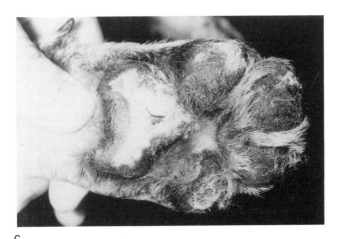
C

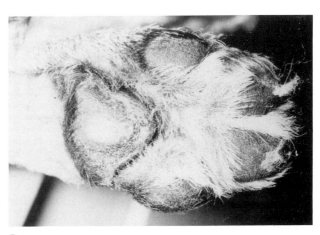
D

FIG. 9-21. Healing of a pad abrasion. A, Digital and metacarpal pad abrasion injuries with epithelial tissue remaining at wound edges (arrows). B through D, Progression of healing of metacarpal pad by re-epithelialization and keratinization.

may come from thermal or chemical sources. With these injuries, bandaging should be the first line of therapy in an effort to stimulate re-epithelializaton of the pads.

If any normal pad epithelial tissue remains at the edge of a pad abrasion or burn injury (Fig. 9-21A), the wound should be treated by bandaging for some time before deciding whether more involved surgical procedures are indicated.

Techniques. The wound should be thoroughly lavaged and debrided of any nonvital tissues (such as eschar) that might occur with a burn. The paw should be dried. A small amount of cotton should be placed between the digits and in the space between the digits and the metacarpal/metatarsal pad to help keep these areas dry. Because re-epithelialization occurs most rapidly between two surfaces (for example, between the wound surface and a bandage), a nonadherent dressing pad should be used to cover the wound. An absorbent wrap followed by porous adhesive tape completes the bandage.

Aftercare. The bandage should be changed daily if wound drainage is copious. As the wound heals and drainage decreases, less frequent bandage changes may be possible. Bandaging should be continued until re-epithelialization and some keratinization have occurred on the wound (Fig. 9-21B through D). Exercise should be restricted while the paw is bandaged, then restricted and gradually increased when bandaging is discontinued. The animal should be kept on a relatively clean, nonabrasive surface for a period after discontinuance of bandaging. This period should be determined by examination of the paw and clinical judgment. Periodic application of a soft boot* during the transition between bandaging and complete discontinuance of any paw cover may be helpful.

Advantages and Disadvantages. The primary advantage of nonadherent bandage therapy is that it provides a good environment for re-epithelialization. The epithelium that resurfaces pads tends to keratinize and withstand friction much better than the epithelium that covers wounds elsewhere on the body. Bandaging also averts more time-consuming and expensive surgical procedures.

REFERENCES AND SUGGESTED READING

1. Posch, A.J., and McDonald, G.: Thermal burns in cats. Mod. Vet. Pract. *58*:937, 1977.
2. Swaim, S.F.: Management and bandaging of soft tissue injuries of dog and cat feet. J. Am. Anim. Hosp. Assoc. *21*:329, 1985.

---

*Fleece Dog Bootie, Sawtooth Mountain Sled Works, Grand Marais, MN 55004.

Replacement: Phalangeal Fillet

Definition and Indications. Phalangeal fillet technique for pad replacement entails the removal of the proximal, middle, and distal phalanges from a digit to free the pad to be used to fill a defect in the metacarpal or metatarsal pad (Fig. 9-22A and B). This technique is indicated when large amounts of the metacarpal or metetarsal pad are missing as a result of trauma and conservative bandaging technique has not resulted in effective healing of the pad.

Techniques. Animals with chronic nonhealing metacarpal or metatarsal pad wounds that have not been caused by trauma should receive a thorough examination before surgery, including cytologic examination, fungal and bacterial culture, and sensitivity and histopathologic examination. If examinations reveal fungal or neoplastic tissue, appropriate medical and surgical therapy should be performed, ranging from limb amputation to amputation and replacement of only the pad (phalangeal fillet technique). If histopathologic examination reveals chronic nonhealing tissue, the wound should be thoroughly debrided because the chronic granulation tissue may have foreign material (such as dirt or sand) embedded in it because the animal has been walking without a bandage.

Palmar/Plantar Fillet. The digit nearest the metacarpal or metatarsal pad defect is selected for filleting. A rectangular segment of skin is removed from the palmar/plantar interdigital skin between the digital pad and the edge of the metacarpal or metatarsal pad defect (Fig. 9-23A). The proximal, middle, and distal phalanges of the digit are removed by incising the joint capsules and ligamentous attachments to the bones. Using blunt dissection as close to the bone as possible, the phalanges and nail are removed (Fig. 9-23B). This leaves the blood and nerve supply intact. The surface and edge of the pad defect are debrided, and the digital pad of the filleted digit is folded back on its neurovascular pedicle of skin to fill the metacarpal or metatarsal pad defect (Fig. 9-23C). The edges of the digital pad are sutured to the edges of the pad defect using 3-0 monofilament nonabsorbable material with simple interrupted or far-near-near-far sutures (Fig. 9-23D).

Dorsal Fillet. An alternate technique is to remove the bones of the digit from a single longitudinal incision on the dorsum of the digit (Fig. 9-24A and B). After removal of the phalanges, the skin is closed with simple interrupted sutures of 3-0 monofilament nonabsorbable suture material, leaving an opening for drainage where the nail was removed (Fig. 9-24C). The paw is bandaged with periodic bandage changes and allowed to heal for 14 days. At this time, the rectangle of palmar/plantar interdigital skin is removed and the digital pad is folded back and sutured into the defect as previously described (Fig. 9-24D through F).

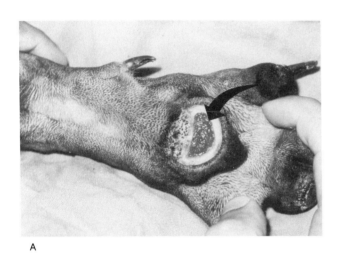
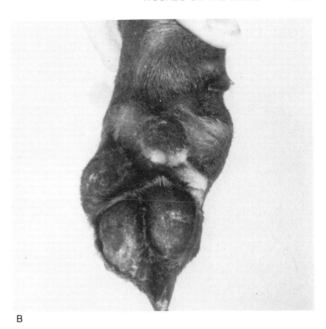

A

B

FIG. 9-22. Phalangeal fillet technique for pad replacement. A, Large nonhealing metacarpal pad lesion. Pad of second digit will be folded back (arrow) to fill defect after bones and nail have been removed from digit 2. B, Completed transposition of pad.

Aftercare. See Lacerations: Suturing, this chapter.

Advantages and Disadvantages. Filleting a digit from the palmar/plantar surface has the advantage of being a one-step procedure. The digit is filleted and transposed at the same operation. The digit, however, is a little more difficult to fillet from this approach than from the digit's dorsum because there is greater potential of injuring the blood supply to the pad. Filleting the digit from its dorsum is simpler; however, the technique takes longer because it is a two-step procedure, with transposition of the digital pad performed 14 days after the bones have been removed.

Digital pad transposition is generally not successful if the pad is transposed into a metacarpal or metatarsal pad wound caused by abnormal paw position as a result of tendon malfunction, bone misalignment, or nerve damage. Unless the underlying cause is corrected, the new pad will wear through as did the original pad.

REFERENCE AND SUGGESTED READING

1. Swaim, S.F., and Garrett, P.D.: Foot salvage techniques in dogs and cats: Options, "Do's" and "Don'ts." J. Am. Anim. Hosp. Assoc. *21*:511, 1985.

Replacement: Pouch Flap (Cats Only)

Definition and Indications. See Mid and Distal Thoracic Limb and Mid and Distal Pelvic Limb, Pouch Flap, this chapter. These flaps may be used to cover skin defects on the dorsum of the paws of dogs and cats. In cats, however, pouch flaps may also be used to replace pad tissue. If the cat is a house cat and will walk primarily on carpets, the skin from the body transposed to the paw as a pouch flap will undergo sufficient metaplasia to function as a pad replacement. Skin from the body should not be used to replace pad skin of the dog. It will not withstand the stress that a dog places on the skin.

Technique. See Mid and Distal Thoracic Limb and Mid and Distal Pelvic Limb, Pouch Flap, this chapter. (see Figs. 9-5A through D and 9-6A through G). If any viable pad tissue remains on the paw, it should be retained. The limb is positioned along the cat's side, and the two parallel dorsoventral incisions are made in the lateral thoraco-abdominal skin. The distance between the incisions is equal to the distance between the remaining pads and the proximal edge of the defect. The skin between the two incisions is undermined to create the flap, the affected paw is placed under the flap, and the edges of the flap are sutured to edges of the defect with simple interrupted 3-0 monofilament nonabsorbable suture (Fig. 9-25A and B).

If no pad tissue remains at the end of the stump, only one incision is made in the thoracoabdominal skin and

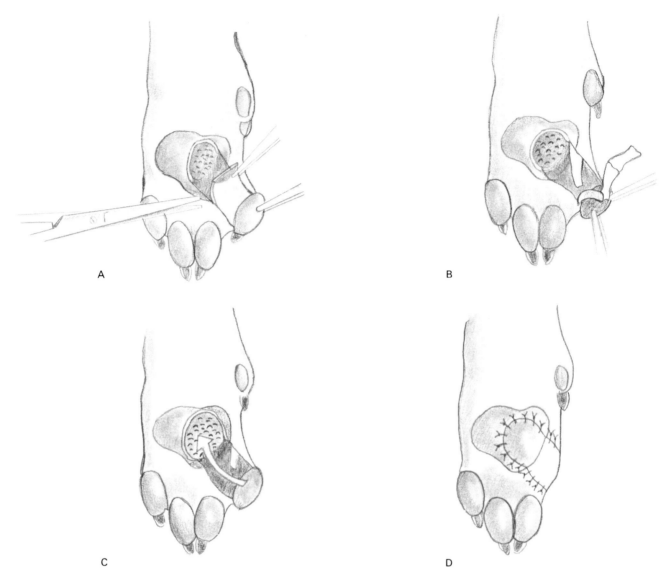

FIG. 9-23. Palmar/plantar phalangeal fillet technique to replace a pad. A, Removing a rectangle of skin between metacarpal and second digital pads. B, Removing proximal, middle, and distal phalanges and nail. C, Second digital pad will be folded back into metacarpal pad defect (arrow). D, Second digital pad sutured in place.

the adjacent skin is undermined to accommodate the paw stump. The edge of the wound is sutured to the edge of the flap as described above (Fig. 9-25E and F).

A small Penrose drain may be placed under the stump/flap area for drainage. Two or three tacking sutures may be used to help immobilize the flap over the defect (Fig. 9-25B and F). At the end of 14 days, the skin is incised from the thoracoabdominal donor area at a sufficient distance from the stump so that it will supply enough skin to cover the medial aspect of the paw stump (Fig. 9-25C, G, D, and H).

Aftercare. See Mid and Distal Thoracic Limb and Mid and Distal Pelvic Limb, Pouch Flap, this chapter.

After the flap has been transposed to the paw, bandaging should be continued until the last suture lines have healed (10 to 14 days). At this time, bandaging should be continued; however, the bandages should be removed from the paw daily for increasingly longer periods each day to allow the new skin to undergo metaplasia gradually until it can function in its new capacity as pad replacement skin. Clinical judgment is necessary in deciding when bandaging can be discontinued.

REFERENCES AND SUGGESTED READING

See Mid and Distal Thoracic Limb and Mid and Distal Pelvic Limb, Pouch Flap, this chapter.

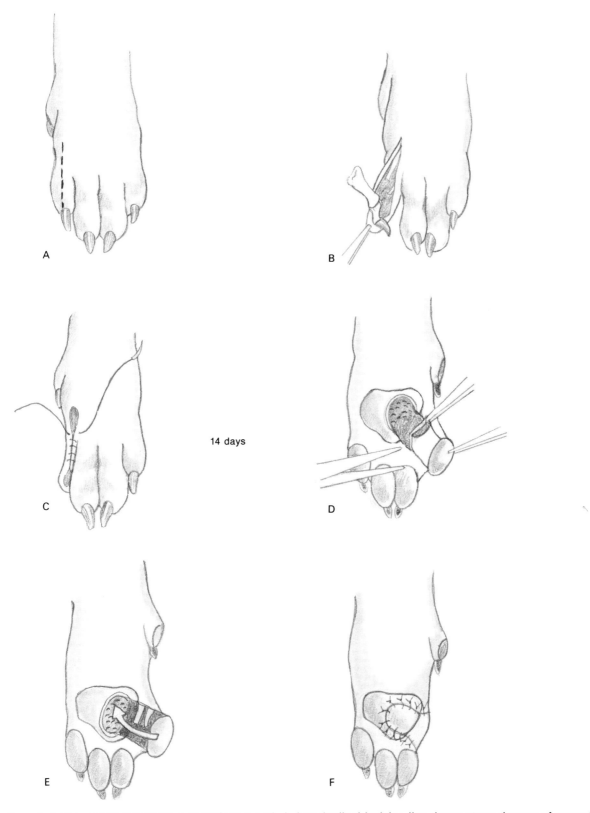

FIG. 9-24. Dorsal phalangeal fillet technique to replace a pad. A, Longitudinal incision line drawn along dorsum of second digit (broken line). B, Removing proximal, middle, and distal phalanges, and nail. C, Closing longitudinal incision. D, Removal of a rectangle of skin between metacarpal and second digital pads. E, Second digital pad will be folded back into metacarpal pad defect (arrow). F, Second digital pad sutured in place.

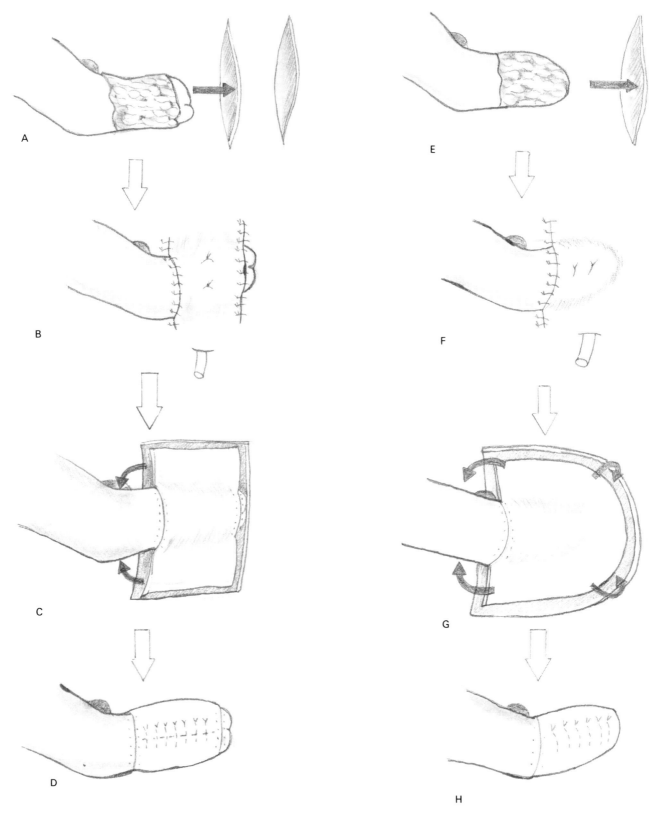

FIG. 9-25. Pouch flaps to replace pads on cats. A, When some pad tissue remains, two parallel incisions are made in lateral thoracic-abdominal skin. Skin is undermined. E, When no pad tissue remains, one incision is made in lateral thoraco-abdominal skin. Skin is undermined. B and F, Paw defect placed under flap and sutured. Drain in place. C and G, Excision of flap from body. D and H, Flap wrapped around paw and sutured.

Replacement: Mesh Graft (Cats Only)

Definition and Indications. See Mid and Distal Thoracic Limb, Mesh Graft, this chapter. Mesh grafts may be used to cover skin defects on the dorsum of the paws of dogs and cats. In cats, however, mesh grafts may also be used to replace pad tissue. If a cat is a house cat and will walk primarily on carpets, the skin of a mesh graft will undergo sufficient metaplasia to function as a pad replacement. Mesh grafts should not be used to replace pad skin of the dog. They will not withstand the stress that a dog places on the skin.

Technique. See Mid and Distal Thoracic Limb, Mesh Graft, this chapter.

Aftercare. See Mid and Distal Thoracic Limb, Mesh Graft, this chapter. After 21 days, the bandaging should be continued; however, the bandage should be removed from the paw daily for increasingly longer periods each day to allow the graft skin to undergo metaplasia gradually until it can function in its new capacity as pad replacement skin. Clinical judgment is necessary in deciding when bandaging can be discontinued.

REFERENCES AND SUGGESTED READING

See Mid and Distal Thoracic Limb, Mesh Graft, this chapter.
1. Swaim, S.F., and Garrett, P.D.: Foot salvage techniques in dogs and cats: Options, "Do's" and "Don'ts". J. Am. Anim. Hosp. Assoc. *21*:511, 1985.

DIGITS AND DORSAL PAW

Resurfacing: Phalangeal Fillet

Definition and Indications. Digital and dorsal paw resurfacing using the phalangeal fillet technique entails removing damaged phalanges and tendons from a digit or digits and using the skin of that digit or digits and any available interdigital webbing skin to resurface adjacent digits and/or the dorsum of the paw when these structures have intact bones and sizeable skin defects (Fig. 9-26A through F). The technique is indicated when trauma to a paw has caused osseous damage to a digit or digits without severe skin deficit of that digit or digits and severe skin deficit without osseous damage to adjacent digit(s) and/or skin damage to the dorsum of the paw.

Technique. After careful debridement of the soft tissues, remaining proximal, middle, and distal phalanges and tendon fragments are removed from the digit(s) with severe osseous damage (Figs. 9-27A, and 9-28A). The skin of this digit or digits and any available interdigital webbing skin are cut and trimmed in such a way that they can be used as a flap or flaps to resurface

adjacent digit(s) with large skin deficits and/or the dorsum of the paw (Figs. 9-27B and C, and 9-28B and C). Care should be taken in cutting and trimming the digital and webbing skin to ensure that sufficient skin and subcutis are left at the base to serve as a pedicle for blood supply to the flap(s). The flap(s) is/are sutured to the remaining skin of the adjacent digit(s) and/or dorsum of the paw using simple interrupted sutures of 3-0 monofilament nonabsorbable suture material (Figs. 9-27D, and 9-28D).

Aftercare. A *small* amount of powder and a small amount of cotton should be placed between remaining intact digits and in the space between the digits and the metacarpal/metatarsal pad to help keep these areas dry. A strip of nonadherent pad should be placed over the suture line. Absorbent wrap and adhesive tape complete the bandage. The amount of absorbent wrap does not have to be as great, and there may be no need for a metal splint as when bandaging a pad laceration or phalangeal fillet to replace a pad.

Bandages should be changed periodically for 7 to 10 days depending on the amount of drainage. The length of time sutures should remain in place, the frequency of bandage changes, and the length of time bandages are needed are factors that vary according to wound tension, wound healing rate, and drainage.

Advantages and Disadvantages. The advantage of the technique is that skin defects of a digit or digits and/or dorsum of the paw can be reconstructed using the locally available skin of an adjacent digit(s) and webbing skin. The disadvantage of the technique is that filleting of digit 3 or 4 leaves a cosmetic defect in the central aspect of the paw. A defect in this area could cause lameness. If digits 3 and 4 have been filleted to resurface digits 2 and 5 and/or the dorsum of the paw, digits 2 and 5 protrude and may be subject to snagging on vegetation or carpets. If the pad(s) of the filleted digit(s) is/are necessary for the resurfacing procedure, they should be used; however, pad tissue in an abnormal location on the digits or dorsum of the paw may not be cosmetically pleasing.

REFERENCE AND SUGGESTED READING

1. Swaim, S.F., and Garrett, P.D.: Foot salvage techniques in dogs and cats: Options, "Do's" and "Don'ts." J. Am. Anim. Hosp. Assoc. *21*:511, 1985.

Digit Amputation

Definition and Indications. Digit amputation is the surgical removal of all or part of one or more digits from an animal's paw. Digit amputation is most commonly

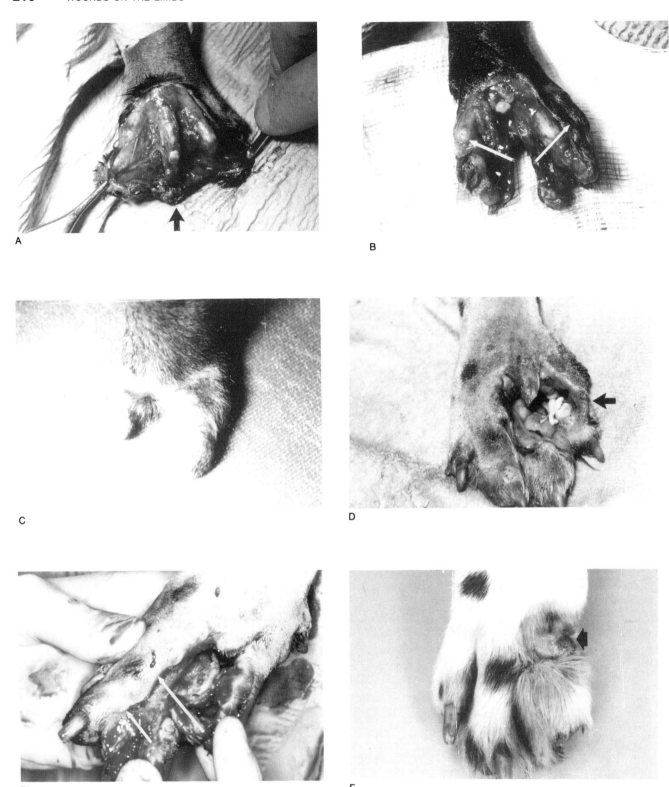

FIG. 9-26. Phalangeal fillet to resurface digits and dorsum of paw. A and D, Digits with damaged bones to be removed (arrows). B and E, All phalanges and nails removed from damaged digits. Skin will cover adjacent digits (B) and dorsum of the paw (E) (arrows). C and D, Digital skin flaps healed. Note pad skin on dorsum of paw (F) (arrow). (A, B, and C courtesy of I. Sanchez.) (D and E from Swaim, S.F.: Management and bandaging of soft tissue injuries of dog and cat feet. J. Am. Anim. Hosp. Assoc. *21*:329–340, 1985).

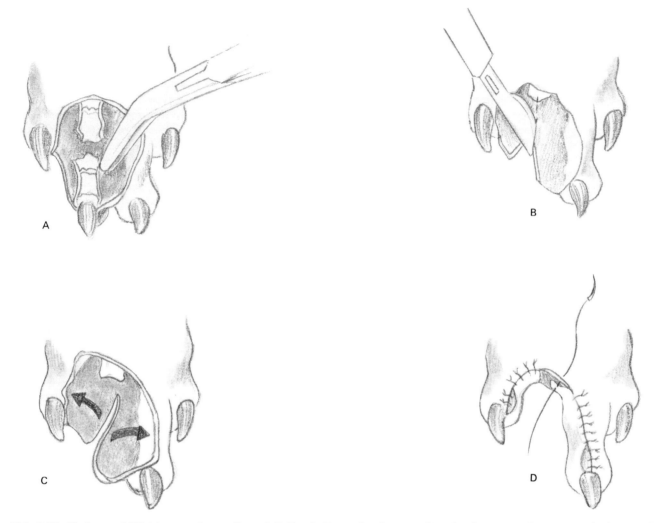

FIG. 9-27. Phalangeal fillet to resurface adjacent digits. A, Removing bone and tendon fragments from severely damaged digit. B, Midline incision made in skin of severely damaged digit creating flaps. C, Rotating flaps to resurface adjacent digits (arrows). D, Suturing flaps in place.

indicated in traumatic injuries such as fractures, luxations, or severe wounds. Neoplasias, chronic osteomyelitis, phlebitis, pressure necrosis from casts or bandages, and arthritis are other indications for digit amputation.

Techniques. *Distal Interphalangeal Amputation.* An encircling incision is made in the skin at the base of the nail (Fig. 9-29A). The distal interphalangeal joint between the middle and distal phalanges is isolated, followed by severance of the extensor and flexor tendons, the collateral ligaments, and the joint capsule. The distal phalanx and nail are removed (Fig. 9-29B). Hemorrhage is controlled by ligation or electrocoagulation. The head of the middle phalanx is removed (Fig. 9-29C). Removal of the distal 1/3 of the middle phalanx may be necessary to provide more soft tissue between the skin

and the bone end. Dead space can be closed with one or two 3-0 simple interrupted absorbable sutures. Simple interrupted sutures of 3-0 monofilament nonabsorbable material are used to close the skin defect (Fig. 9-29D). "Dog ears" are removed as necessary.

Proximal Interphalangeal and Metacarpophalangeal/Metatarsophalangeal Amputation. For amputations of the third and fourth digits, an encircling incision is made at the base of the digit with a short longitudinal incision on the dorsum of the paw adjoining the encircling incision (Fig. 9-30A). For amputation of the second and fifth digits, the incisions are made similarly; however, the longitudinal incision is made on the side of the paw. The skin and underlying soft tissues are reflected to expose either the proximal interphalangeal joint or the metacarpophalangeal/metatarso-

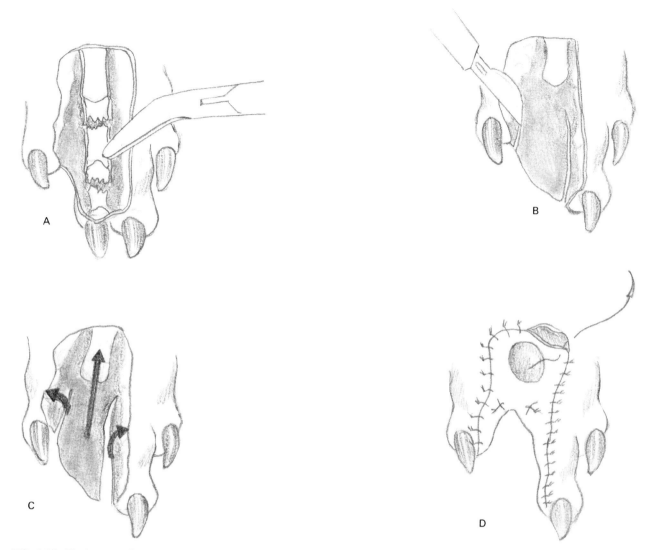

FIG. 9-28. Phalangeal fillet to resurface dorsum of paw and adjacent digits. A, Removing bone and tendon fragments from severely damaged digit. B, Two skin incisions made in skin of severely damaged digit, creating flaps. C, Rotating flaps to resurface adjacent digits and dorsum of paw (arrows). D, Suturing flaps in place.

phalangeal joint. The dorsal (axial and abaxial) common digital or proper digital vessels are ligated and severed and the matching nerves are cut. The extensor tendons and collateral ligaments are then severed, and the joint capsule is incised. The sesamoid ligaments are cut and the sesamoid bones are removed, with amputation at the metacarpophalangeal and metatarsophalangeal joint. This is followed by ligation and severance of the palmar/plantar (axial and abaxial) common or proper digital vessels along with severance of the associated nerves and cutting of the flexor tendons. After removal of the digit, the head of the proximal phalanx is removed if the amputation was performed at the proximal interphalangeal joint. The head of the metacarpal/metatarsal bone is removed if the amputation was at the metacar-

pophalangeal or metatarsophalangeal joint (Fig. 9-30B and C). Simple interrupted absorbable sutures of 3-0 material are used to close dead space. The skin is sutured with simple interrupted sutures of 3-0 monofilament nonabsorbable suture material (Fig. 9-30D).

Proximal Pandigital Metacarpophalangeal/Metatarsophalangeal Amputation. If it is suspected that the digits have lost or are losing their viability as a result of pressure necrosis, phlebitis, trap injuries, or other sources of trauma, they should be evaluated to determine if amputation is needed. Signs of impending avascular digit loss include (1) hair that epilates from the digit easily, (2) digital skin that has lost its normal turgor (becomes extremely soft and moist or hard), (3) nails that can be pulled off nail beds easily, and (4)

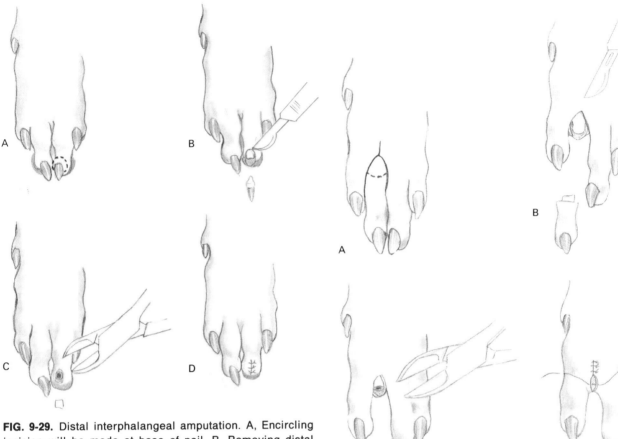

FIG. 9-29. Distal interphalangeal amputation. A, Encircling incision will be made at base of nail. B, Removing distal phalanx and nail. C, Removing the distal head of the second phalanx. D, Skin defect sutured.

FIG. 9-30. Proximal interphalangeal and metacarpophalangeal/metatarsophalangeal amputations. A, Encircling incision at base of third digit with a short longitudinal incision on dorsum of paw. B, Removing third digit. C, Removing distal head of proximal phalanx or metacarpal/metatarsal bone. D, Suturing skin defect.

insertion of a large gauge needle (18 guage) into the digital pad or trimming the nail into the quick with no signs of discomfort or hemorrhage.

A transverse incision is made in the skin on the dorsum of the paw over the metacarpophalangeal/metatarsophalangeal articulation. Where a sharp line of demarcation exists between the viable and nonviable tissue, the incision is made in viable tissue approximately 3 mm proximal to the demarcation line (Figs. 9-31A and 9-32A). The incision is continued on to the palmar/plantar surface of the paw, incising at the junction of the metacarpal/metatarsal pad with the skin between the digits and this pad (Fig. 9-32B). If there is a line of demarcation in this skin cranial to the metacarpal/metatarsal pad, the incision should be approximately 3 mm proximal to the line in viable skin.

Working from the dorsum of the paw, the skin is reflected and dorsal axial and abaxial common or proper digital vessels are ligated with 3-0 absorbable ligatures and severed distal to the ligations. Associated nerves are also severed. Extensor tendons, collateral ligaments, and

metacarpophalangeal/metatarsophalangeal joint capsules are severed. On the palmar/plantar surface of the limb, the sesamoid ligaments are cut and the sesamoid bones removed. The palmar/plantar common or proper digital vessels are ligated and severed along with severance of the associated nerves and the flexor tendons are cut. The digits are removed (Figs. 9-31B and 9-32C).

If the area is not infected, bone rongeurs should be used to remove the heads of the metacarpal/metatarsal bones. Metacarpals/metatarsals 3 and 4 may be trimmed so that they are the same length as metacarpals/metatarsals 2 and 5 (Fig. 9-32D). If infection is present, the heads should not be removed at this time to avoid the possibility of infection ascending into the marrow cavities of the bones. After infection has been

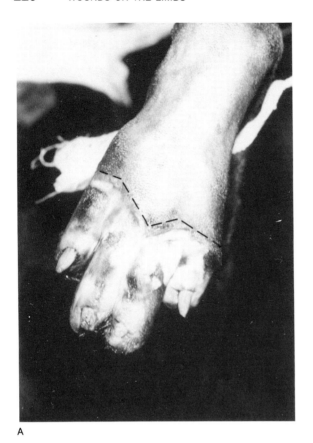

A

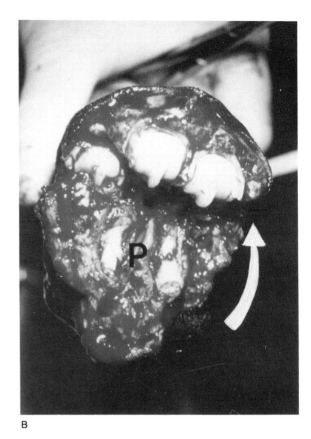

B

C

FIG. 9-31. Proximal pandigital metacarpophalangeal/ metatarsophalangeal amputation. A, Necrotic digits. Proposed incision line (broken line). B, Following digit removal, metacarpal pad (P) is rotated (arrow) to cover ends of metacarpal bones. C, Metacarpal pad sutured in place, with Penrose drain to allow for drainage.

controlled, the area may be reoperated on to remove heads and trim bones.

Because the metacarpal/metatarsal pad has been salvaged, it is folded cranially over the ends of the metacarpal/metatarsal bones after a 1/4" Penrose drain has been placed between the pad and ends of the bones. Interrupted horizontal mattress sutures of 3-0 absorbable suture material are used to join the subcutaneous tissue of the cranial edge of the metacarpal/metatarsal pad to the subcutaneous tissue overlying the

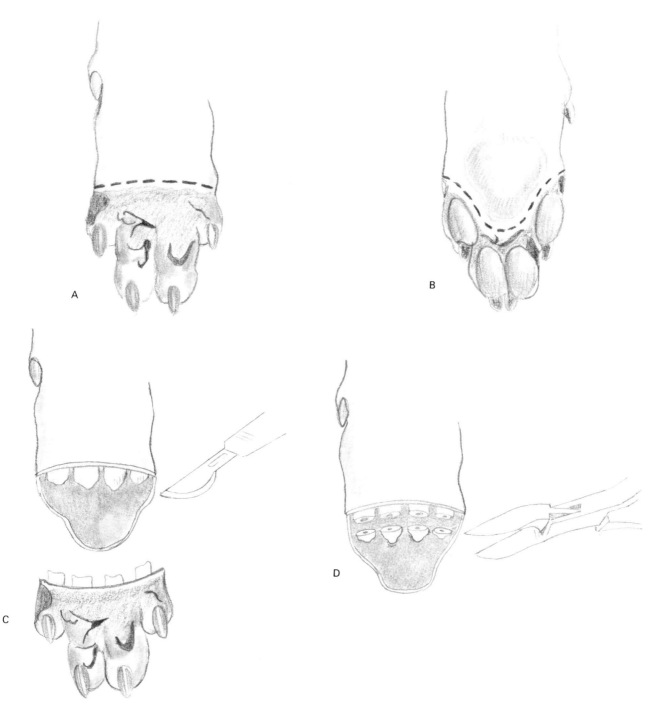

FIG. 9-32. Proximal pandigital metacarpophalangeal/metatarsophalangeal amputation. A, Transverse incision on dorsum of paw just proximal to demarcation line (broken line). B, Incision on palmar/plantar surface at junction of metacarpal/ metatarsal pad with interdigital skin (broken line). C, Removing all digits. D, Removing distal heads of metacarpal/ metatarsal bones.

fistulous tract and foreign body are isolated (Fig. 9-34A). It is necessary to extend the skin incision or excise tissue associated with the tract for adequate exposure. The subcutis is closed with 4-0 absorbable simple interrupted sutures, and the skin incision is closed with simple interrupted sutures of 3-0 monofilament nonabsorbable suture material. The most distal portion of the wound is left open to allow drainage as the wound heals (Fig. 9-34B). A bandage is applied.

Chronic Unresponsive Interdigital Lesions. Dorsal and palmar/plantar skin incisions are made at the junction of interdigital skin with the two adjacent digits (Fig. 9-35A and B). All interdigital skin between the incisions is excised. Electrocoagulation or ligatures of 3-0 absorbable suture material are used to control hemorrhage. The same suture material is used to close dead space between the skin edges, taking care not to damage the blood supply to the digits. The dorsal wound edge may be sutured to the palmar/plantar wound edge using 3-0 monofilament nonabsorbable simple interrupted sutures (Fig. 9-35C and D). If insufficient skin is available to suture the dorsal wound edge to the palmar/plantar wound edge of each digit, the palmar/plantar skin edges of the adjacent digits may be sutured together. This is followed by suturing the dorsal skin edges of the adjacent digits together. This fuses the 2 digits together with no interdigital space (Fig. 9-35E and F).

Aftercare.   See Lacerations: Suturing, this chapter. A *small* amount of powder and cotton should be placed between all digits except those between which surgery has been performed. Powder and cotton are also placed between the digits and the metacarpal/metatarsal pad. A piece of nonadherent bandage material should be placed over the suture line where an interdigital web has been removed. Absorbent wrap and adhesive tape complete the bandage. Heavy padding and splints are generally not necessary.

Bandages should be changed periodically, depending on the amount of drainage that occurs. Bandaging is continued for approximately 7 to 10 days or until healing is considered adequate.

Advantages and Disadvantages.   Once foreign bodies have been removed, the wounds heal uneventfully; however, if any foreign material remains in the tissue, the wounds do not heal or they heal and later break open to drain. This is an example of "tissue intelligence"—the tissues do not heal as long as a reactive foreign body is present. Such wounds need to be reoperated on.

Removal of the interdigital web may result in closer than normal apposition of the two adjacent digits.

REFERENCES AND SUGGESTED READING

1. Anderson, R.K.: Canine Pododermatitis. Compend. Contin. Educ. 2:361, 1980.
2. Krahwinkel, D.J., and Bone D.L.: Surgical management of specific skin disorders. *In* Textbook of Small Animal Surgery. Edited by D.H. Slatter. Philadelphia, W.B. Saunders, 1985.
3. Manning, T.O., Walton, D.K., and Ford, R.B.: Canine pododermatitis. Dermatol. Rep. 2:1, 1983.
4. Muller, G.H., Kirk, R.W., and Scott, D.W.: Small Animal Dermatology. 3rd ed. Philadelphia, W.B. Saunders, 1983.

10

SKIN TUMORS

STAGING CUTANEOUS NEOPLASMS

Definitions and Indications. Staging is not unique to neoplasia. Accurate prognosis and therapy of any disease process are based on knowledge of the extent of the disease. In oncology, "staging" denotes efforts to discover the extent of spread of neoplastic disease. The reason for examining for distant spread of neoplasia is that, if a neoplasm has spread regionally or systemically, local forms of treatment such as surgery and radiation are insufficient if used alone. To be appropriate, the therapy must be matched to the extent of spread. The data obtained from staging is also used to compare the results of therapy of different investigators.

Technique. Official World Health Organization (WHO) staging protocol varies according to the body system and the biologic activity of the neoplastic process being investigated. In tumors of the skin and subcutis, which are considered together, sequential evaluation of the tumor (T), lymph nodes (N), and presence of metastasis (M) is recommended. Separate staging forms are in use for mast cell tumors (see Canine Mast Cell Tumor, this chapter), mammary gland tumors of dogs and cats (see Canine Mammary Neoplasia, this chapter); and lymphosarcoma, which is usually considered a systemic disease. The form used is not essential, but staging (Table 10-1) is essential.

If standard WHO forms are not available, staging information is written in the record. The exact location of the primary tumor (T) is drawn on a topography map of a "generic animal" to locate the tumor relative to the animal's body surface (Fig. 10-1A). The physical characteristics of the primary tumor are recorded. These include attachments to skin and muscle fascia, inflammation, ulceration, or thickened cords of tissue present between the primary tumor and deeper tissue or lymph nodes. The tumor is then measured with ruler or calipers in two or three orthogonal dimensions (depending on the anatomical location) for use in calculating tumor volume (Fig. 10-1B). The measurement of thickness or depth is difficult to obtain if the tumor is fixed, so this value is guessed as closely as possible (Fig. 10-1B inset). If a WHO form is being used, the largest measurement is used to assign a "T" value to the primary tumor.

Based on the expected lymphatic drainage of the tumor bed, the lymphatics are examined for cording and local and more distant regional lymph nodes (N) are examined for symmetry, enlargement, and fixation to adjacent tissue (Fig. 10-1C). These findings are used to establish the "N" value. The lymphatics and nodes distal to the tumor should also be evaluated to detect the unusual, but possible, occurrence of retrograde or intransit metastases. This type of lymphatic metastasis occurs when the afferent lymph node becomes obstructed by tumor emboli and growth, and the flow of lymph reverses toward collaterals, carrying neoplastic cells through the efferents to seed skin, subcutis, (in transit) and distal lymphactics and nodes (retrograde).

After the primary tumor and lymph nodes have been evaluated, the patient is examined for metastatic foci (M) and other primary tumors. To some extent, knowledge of the type of tumor allows prediction of metastasis to, and examination of, the more common sites. In general, carcinomas metastasize along lymphatic channels to

225

Table 10-1. Clinical Stages (TNM) of Canine or Feline Tumors of Epidermal or Dermal Origin (Excluding Lymphosarcoma and Mastocytoma)

T   Primary Tumor
   Tis Preinvasive carcinoma (Carcinoma in situ)
   T0   No evidence of tumor
   T1   Tumor <2 cm maximum diameter, superficial or exophytic
   T2   Tumor 2 to 5 cm maximum diameter, or minimally invasive, irrespective of size
   T3   Tumor >5 cm maximum diameter or invading subcutis irrespective of size
   T4   Tumor invading other structures such as fascia, muscle, bone, or cartilage

N   Regional Lymph Nodes (RNL)
   N0   No evidence of regional lymph node involvement
   N1   Movable ipsilateral nodes
      N1a Nodes not considered to contain growth*
      N1b Nodes considered to contain growth*
   N2   Movable contralateral or bilateral nodes
      N2a Nodes not considered to contain growth†
      N2b Nodes considered to contain growth†
   N3   Fixed nodes

M   Distant Metastasis
   M0   No evidence of distant metastasis
   M1   Distant metastasis detected at specified sites

*(−) = histologically negative, (+) = histologically positive.
†Including lymph nodes beyond the region in which the primary tumor is situated.
(Reprinted with permission from World Health Organization: Report of the Second Consultation on the Biological Behavior and Therapy of Tumors of Domestic Animals. WHO, Geneva, 1978.)

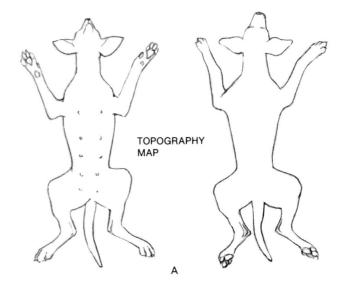

A

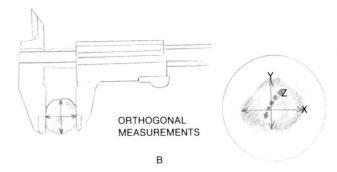

B

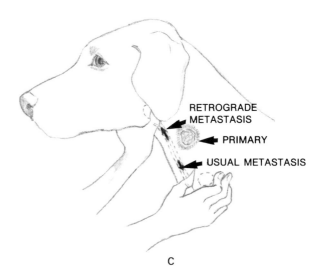

C

FIG. 10-1. Staging skin tumors. A, Body surface topography for plotting tumor location. B, Caliper measurement of tumor. Orthogonal measurements (inset). C, Examination of local lymphatic drainage and nodes showing usual and retrograde metastatic routes.

lymph nodes, and by blood to the lungs. Sarcomas frequently bypass lymphatics, metastasizing by blood to the lungs. Besides distant lymph nodes and the lung, many other organs are potential sites of metastasis such as bone, brain, kidney, and liver. Clinical signs or biochemical abnormalities direct detailed testing of these and other organs. Survey radiographs of the thorax (in three apposing views—VD, DV, and right and left laterals), abdomen (two apposing views—VD and lateral), and bone (lateral view of each long bone) are useful for routine screening. Depending on the malignancy suspected, other methods of detecting metastasis are bone marrow examination, serum electrophoresis, occult fecal blood, ultrasound, thermography, endoscopy, and special imaging techniques such as contrast radiography, scintigraphy, and computed tomography. The finding of a mass may not be adequate to document metastasis. The mass may represent metastasis, an additional primary tumor, or an inflammatory process. Ideally, suspected metastatic lesions should be confirmed with histopathologic analysis of tissue. The summary of these findings is used to establish the "M" value.

Aftercare. Staging is repeated at follow-up examinations, which in the case of surgical treatments are usually conducted at 7 to 10 days with suture removal and then at 1, 3, 6, 9, 12, 18, and 24 months from the most recent treatment. Specific aftercare may be required for some staging examinations such as biopsy.

Advantages and Disadvantages. Staging is a must. It affords the clinician the only realistic basis on which therapy may be formulated and helps prevent attempted local treatment (surgery) of a disease that is already systemic.

REFERENCES AND SUGGESTED READING

1. Henderson, R.A., and Core, D.C.: Skin—Oncology Section. *In* Textbook of Small Animal Surgery. Edited by D.H. Slatter. Philadelphia, W.B. Saunders, 1985.
2. Madewell, B.R., and Theilen, G.H.: Tumors of the skin and subcutaneous tissue—Introduction. Veterinary Cancer Medicine. Edited by B.R. Madewell and G.H. Theilen. Philadelphia, Lea & Febiger, 1987.
3. Owen, L.N.: TNM classification of tumors in domestic animals. WHO Bulletin, VPH/CMO/80.*20*:12, 1980.

ASPIRATION AND "INCISION" BIOPSIES

Definitions and Indications. The use of a thin needle to remove fluid and cells from tissues is termed aspiration. Most tumors are amenable to fine needle aspiration as an initial diagnostic method. The cytologic characteristics of many tumors are diagnostic, but in other instances biopsy is needed.

Harvesting tissue for the determination of its cellular morphology is termed biopsy. Complete specimen removal, also known as "excision" biopsy (see Excision Biopsies and Principles of Tumor Excision, this chapter), is preferable in most instances. Partial removal of a lesion for sampling analysis is called incision or invasive biopsy. Invasive biopsy is preferred when inadequate surrounding tissue is available to perform a simple reconstruction of the excision biopsy defect, when vital structures would be jeopardized, or when a tumor that may respond to nonsurgical treatment is suspected. An invasive biopsy of a subcutaneous tumor should be located so that the wound may be excised with the tumor if excision is opted; otherwise, viable cancer cells inoculated into the biopsy incision bed may be left and cause local recurrence.

The most common invasive biopsy techniques used by the authors on skin and subcutaneous neoplasms are needle biopsy when the tumor is covered by skin, biting biopsy when the tumor is ulcerated or exophytic, and incision biopsy when larger diagnostic samples are preferred. Contraindications for biopsy are the presence of severe coagulation disorders and inadequate equipment

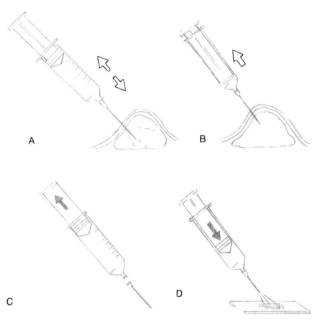

FIG. 10-2. Fine needle aspiration. A, Syringe movement to redirect the needle during fine needle aspiration (open arrows). B, Vacuum in syringe released before withdrawal from tumor (open arrow)..C, Needle removed before moving plunger (dark arrow) to fill syringe with air. D, Needle reattached and plunger (dark arrow) expelling cells onto slide.

or experience. Failure to obtain the correct diagnosis with aspiration or biopsy must be considered a surgical failure.

Technique. Fine needle aspiration. A 23 gauge needle is inserted into the tumor, and maximum vacuum is applied to the needle using a 10 ml syringe. The needle is moved back and forth within the tumor, slightly changing direction with each forward thrust (Fig. 10-2A). Ideally, a cellular aspiration should remain confined in the needle bore and hub. For this reason, the vacuum in the syringe is released before the needle is withdrawn from the tumor (Fig. 10-2B). The transfer of the cells onto a slide is accomplished by removing the syringe from the needle, filling it with air (Fig. 10-2C), reattaching it to the needle, and expelling the cells onto a glass slide (Fig. 10-2D). The cells are spread and stained.

A 23 gauge needle is used first, but if a bloody sample is obtained, the aspiration is repeated with a 25 gauge needle. Conversely, if no cells or blood are obtained, a larger needle is used to repeat the aspiration. Aspiration of blood is avoided when possible because blood dilutes the concentration of tumor cells and makes interpretation more difficult. A sample containing blood should still be examined because some tumors are highly vascular, and tumor cells can still be found.

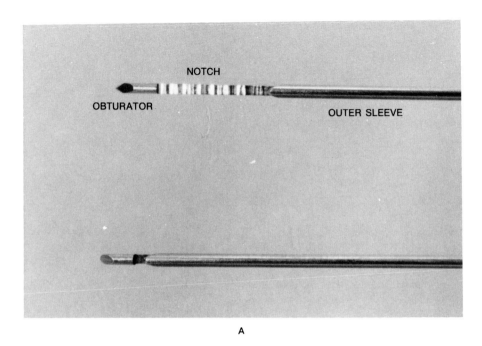

A

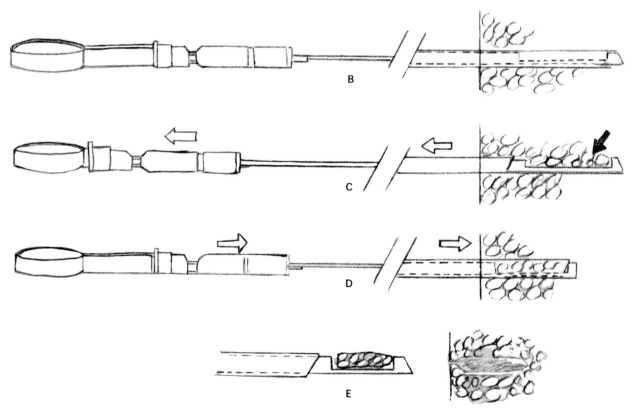

FIG. 10-3. Needle biopsy. A, Tip of biopsy instrument: open and partially closed. (Actual size 11.4 cm length, 2.0 cm specimen notch.) B, Closed instrument in tumor. Inner obturator and cutting notch (broken line) covered by outer sleeve (tip magnified for detail). C, Outer sleeve retracted (open arrow) allows tumor to enter cutting notch (dark arrow). D, Outer cutting sleeve thrust forward (open arrow) capturing biopsy in notch. E, Instrument removed from tissue with outer sleeve retracted, revealing specimen.

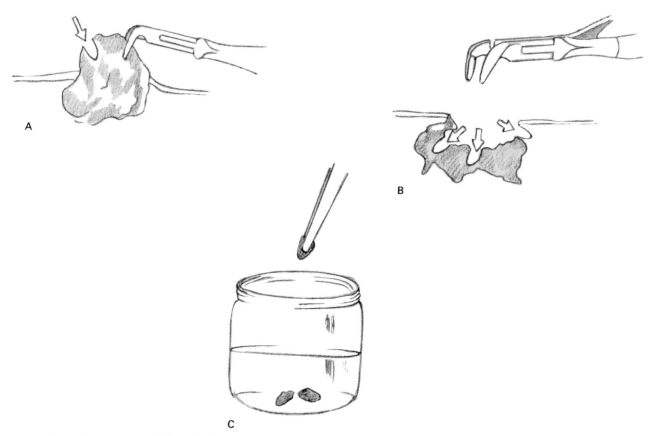

FIG. 10-4. Biting biopsy technique. A, Rongeur biopsy of exophytic mass. Biopsy site (open arrow). B, Rongeur biopsy of ulcerated mass. Biopsy sites (open arrows). C, Biopsy specimens transferred to fixation medium.

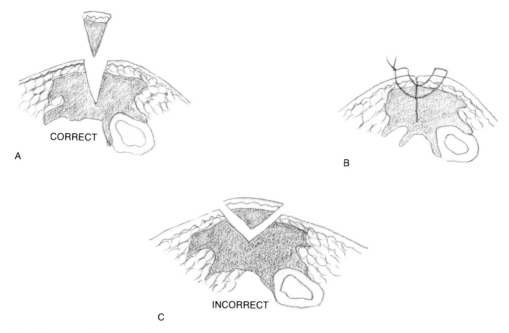

FIG. 10-5. Incision biopsy technique. A, Correct deep, narrow-wedge incision. B, Deep-wedge incision biopsy closed with vertical mattress. C, Incorrect wide, shallow-wedge biopsy.

Needle biopsy. The authors prefer a 19 gauge disposable biopsy needle.* The outer cutting sleeve of this particular instrument contains a slightly pointed obturator that has a specimen notch machined into its side (Fig. 10-3A). Because the obturator is only slightly pointed, it is necessary to nick the skin with a scalpel blade to allow passage of the needle through the skin. The closed needle (cutting sleeve forward) is placed in the mass (Fig. 10-3B) and the cutting sleeve is retracted to expose the notched obturator (Fig. 10-3C). The surrounding tissue presses into the notch and the tissue in the notch is sliced free and trapped in the slot by quickly advancing the cutting sleeve back over the obturator (Fig. 10-3D). The needle is withdrawn and the tissue removed from the notch with a hypodermic needle for processing (Fig. 10-3E). A 17 gauge biopsy needle with a hollow obturator for aspiration is also available.†

Biting biopsy. The authors prefer sharp-angled mastoid rongeurs over uterine or intestinal biopsy forceps for biting biopsy because the specimen harvested with rongeurs is larger. These bone rongeurs are kept sharp by restricting their use to soft tissue biopsies. The tips of the rongeurs are forced into the tissue or placed over an edge of tissue and the specimen is quickly bitten off and placed in formalin (Fig. 10-4A through C).

Incision biopsy. A wedge of tissue may be harvested using a scalpel. The wedge should be deep and narrow (Fig. 10-5A). The resulting deep wedge defect can be closed with a series of vertical mattress sutures (Fig. 10-5B). The most common error is making too wide and shallow a biopsy (Fig. 10-5C). A shallow, wide wedge removed from the tissue may miss the majority of the tumor and the resulting defect cannot be closed with sutures, which increases the potential for continued hemorrhage.

Aftercare. Usually no special aftercare is necessary. A padded absorbent bandage may be required after some biopsies for hemostasis and inhibition of secondary contamination and self-mutilation.

Advantages and Disadvantages. The biopsy tract or incision bed may be a site of local tumor spread (Fig. 10-6), but biopsy-induced metastasis to distant organs is not considered a significant danger. Vigorous tumor manipulation is more apt to cause metastasis than incision or sharp probing. With invasive biopsy samples, only a portion of the tumor may be obtained,

---

*Tru-cut Disposable Biopsy Needle, Travenol Laboratories, Deerfield, IL.

†Tru-cut Disposable Biopsy/Aspiration Needle, Travenol Laboratories, Deerfield, IL.

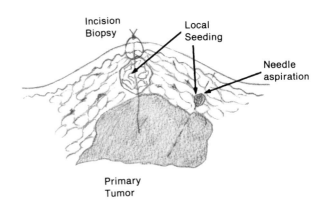

FIG. 10-6. Inoculation of biopsy tracts with tumor cells. Both incision biopsy and needle biopsy tracts contain viable tumor.

thus leading to misdiagnosis. If one highly representative sample is not obtained, multiple specimens should be taken. The authors usually obtain three samples of each lesion with needle and biting biopsy techniques.

Needle aspiration defines the content of masses (solid or cystic), and some cell types (white blood cells, mast cells, melanoma cells) are recognizable even to persons not trained in cytology. The small sample size and skill required for recognition of cells are the principal disadvantages.

An advantage of needle biopsy is that nearly any tissue that can be palpated and immobilized may be biopsied. Others are that the potential for hemorrhage is reduced because of the small biopsy tract and that, normally, only a local anesthetic is necessary. Also, the instruments are relatively inexpensive, and although marketed as disposable, they may be cleaned and reused several times. The principal disadvantage of the instrument is that it obtains a small specimen relative to the tissue in question.

Biting biopsy of superficial, ulcerated tumors can frequently be accomplished without anesthesia because tumors usually do not contain nerves. This means that a patient with compromised major organ reserves may sometimes be biopsied without an in-depth workup delaying submission of the sample, and even on an outpatient basis. The more rapid harvesting of tissues hastens the time to diagnosis, but the technique is limited to superficial lesions.

Incision biopsy harvests the largest and most representative tissue volume, which in some instances increases diagnostic accuracy. Incision is accompanied by greater operative morbidity and the possibility of more serious complications such as hemorrhage or inadvertent injury to important structures; however, complications are unusual with this or any other properly performed biopsy technique.

REFERENCES AND SUGGESTED READING

1. Henderson, R.A., Swaim, S.F., and Hankes, G.H.: The surgical management of cancer. Mod. Vet. Pract. *8:*615, 1984.
2. Withrow, S.J., and Lowes, N.: Biopsy techniques for use in small animal onocology. J. Am. Anim. Hosp. Assoc. *17:*889, 1981.

EXCISION BIOPSIES AND PRINCIPLES OF TUMOR EXCISION

Definitions and Indications. Biopsy is the harvesting of tissue for the purpose of determining the cellular morphology and activity. Excision is the preferred biopsy technique because its intent is surgical cure (removal of all gross tumor and a margin of adjacent normal tissue). Excision is absolutely indicated over invasive biopsy when tissue to repair the defect is available, danger to vital structures in the surgical field is minimal, and there is little probability of obtaining a diagnosis of a tumor that would respond to nonsurgical treatment. Circumstances that may contraindicate excision include severe coagulation disorders, inappropriate equipment, and inadequate experience.

Technique. A minimum of 1 cm and preferably a 2 to 3 cm "margin" of normal tissue must be excised with the neoplastic tissue to achieve curative intent. Before the incision is begun, the margin to be excised should be marked using a ruled scalpel handle and multiple punctate incisions or other skin-marking technique (Fig. 10-7A and inset). Because normal skin and subcutis must be conserved for reconstruction of wounds with unexpected tension lines or the need for additional excision, the initial incision should surround only the neoplasm and desired normal tissue margin rather than creating the entire wound to be reconstructed. After the tumor is excised, the resulting wound may be modified by additional incisions or excisions to create a wound of a shape that is more easily closed (see Closure of Various-Shaped Wounds, Chapter 7).

The incision should be perpendicular to the skin to the level of the muscle fascia (Fig. 10-7B). The margin of the deep surface of the tumor is the one most frequently neglected. Although malignant tumors invade fascia, fascia frequently functions to slow the deep invasion of a tumor. When the physical findings or cytologic morphology suggest the possibility of a malignant tumor, fasciectomy/fasciomyectomy (Fig. 10-7B), myectomy (Fig. 10-7C) or even full-thickness body wall excision (Fig. 10-7D) should be performed. Suction, electrosurgical dissection, and judicious use of ligatures improve the dissection through improved visualization and thus help to prevent accidental incision of the neoplasm. If surgical excision has been performed previously, fibrous "scar

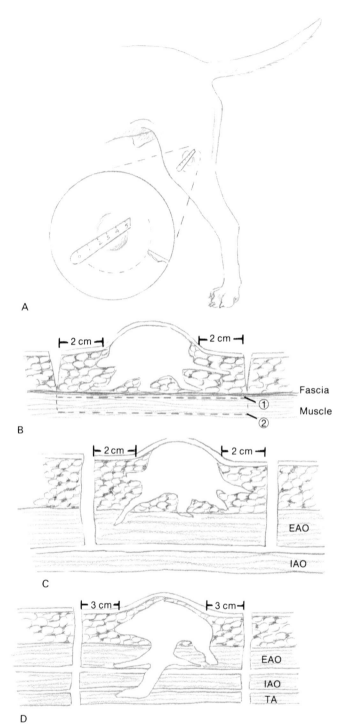

FIG. 10-7. Principles of excision of cutaneous neoplasms. A, Marking quantity of normal tissue margin to be removed (2 cm in this instance) with multiple punctate incisions (inset). B, Perpendicular incisions including fascia for fasciectomy (1) and fasciomyectomy (2) (broken lines indicate incision depth). C, Incision for margins including myectomy of abdominal wall (EAO and IAO = External and internal abdominal oblique muscles, respectively). D, Incision of multiple fascial and muscular planes to encompass full-thickness body wall (TA = transversus abdominis).

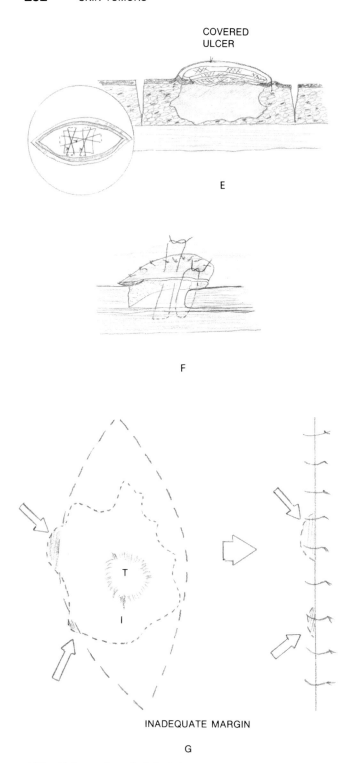

COVERED
ULCER

E

F

INADEQUATE MARGIN

G

FIG. 10-7 continued. Principles of excision of cutaneous neoplasms. E, Suturing gauze over an ulcerated neoplasm to protect wound from exfoliation of cells. Surface view (inset). F, Suturing mesh to support fasciectomy/myectomy site. Mesh folded under at edge. Mattress sutures. G, Tumor (T) and zone of infiltration (I, inside dotted line) with inadequate tumor excision (broken line, arrows). Tumor will recur from sites at arrows in sutured wound.

tissue" must be suspect because it is indistinguishable from neoplastic tissue, and is also removed with a margin of normal tissue. Lymph nodes are excised when enlarged or known to contain neoplastic cells. Preferably, the nodes are removed in conjunction with the primary tumor and the intervening lymphatics, which is termed "en bloc" excision.

Tumor cell exfoliation and subsequent growth in surgically wounded tissue should be prevented by covering any ulcerated tissue with gauze and "basket" retention sutures before beginning surgery (Fig. 10-7E and inset). Additionally, incised tumor encountered during the operation should be covered and the surgical field regarded as a "contaminated" wound and irrigated frequently. Instruments and gloves should be washed or changed whenever they become contaminated with tumor cells. Hematogeneous or lymphatic metastasis is a greater risk if tumor emboli are dislodged by rough manipulation or compression of the tumor, so gentle technique and early ligation of the venous drainage of a neoplasm are desirable. If a tumor must be manipulated during surgery, it should be handled with a tenaculum or towel forceps, which grip without compressing the tumor. Alternately, a bridle suture may be passed through the tumor and tied loosely for application of traction and to assist exposure.

Nerves, arteries, veins, muscle bellies, and other structures may variably become a portion of a necessary excision. The extent of reasonable and tolerable functional impairment that might result from tumor excision must be considered preoperatively. The reconstructive plan(s) are based on the greatest probable excision, in which circumstance a smaller reconstruction could also be done. Conceptually, then, once a reconstructive option is conceived for the largest defect likely, the excision is performed with little regard for the resulting defect. The possibility of excision or injury of nerves is a major consideration. Major nerves must be spared whenever possible. Extensive collateral circulation in the dog and cat allows most vessels to be ligated and excised when necessary. Muscle defects may be left unsutured or sutured closed if support is needed. If muscle cannot be apposed and the supportive musculature is inadequate, as with partial body wall excision, the muscle may be reinforced with polypropylene mesh* (Fig. 10-7F).

Aftercare. Postsurgical care depends on the surgical wound created and whether it requires bandaging, drainage, etc., and the reader is directed to other sections in this book that relate to these particular procedures. Any abnormal tissue should be submitted for histopathologic examination (see Preparation of Specimens for

---

*Marlex, Davol Rubber Company, Providence, RI.

Histopathologic Examination, this chapter). The finding of tumor cells in a surgical margin requires immediate re-excision of the previous wound to remove the residual tumor, or the use of adjuvant chemotherapy or irradiation if appropriate. Surveillance of the site for recurrence should be conducted at appropriate intervals such as the time of suture removal, and then 1, 3, 6, 9, 12, 18, and 24 months after treatment.

Advantages and Disadvantages. The potential resectability of a tumor varies because the skill and imagination for reconstruction varies between surgeons. Simpler reconstructive techniques such as moving local skin and shifting skin flaps have the inherent advantage of being more successful when properly employed; however, simple techniques are not useful when local skin is limited. More complicated reconstructive techniques should be reserved for cases in which simple, economical techniques are inadequate. As the reconstructive plan becomes more elaborate, the risk of surgical failure increases and an alternate therapy or referral should be considered.

The tendency toward conservative excision to facilitate reconstruction is perhaps the most frequent cause of inadequate excision, which results in recurrence and surgical failure (Fig. 10-7G).

REFERENCES AND SUGGESTED READING

1. Henderson, R.A., Swaim, S.F., and Hankes, G.H.: The surgical management of cancer. Mod. Vet. Pract. *8*:615, 1984.
2. Henderson, R.A.: Recent advances in the surgical control and management of neoplasia. Contemporary Issues in Small Animal Practice. Edited by N. Gorman, New York, Churchill Livingstone, *6*:45, 1986.
3. Schrock, T.R.: Principles of surgical oncology. *In* Principles of Cancer Treatment. New York, McGraw-Hill, 1982.

PREPARATION OF SPECIMENS FOR HISTOPATHOLOGIC EXAMINATION

Definitions and Indications. Proper preparation of biopsies for histopathologic examination is the orderly sequence of tissue preservation or "fixing" to prevent necrosis, marking of interest points for the pathologist, and packing of specimens for transport. Histopathologic examination of biopsy-derived specimens is necessary to determine cell type and interaction of the abnormal tissue with the surrounding tissue for the purpose of prognosis and treatment. Therefore all abnormal tissues removed from animal patients should be properly prepared to be submitted for histologic evaluation.

Technique. Formalin can penetrate tissues only to a depth of about 0.5 cm. Deeper than this, the tissues begin to undergo autolysis. Because the formalin penetrates from both sides, the tissue may be sectioned up to 1 cm thickness. If the entire tumor is to be submitted, it should be partially sectioned serially (scored) so that one dimension of each portion is no greater than 1 cm in thickness (Fig. 10-8A). If the entire tumor is not to be submitted, it is serially sectioned and grossly examined for homogeneity. If the tumor is not homogeneous, several representative sections are selected for submission from each different area based on color, texture, and other features.

In some instances, it is important to mark the tissue edges of an "en bloc" excision to determine if neoplastic cells extend beyond the surgical margin. Sutures may be placed at the areas that the surgeon believes are most likely to contain tumor cells or that need to be marked for other reasons (Fig. 10-8B).

The pathologist must be given instructions that describe any special techniques of preparation, as well as for what purpose the marking sutures were placed.

Another method for marking tumor margins is "painting" the cut margins of the tissue with India ink (Fig. 10-8B). The ink is allowed to dry and the tissue is fixed whole or processed with routine serial sectioning and fixation and then submitted to the pathologist with instructions including what has been done and the intended purpose of the India ink. This method fixes the margin of the excision with an indelible contrasting ink that is visible microscopically, and if the pathologist finds neoplastic cells in contact with India ink in the tissue block margin, the surgical excision was not complete and additional therapy, including further excision, should be considered (Fig. 10-8C).

For routine processing, the tissue specimens are fixed in 10% buffered formalin overnight at a ratio of 1 volume of tissue to 20 volumes of fixative. The tissue may be stored or mailed in a smaller ratio of tissue to formalin (1:1) after it has fixed thoroughly (Fig. 10-8D).

Aftercare. Before fixing, the tissue is soft and flexible enough to fit into a container with a small opening, but after fixing, the tissue is rigid and the container may have to be broken to retrieve the specimen. Therefore, the container in which the specimen is fixed should have a wide mouth. In addition to animal identification, complete descriptions and measurements of the tissue should be provided for the pathologist, especially if the tumor is marked with suture or India ink. Labels should be attached to the container rather than the lid to reduce laboratory error. Labels and accompanying letters should be written in permanent ink. Otherwise, moisture in the packing may render the sample unidentifiable. When submitting samples, it is wise to submit only one-half of the tissue and retain and store the other half. It may be used if the first is

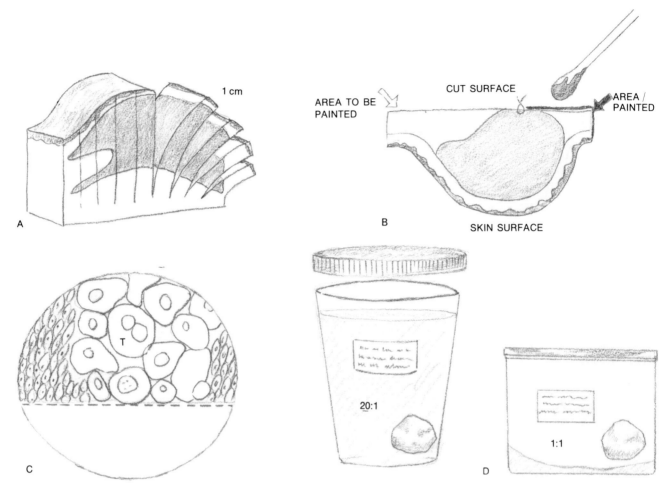

FIG. 10-8. Technique for preparing histological specimens. A, Serial section of whole neoplasm for submission. B, Tumor placed with cut surface up. Painting cut edges of specimen with India ink and marking area of interest with a suture. C, "Dirty" surgical margin. Neoplastic cells (T) contact India ink (represented by broken line), tumor excision incomplete. D, Formalin to tissue ratio at 20:1 for fixation (wide-mouth vessel), storage or shipment 1:1 ratio (zip-locked plastic bag).

lost or if an additional histopathologic opinion from another laboratory is desired.

Advantages and Disadvantages. Improperly prepared tissues are worthless. The general tumor size and shape may be maintained by using the technique of partial serial sectioning from which the pathologist may reconstruct the tumor. The accuracy of examination of margins may be enhanced if the India ink preparation is combined with the placement of sutures at the points of concern.

Some veterinarians have suggested to the authors that owners are often unwilling to pay for examination of tissues. We suggest that, if this seems to be a persistent problem, the tissue processing fee should be included in the surgical fee. Tissue diagnosis may have a bearing on the long-term health of the animal and has medico-legal implications.

REFERENCES AND SUGGESTED READING

1. Veit, H.P., Walton, A.M.: Mistakes to avoid when submitting tissue for histologic evaluation. Vet. Med. Sm. Anim. Clin. *76*:1143, 1981.
2. Withrow, S.J.: Personal communication (India ink). First European Surgical Forum, Frankfurt, June 1986.

SURGICAL EXCISION OF SOFT TISSUE SARCOMA

Definitions and Indications. Soft tissue sarcoma is a collective term applied to a group of tumors that arise from nonosseus mesenchymal tissue and are characterized by a combination of locally agressive and invasive behavior as well as an expanding mass, but that exhibit delayed systemic metastasis. Because of the late metastasis of these tumors arising in the skin and sub-cutis, aggressive surgery is indicated. Some examples of tumors in this group include fibro-, neuro-, rhabdo-, leiomyo-, osteo-, chondro-, and liposarcomas, malignant melanoma, and mast cell tumors. Hemangiopericytoma is usually included in discussions of these tumors because of its infiltrative growth pattern; however, it rarely metastasizes. Though canine hemangiosarcoma (HSA) is managed surgically by the same techniques as other soft tissue sarcomas, it is considered to have early metastasis and is not expected to be treated curatively by surgery. Feline HSA originating in the subcutaneous tissue is less likely to metastasize than canine HSA and may be responsive to aggressive surgery. The treatment of mast cell sarcoma is discussed in another section.

With the exception of malignant melanoma and mast cell sarcoma, it is unusual to detect local and regional lymph node involvement when staging these tumors. Surgery is indicated as the sole treatment only when systemic metastasis is not detected and complete excision is expected (see Staging Cutaneous Neoplasms, this chapter). If systemic metastasis is seen, a multi-modal therapeutic approach is recommended that may include surgery, irradiation, chemotherapy, hyperther-mia, or immunomodulation. An oncologist should be consulted for a protocol.

Technique. Tumor aspiration and cytologic exami-nation are valuable components of the preoperative planning. When the cytologic characteristics of malig-nancy are observed, much more liberal surgical margins should be planned. It may be difficult to obtain cells from these neoplasms. When found, the cells are charac-terized by the spindle shape of the fibroblast. The possible and notable exceptions are the mast cell tumor and the epithelioid variety of malignant melanoma, which are more likely to be round cells.

The most important surgical feature of these soft-tissue sarcomas is the apparent capsule formed by the combination of infiltrative and expansile growth (Fig. 10-9A). The sarcomatous cells directly infiltrate and displace surrounding tissues, but the growth from the tumor core compresses the thin sheets of invasive tissue circumferentially, forming concentric lamella like an onion's skin. The term "pseudocapsule" accurately de-scribes this mode of growth (Fig. 10-9B and inset). The pseudocapsule forms a convenient though unfortunate dissection plane that results in the surgical "shelling out" of the neoplastic core, leaving the infiltrative interface of tumor and normal tissue and thus leading to local recurrence. This highly characteristic mode of tumor growth mandates wide surgical margins.

These tumors require circumferential margins from 2 to 4 cm and fasciectomy or myectomy at the deep margin (Fig. 10-9C). Because of the infiltrative nature of

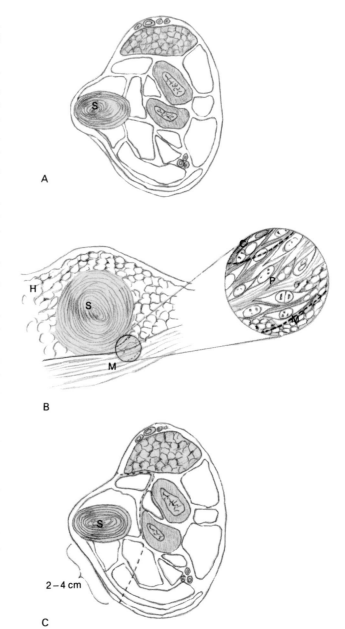

FIG. 10-9. Surgical considerations for soft tissue sarcoma. A, Whorled growth pattern of soft tissue sarcoma (S) in medial antebrachial tissues. B, Microscopic representation of sarcoma (S) in hypodermis (H) adjacent to muscle (M), and close-up of sarcoma/muscle interface demonstrating tumor core (C) compression, infiltration and "pseudo-capsule" lamella (P) invading adjacent muscle (M) (inset). C, Excision of sarcomas must include 2 to 4 cm normal tissue, muscle, fascia, and skin in this instance (broken line).

these tumors, if the underlying muscle and fascial sheet are thin, additional deep margin is desirable; this may include additional muscle belly or, in some areas, full-thick-ness excision of the body wall. Wound reconstruction must be based on the nature and location of the excision.

Aftercare. No special aftercare peculiar to soft tissue sarcomas is required if excision is deemed complete. If excision is thought to be incomplete, re-excision or tumor irradiation is recommended. Prognosis should be based on completeness of the surgical excision by examination of surgical margins. The number of mitoses seen per 10 high power fields has been suggested to be prognostic. Sarcomas with 9 or more mitoses per 10 fields have been associated with higher recurrence rates and shorter survival times. Though hemangiopericytomas were also thought to follow this prognostic rule, recent studies have not supported the theory. Regular, periodic recheck examinations should be scheduled.

Advantages and Disadvantages. The advantage of surgical excision is that no other form of therapy has been shown to have consistent therapeutic value, but complete surgical excision is able to provide cure. The principal disadvantage of managing soft-tissue sarcomas by surgery is that the wide margins required for curative intent frequently require more complex reconstructive procedures.

REFERENCES AND SUGGESTED READING

1. Bostock, D.E., and Dye, M.T.: Prognosis after surgical excision of canine fibrous connective tissue sarcomas. Vet. Pathol. *17*:581, 1980.
2. Brown, N.O., Patnaik, A.M., and MacEwen, E.G.: Canine hemangiosarcoma: Retrospective analysis of 104 cases. J. Am. Vet. Med. Assoc. *186*:56, 1985.
3. Graves, G.M., Bjorling, D.E., and Mahaffey, E.: Canine Hemangiopericytoma: 23 cases (1967–1984). J. Am. Vet. Med. Assoc. *192*:99, 1988.
4. Henderson, R.A., and Core, D.C.: Skin—Oncology Section. *In* Textbook of Small Animal Surgery. Edited by D.H. Slatter. Philadelphia, W.B. Saunders, 1985.
5. Madewell, B.R., and Theilen, G.H.: Tumors of the skin and subcutaneous tissues—Introduction. *In* Veterinary Cancer Medicine. Edited by B.R. Madewell and G.H. Theilen. Philadelphia, Lea & Febiger, 1987.
6. Pories, W.J., Murinson, D.S., and Rubin, R.: Soft-tissue sarcoma. *In* Clinical Oncology for Physicians and Medical Students. Edited by P. Rubin. American Cancer Society, 1983.
7. Postovino, N.C., Berg, R.J., and Powers, B.E.: Prognostic Variables for Canine Hemangiopericytoma: 50 cases (1979–1984). J. Am. Anim. Hosp. Assoc. *24*:501, 1988.
8. Scavelli, T.D., Patnaik, A.M., and Mehlhaff, C.J.: Hemangiosarcoma in the cat: Retrospective evaluation of 31 surgical cases. J. Am. Vet. Med. Assoc. *187*:817, 1985.

CANINE MAMMARY NEOPLASIA

The natural history of canine mammary neoplasia is associated with complex interrelationships of multiple benign and malignant cell types, hormonal influences, prognostic factors, and personal prejudices regarding optimum treatment. Surgeons agree that adequate excision is the single most important factor in management of mammary tumors; however, the quantity of tissue defined as "adequate" is controversial. The authors recommend an excision that includes all neoplastic tissue plus a margin of normal tissue. Unless specifically stated as concerning cats, all the recommendations and discussions that follow are for dogs.

STAGING CANINE AND FELINE MAMMARY NEOPLASMS

Mammary tumors are staged by palpation of the primary tumors and regional, inguinal, and axillary lymph nodes (Table 10-2). The pulmonary parenchyma and sublumbar nodes are evaluated radiographically (see Staging Cutaneous Neoplasms, this chapter). Surgical intervention is contraindicated as a sole treatment if metastasis is discovered.

Table 10-2. Clinical Stages of Canine (Feline) Mammary Tumors

T Primary Tumor
 T0 No evidence of tumor
 T1 Tumor <3 cm [<1 cm] maximum diameter
 T2 Tumor 3 to 5 cm [1–3 cm] maximum diameter
 T3 Tumor >5 cm [>3 cm] maximum diameter, muscle fixation
 T4 Tumor of any size, inflammatory carcinoma locally invading skin without infection or trauma as the cause.

N Regional Lymph Nodes (RLN) (axillary, superficial inguinal)
 N0 No RLN involved
 N1 Ipsilateral RLN involved
 N2 Bilateral RLN involved
 N3 Distant LN involved
 NR LN previously removed
   a. not fixed
   b. fixed

M Distant Metastasis
 M0 No evidence of lung metastasis
 M1 Distant metastasis including distant nodes

(Reprinted with permission from World Health Organization: Report of the Second Consultation on the Biological Behavior and Therapy of Tumors of Domestic Animals. WHO, Geneva, 1978.)

NODULECTOMY

Definitions and Indications. Nodulectomy is the removal of a small mammary tumor in conjunction with a margin of normal mammary tissue. It is indicated in certain circumstances when only a few tumors of 1 cm or smaller size are detected in the mammary glands. Nodulectomy in one site may also be used in conjunction with, and following, a mastectomy of another site when the nodule is isolated from the mastectomy site (see Mastectomy, this chapter) such as a nodulectomy of gland 2 on the right side in conjunction with a mastectomy of glands 4 and 5 on the left side. Nodulectomy may be used as an excision biopsy, and may spare patients an extended anesthesia period if they suffer compromised function or reserves of a major organ such as the heart, lungs, liver, or kidneys. Nodulectomies should not be performed in cats.

Technique. Local anesthesia is not recommended because, if the tumor margin is infiltrated, the tumor cannot be palpated, and the injection of fluid into the nodule may hydraulically force exfoliated tumor cells through the tissues, causing local spread. Despite this, the use of local analgesia may be desired because of concomitant medical conditions that preclude sedation or general anesthesia. In these instances, care should be taken not to infiltrate the mammary tissue adjacent to the tumor.

If the mammary tumor is not fixed to the skin, the skin directly over the nodule is incised for a length approximately twice the diameter of the nodule (Fig. 10-10A). If a vessel is visible that is likely to be incorporated by the excision, the vessel is ligated in situ at either end of the wound before excising the tumor (Fig. 10-10B). Otherwise, hemostasis is ignored until the excision is complete. During excision, the glandular tissue adjacent to the tumor is grasped and the tumor and adjacent gland are elevated and excised (Fig. 10-10C and D). The tumor is NOT dissected at the tumor mammary tisssue junction. If the tumor is fixed to the skin, the skin is grasped to manipulate the tumor and an ellipse of skin is excised with the tumor and adjacent glandular tissue (Fig. 10-10E and F).

Usually the dead space may be obliterated and the skin apposed simultaneously by using vertical mattress sutures of 3-0 monofilament suture (Fig. 10-10G). If deeper appositional sutures seem necessary, they should be of 3-0 or 4-0 absorbable suture with minimum tissue incorporated in the placement. The excised nodules are

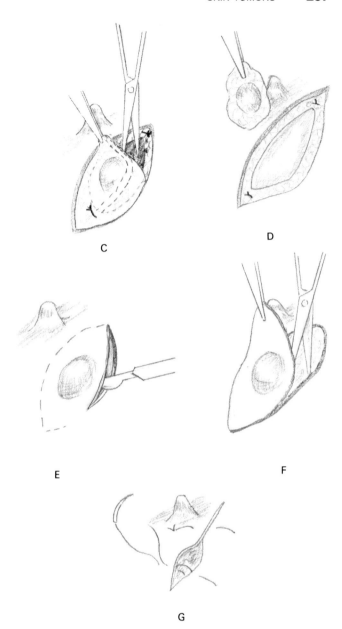

FIG. 10-10. Nodulectomy for mammary tumors 1 cm and smaller. A, Incision over nodule 2 times size of nodule. B, Ligating adjacent vessel in situ. C, Grasping adjacent glandular tissue during excision. D, Completed excision. E, Elliptical skin incision when tumor is fixed to skin. F, Grasping skin during excision. G, Closure with vertical mattress sutures.

submitted for histopathologic examination (see Preparation of Specimens for Histopathologic Examinations, this chapter).

Aftercare. Nodulectomies may be performed on an outpatient basis. If the pathologist reports a malignancy, but the margin appears free of tumor, the site is inspected monthly for recurrence during the first 3 months

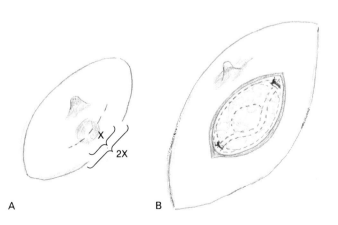

and every 3 months thereafter. If the margin contains neoplastic cells, mastectomy is recommended.

Advantages and Disadvantages. Nodulectomies are less traumatic than mastectomies. Our reasoning in performing nodulectomies is that up to 50% of mammary nodules are benign tumors or dysplastic tissue, and aggressive excision of larger quantities of mammary tissue has not been shown to decrease occurence (or recurrence) of mammary neoplasia. The principal disadvantage of this technique is the risk of incomplete excision. This is compounded because of the potential for abuse of this technique through failure to strive for an adequate margin or inappropriate tissue examination.

REFERENCES AND SUGGESTED READING

1. Allen, S.W.: Surgery for Canine Mammary Cancer: Removal of the diseased tissue only. Vet. Med. Report *1*:104, 1988.
2. Henderson, R.A., Swaim, S.F., and Hankes, G.H.: The surgical management of cancer. Mod. Vet. Pract. *8*:615, 1984.
3. Henderson, R.A.: Recent advances in the surgical control and management of neoplasia. *In* Contemporary Issues in Small Animal Practice. Edited by N. Gorman. New York, Churchill-Livingstone, *6*:45, 1986.
4. Johnston, S.D.: Female Reproductive System—Oncology. *In* Textbook of Small Animal Surgery. Edited by D.H. Slatter. Philadelphia, W.B. Saunders, 1985.

MASTECTOMY

Definitions and Indications. The authors define mastectomy as the removal of a single mammary gland "unit" including the subcutis, glandular tissue, overlying skin, and nipple (Fig. 10-11A). Subtotal mastectomy is the removal of multiple mammary gland units in the dog based on lymphatic or blood vascular flow (Fig. 10-11B). Removal of all glands of one chain is a unilateral mastectomy and removal of both chains is a bilateral or total mastectomy (Fig. 10-11C and D). The term "radical" mastectomy denotes that muscle of the thoracic or abdominal wall is excised to obtain an adequate deep margin regardless of the quantity of mammary tissue removed.

As with all surgery for malignant tumors, the minimum excision should include all neoplastic tissue. This is accomplished by also removing a margin of normal tissue. For tumors larger than 1 cm, the authors prefer to perform a mastectomy. A solitary mastectomy may be performed; however, glands 1 to 3 and 4 and 5 are frequently excised together as subtotal mastectomies for the sake of convenience and because they share blood and lymphatic vessels. Unilateral mastectomy (glands 1 through 5) may be performed when both subtotal units (1 to 3 and 4 and 5) are involved on one side. Bilateral

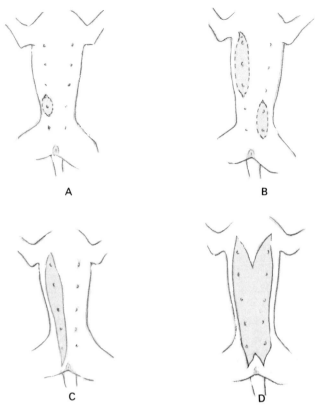

FIG. 10-11. Mastectomy incisions (broken lines). A, Incision for mastectomy. B, Incisions for subtotal mastectomy. C, Incision for unilateral mastectomy. D, Incision for bilateral mastectomy.

mastectomy is reserved for use when the mammary tissue is bilaterally and diffusely involved and when necessary skin is available for reconstruction. Combining subtotal or unilateral mastectomy with nodulectomy(ies) is useful when tumors on one side are large or diffuse, but only a few small nodules are present on the contralateral side. Bilateral involvement may also be managed by staged unilateral mastectomies performed with a 2 week interval between surgeries. Axillary lymph nodes are removed if they are enlarged or neoplastic; however, the inguinal lymph node is always removed with the caudal gland because it lies in the gland substance.

All mammary tumors are staged (see Staging Cutaneous Neoplasms and Staging Canine and Feline Mammary Neoplasms, this chapter). Surgical intervention is indicated when neoplasia is localized to the gland(s) and local lymph nodes. A specific behavior pattern of mammary carcinoma characterized by cutaneous ulceration with warmth and edema of the glands caused by intralymphatic growth is termed "inflammatory carcinoma." Surgery is not recommended for this condition. Other causes of ulceration are infection and trauma. These should be distinguished from inflammatory carcinoma because they do not preclude surgical treatment.

In dogs, tumor size of less than 5 cm, slow growth, encapsulation, and absence of distant metastases are all positive prognostic findings. The location of the tumor, duration of its presence, and type of previous mammary excision performed are of no prognostic significance. The prognosis is adversely affected if tumors have exhibited ulceration, inflammation, or recent rapid growth; are 5 cm or greater in size (clinical stage III); and/or have an infiltrative mode of growth as seen on gross surgical specimens.

In cats, prognosis is not affected by age or breed. Cats with small tumors (1 to 8 cm^3) have the best prognosis. Conservative surgery (removal of the affected gland and one adjacent gland on each side) does not decrease survival when compared to unilateral mastectomy (all four glands removed if any portion of the chain is involved), but the time to recurrence is shorter with conservative surgery. Unilateral mastectomy is therefore recommended as the only surgical procedure for cats.

Technique. The ventral and lateral thorax and abdomen are clipped and prepared for aseptic surgery. The mammary glands should be palpated again after surgical preparation with the dog lying in dorsal recumbency. The added tenseness of the skin and flattening of the glands frequently reveal the presence of additional nodules not discovered on physical exam.

After draping, the skin surrounding the mammary glands to be excised is tented to determine how much tension is likely after excision. Any exposed neoplastic cell (such as ulcers caused by trauma, infection or avascular necrosis) or mammae with significant discharge are covered by suturing sterile gauze over the area to prevent exfoliative seeding of the tissues during surgery. A 2 cm margin of normal tissue is optimum (Fig. 10-12A). The skin and subcutis are incised to the external fascia of the body wall, and the gland(s) to be excised is(are) undermined. The tissue is elevated as the subcutis is dissected completely, leaving only the muscle fascia at the deep margin (Fig. 10-12B). If the mammary tumor had been found to be fixed to muscle fascia in the presurgical examination, the fascia and muscle layer(s) should be excised so that a minimum 2 cm normal lateral margin of each known involved muscle (and fascia) is removed with the glands.

Major blood vessels are ligated as they are encountered. Cranially, these are the perforating intercostals and the cranial superficial epigastric at the costal arch. Caudally, the external pudendal at the inguinal canal and its continuation caudally are the principal vessels. Electrocoagulation speeds hemostasis of smaller subcutaneous vessels. When the excision is complete, the wound is irrigated to remove exfoliated cells.

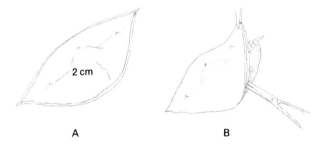

FIG. 10-12. Subtotal mastectomy. A, Incision for subtotal mastectomy. B, Elevation of tissue by dissection.

Mastectomy wounds are sutured using combinations of subcutaneous, "walking", and skin sutures. The inguinal area is the most difficult to suture. In this area, "walking" and other sutures used to close the dead space must avoid the femoral vessels. Tension sutures are used as needed. Though rarely used, drains may be placed when dead space cannot be obliterated with sutures or bandages (see Drains, Chapter 2, and Management of Skin Tension, Chapter 5).

Ovariohysterectomy is reported as having no therapeutic merit; however, a subset of up to 60% of mammary carcinomas has been found to contain estrogen receptors. Tentatively, this presents reasonable evidence to recommend ovariohysterectomy in conjunction with mastectomy; however, correlation with reduced recurrence and improved survival has not been proven.

Aftercare. Antibiotics are usually not used. Compression bandages are helpful in obliterating dead space if properly applied. Larger-volume mastectomies require enforced rest in a cage or home confinement while wound healing progresses. Recheck examinations are required for restaging at 3, 6, 9, 12, 18, and 24 months after surgery.

Approximately 50% of canine mammary tumors will recur or metastasize. Adjuvant radiation may be attempted if the lesion is localized and not resectable. Doxorubicin hydrochloride* used as a single agent has achieved partial remission or stabilized disease in 6 of 8 cases. In cats with recurrent mammary neoplasia, 5 of 11 had complete or partial regression following the administration of doxorubicin and cyclophosphamide†.

Advantages and Disadvantages. There is controversy as to whether excision of multiple glands is an advantage over solitary mastectomy or nodulectomy. A fact that favors multiple gland excision is that, when multiple tumors are detected, 75% are located in adjacent glands and 66% of those are malignant. Aggressive

---

*Adriamycin, Adria Laboratories Inc., 5000 Post Road, Dublin, OH.

†Cytoxin, Mead Johnson Pharmaceutical Division, 2404 W. Pennsylvania St., Evansville, IN.

excision of quantities of mammary tissue much larger than that which contains tumor does not, however, decrease occurrence (or recurrence) in that site, possibly because of the diffuse distribution of mammary tissue. Large excisions are more likely to be associated with surgical complications such as hematoma/seromas, wound disruption, and pelvic limb edema. Poorly placed bandages may further compromise lymphatic and venous drainage from the pelvic limbs.

REFERENCES AND SUGGESTED READING

1. Brody, R.S., Goldschmidt, M.H., and Roszel, J.R.: Canine mammary gland neoplasms. J. Anim. Hosp. Assoc. 19:61, 1983.
2. Fanton, J.W., and Withrow, S.J.: Canine mammary neoplasia: An overview. Calif. Vet. 7:12, 1981.
3. Jeglum, K.A., deGuzman, E., and Young, K.M.: Chemotherapy of advanced mammary adenocarcinoma in 14 cats. J. Am. Vet. Med. Assoc. 187:157, 1985.
4. McEwen, E.G., Patnaik, A.K., and Panko, W.B.: Estrogen receptors in canine mammary tumors. Cancer Res. 42:2255, 1982.
5. McEwen, E.G., Hayes, A.A., Harvey, H.J., Patnaik, A.K., Mooney, S., and Passe, S.: Prognostic factors for feline mammary tumors. J. Am. Vet. Med. Assoc. 185:201, 1984.
6. Misdorp, W., and Hart. A.A.M.: Canine mammary cancer. I. Prognosis. J. Small Anim. Pract. 20:385, 1979.
7. Misdorp, W., and Hart, A.A.M.: Canine mammary cancer. II. Therapy and causes of death. J. Small Anim. Pract. 20:395, 1979.
8. Ogilvie, G.K., Reynolds, H.A., Richardson, R.A., Withrow, S.J., Norris, A.M., Henderson, R.A., Klausner, J.S., Fowler, J.D., and McCaw, D.: Phase II evaluation of doxorubicin for treatment of various canine neoplasms. J. Am. Vet. Med. Assoc. 195:1580, 1989.
9. Susaneck, S.J., Allen, T.A., Hoopes, J., Withrow, S.J., and Macy, D.W.: Inflammatory mammary carcinoma in the dog. J. Am. Anim. Hosp. Assoc. 19:971, 1983.

CANINE MAST CELL TUMOR

CANINE MAST CELL TUMOR STAGING

A special staging format is used for mast cell tumors. Staging is accomplished by examining the primary

Table 10-3. Clinical Stages of Canine Mastocytoma

Stage I	One tumor confined to the dermis with no regional lymph node involvement
Ia	Without systemic signs
Ib	With systemic signs
Stage II	One tumor confined to dermis with regional lymph node involvement
Stage III	Multiple dermal tumors or large infiltrating tumor with or without regional lymph node involvement
IIIa	Without systemic signs
IIIb	With systemic signs
Stage IV	Any tumor with distant metastasis or recurrence with metastasis (including blood and/or bone marrow)

(Reprinted with permission from World Health Organization: Report of the Second Consultation on the Biological Behavior and Therapy of Tumors of Domestic Animals. WHO, Geneva, 1978.)

tumor(s) and lymph nodes and examining for metastasis. Additional staging examinations include occult fecal blood and buffy coat and bone marrow cytology. Mast cell tumors are unusual in that they do not metastasize to the lungs.

CANINE MAST CELL TUMOR SURGICAL EXCISION

Definitions and Indications.   Mast cell tumors are mesenchymal neoplasms that may have a benign or malignant clinical course. The classic description of a mast cell tumor is that of a red, raised nodule about 1 cm in diameter, but mast cell tumors may grossly resemble nearly any other tumor. Malignant mast cell tumors may cause severy systemic illness including peptic ulceration, inflammation and occasionally shock or clotting abnormalities through production of histamine, heparin, and other vasoactive substances.

All tumors should be cytologically inspected before surgery because many mast cell tumors can be easily identified cytologically, and when found, mast cell tumors are staged and surgically managed differently than other skin tumors.

Solitary mast cell tumors with no lymph node involvement (clinical stage I) are most likely to respond to surgery alone. The margins should be histopathologically inspected and re-excised if tumor is present (see Excision Biopsies and Principles of Tumor Excision, this chapter). Surgery alone is less effective if lymph nodes are affected (stage II), and surgery alone is of no value if multiple tumors are present (stage III), or when distant metastasis is present (stage IV). Stages III and IV are considered to be of systemic nature. Systemic signs of mast cell tumors are hyperhistaminemia-induced gastroenteritis and possibly ulceration. Anemia and mastocythemia may result from blood or bone marrow involvement.

Technique.   Preoperative medications such as corticosteroids and antihistamines are not used routinely. They may, however, be used in the presence of larger tumors or when systemic signs such as hematemesis or melena are present. All mast cell tumors should be handled gently, not only to reduce the possibility of metastasis but also to decrease the chance of inducing degranulation of the tumor and systemic shock.

All mast cell tumors should be excised with a large margin of normal tissue, up to 4 cm if possible. Large margins are not always obtained, however, because of tumor location or because a malignant diagnosis was unexpected. This could occur, for example, if, after a cystotomy, a small cutaneous abdominal tumor was excised that had gone unnoticed until surgical preparation for the cystotomy. The tumor was submitted for analysis after excision and reported to be a mast cell tumor. Additional surgery in the form of re-excision

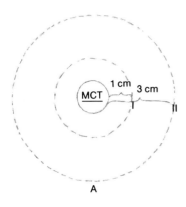

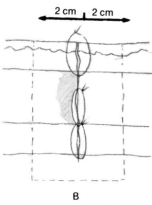

FIG. 10-13. Surgical management of canine mast cell tumor. A, Mast cell tumor excision zones. Tumor (MCT), 1 cm margin for well differentiated tumors (type I), 3 cm margin for less differentiated tumors (types II and III). B, Re-excision of wound because of incomplete excision. Margin of 2 cm lateral and deep enough to include all of previous wound.

may be required. The guidelines that should be followed in this instance are based on the descriptive histopathology of the mast cell tumor and the actual surgical margin. Mast cell tumors that are histopathologically characterized by abundant numbers of metachromatic granules, uniformity of cell shape and size, and absence of mitotic figures are considered well differentiated and are termed histologic "grade I." Such tumors are considered the least malignant and are believed to be surgically curable with a 1 cm margin lateral to the obvious tumor, and the inclusion of a layer of deep fascia would be preferable. Mast cell tumors with intermediate to poor cellular differentiation (histopathologic grades II and III) are more invasive and should be excised with a circumferential margin of normal tissue of 3 cm or more, and a deep margin that includes fascia and muscle (Fig. 10-13A) (see Excision Biopsies and Principles of Tumor Excision and Surgical Excision of Soft Tissue Sarcoma, this chapter). Although not always conclusive in itself, finding no tumor cells in the excised tissue margin may lead to decisions not to re-excise even when margins

less than 3 cm were obtained for Grade II or III tumors (see Preparation of Specimens for Histopathologic Examination, this chapter). If doubt exists as to the histologic grade, the more aggressive surgical procedure should be performed. The histologic grade of most mast cell tumors is not known preoperatively to assist in determining the correct margin because most are not biopsied preoperatively. Therefore, in some instances, additional excision is necessary when the grade becomes known.

Aftercare. No additional treatment is needed if the surgical margins are clean. If the surgical margins contain tumor cells, immediate reoperation is recommended. The new excision should include the entirety of the old incision plus a 2 cm lateral margin and additional deep fascial excision when possible (Fig. 10-13B). Mast cell tumors have been associated with a 30% recurrence rate after surgery. If re-excision is not possible, adjuvant therapy of radiation or oral prednisolone (0.5 mg/kg/day) may be used. Cimetidine.* is included (4 mg/kg by mouth two or three times a day) in the medical management of large tumors, but prednisolone is usually used alone with smaller tumors. Intralesional triamcinalone† has been used instead of prednisolone. Medical therapy is continued as long as the tumor remains in remission. At this time, no other antineoplastic has proven effective.

Advantages and Disadvantages. Local recurrence is common because of incomplete excision. The prognosis of mast cell tumor was correlated to the histologic degree of cellular differentiation more than 10 years ago, and this finding has been recently confirmed. Because poorly differentiated tumors (grade III) are associated with a mean survival time of 18 weeks, compared to 28 weeks for intermediate differentiation (grade II) or 51 weeks for well differentiated tumors (grade I), the surgical oncologist must seek a pathologist who will grade the tumor or provide a description of the tumor.

---

*Tagamet, Smith, Kline and French Laboratories, 1500 Spring Garden St., Philadelphia, PA.

†Vetalog, E.R. Squibb and Sons. P.O. Box 4000, Princeton, NJ.

REFERENCES AND SUGGESTED READING

1. Bostock, D.E.: Prognosis following mastocytoma removal. J. Small Anim. Pract. 14:27, 1973.
2. Henderson, R.A., and Core, D.M.: Oncology—Skin. In Textbook of Small Animal Surgery. Edited by D.H. Slatter. Philadelphia, W.B. Saunders, 1985.
3. Patnaik, A.K., Ehler, W.J., MacEwen, E.G.: Canine cutaneous mast cell tumor: Morphologic grading and survival time in 83 dogs. Vet. Pathol. 21:469, 1984.
4. Tams, T.R., and Macey, D.W.: Canine mast cell tumors. Compend. Contin. Ed. 10:869, 1981.

PERIANAL TUMORS

STAGING AND EXCISION

Although many tumor types may be associated with the perianal tissue, two principal types are of greatest clinical importance, perianal adenomas/carcinomas and apocrine gland adenocarcinoma of the anal sac.

Definitions and Indications. Arising from the cutaneous perianal glands, perianal adenomas and carcinomas are found most frequently in intact male dogs. Adenocarcinoma of the apocrine glands of the anal sac is reported only in bitches, and although other tumors of the peraneal area may also be present, malignancy should be considered a likely possibility in all perianal tumors in intact females.

Cytology is useful in revealing the type of perianal tumor present. Perianal tumors are staged using the TNM system (see Staging Cutaneous Neoplasms, this chapter). The sacral, hypogastric (intrapelvic), and medial iliac (caudal sublumbar) lymph nodes are the local and regional nodes that should be inspected by rectal palpation and radiographs in addition to a systemic search for metastasis to stage this tumor accurately. The authors use the interpretation of cytology obtained by fine needle to direct the type of excision to be performed. If the well differentiated uniform hepatoid cells characteristic of perianal adenoma are present, the tumor is excised with little normal tissue margin. If the cellular population is not uniform in size and shape, and has multiple nucleoli or mitotic figures, the suspected diagnosis is a perianal adenocarcinoma in the male and apocrine gland adenocarcinoma of the anal sac in the bitch, and the surgical objective is to excise the tumor intact with a margin of normal tissue.

Techniques

Cytologically Benign Tumor. If castration is to be performed, it is performed first. For subcutaneous tumors, perianal skin incisions (excisions) may be tangential curvilinear or radial (Fig. 10-14A and B). Because of tension lines, the curvilinear tangential incision tends to be better as the anal tumor is nearer the middle periphery of the anal sphincter. The radial incision tends to be better when the tumor is nearer the anal orifice. The skin is incised over the tumor. The dissection plane of benign tumors is at the tumor margin—tissue interface. Grasping these tumors frequently causes rupture because the tumors are usually friable. For this reason, a traction suture aids in manipulation of the tumor during dissection (Fig. 10-14C). If, despite precautions, the tumor capsule ruptures, the tumor will begin fragmenting with each added manipulative effort. In this case, the tumor content and margin are obliterated by curettage with a curette or the edge of the scalpel blade (Fig. 10-14D).

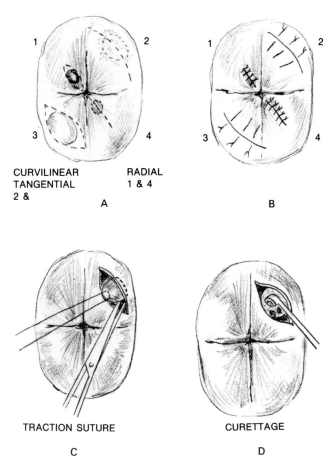

CURVILINEAR TANGENTIAL 2 &

RADIAL 1 & 4

A

B

TRACTION SUTURE

C

CURETTAGE

D

FIG. 10-14. Surgical management of perianal tumors (benign cytology). A, Use of radial or tangential incisions (broken lines) for perianal tumors: 1) Small tumor, near anus, fixed to skin, radial excision; 2) Larger tumor, away from anus, not fixed to skin, tangential incision; 3) Larger tumor, away from anus, fixed to skin, curvilinear tangential excision; 4) Small tumor, near anus, not fixed to skin, radial incision. B, Resulting suture lines after excising tumors. C, Traction suture to aid dissection. D, Curettage of ruptured tumor.

The cavity is then irrigated and the wound is sutured. For superficial tumors removed from near the anal orifice, the skin is apposed and wound cavity obliterated simultaneously if possible, using 3-0 monofilament vertical mattress sutures (Fig. 10-14B). Tumors fixed to the skin must be removed with an ellipse of skin.

Cytologically Suspicious or Malignant Tumor Type. For curative intent (no metastases found), the tumor (with skin if the tumor is fixed to the skin) and 0.5 to 1 cm of normal tissue margin are excised (Fig. 10-15A). Larger tumors usually have the potential to be more invasive and should be excised along with larger margins. The incision should be made without regard for saving involved anal sphincter (Fig. 10-15B). When the anal

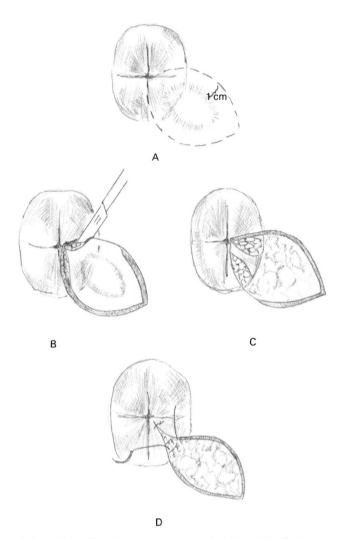

A

B

C

D

FIG. 10-15. Surgical management of perianal tumor (suspect or known malignant cytology). A, Segmental excision plan with 1 cm margin of normal tissue. B, Radial incision of anal sphincter and sac to maintain margin. C, Completed excision. D, Suture apposition of anal sphincter prior to skin closure.

sphincter must be partially excised to help provide a margin of normal tissue around a malignant tumor, it may be radially incised or its fibers may be divided. Segments of the anal sphincter may be resected to provide adequate margins of normal tissue adjacent to malignant tumors (Fig. 10-15C). The incised edges of a resected anal sphincter are reapposed when possible (Fig. 10-15D), but this is not essential because scar tissue will fill the void and anal function will continue. Excision of the motor innervation of the anus (caudal rectal branch of the external pudendal nerve) may be necessary when it is incorporated in a malignant tumor. Unilateral excision of the innervation does not cause incontinence if the contralateral nerve is preserved and functional. As with all

surgery in which the surgical excision is determined during the procedure, familiarity with anatomical topography is invaluable. Every effort is made to avoid incision of the tumor, which may cause exfoliative seeding of the wound and recurrence (see Excision Biopsies and Principles of Tumor Excision, this chapter). Approximately 30 to 50% of these malignancies mestastasize to the lumbar lymph nodes, lungs, liver, and spleen. If metastases are found in lymph nodes, they should be excised by laparotomy. Alternately, intraoperative radiation may be administered if available. Long-term survivals have been obtained with these treatments.

Aftercare. Perianal tissues heal quickly and infection is uncommon. If surgical margins contain malignant cells, either re-excision or local irradiation is indicated. The hypercalcemia present with some perianal tumors falls to normal levels with complete excision, but persistence of hypercalcemia indicates possible metastasis. Tumor recurrence is associated with recurrence of the hypercalcemic state.

Advantages and Disadvantages. Surgical removal of adenomas has the advantage of avoiding the complications and expense associated with other forms of therapy such as estrogens and tumor irradiation. Estrogens have been used to control perianal adenomas in male dogs; however, the potential complications of estrogen therapy in dogs are severe, including fatal aplastic anemias, and the authors strongly discourage their use.

The authors recommend castration of intact male dogs with either perianal adenoma or carcinoma because castration may be additive to the therapy in both instances. Because most perianal adenomas tend to regress following castration, some veterinarians castrate the dog but do not excise the perianal tumor for analysis. This is not a good procedure because other tumors that may not respond to castration also occur in this area.

REFERENCES AND SUGGESTED READING

1. Goldschmidt, M.H., and Zoltowski, C.: Anal sac adenocarcinoma in the dog: 14 cases. J. Small Anim. Pract. *22*:119, 1981.
2. Hause, W.R., Stevenson, S., Meuten, D.J., Capen, C.C. and Capen, C.C.: Pseudohyperparathyroidism associated with adenocarcinomas of anal sac origin in four dogs. J. Am. Anim. Hosp. Assoc. *17*:373, 1981.
3. McGavin, M.D., and Fishburn, F.: Perianal adenoma of apocrine origin in a dog. J. Am. Vet. Med. Assoc. *166*:388, 1975.
4. Meuten, D.J., Segre, G.V., Capen, C.C., Kociba, G.J., Voelkel, E.F., Levine, L., Tashjian, A.H., Chew, D.F., and Nagode, L.A.: Hypercalcemia in dogs with adenocarcinoma derived from apocrine glands of the anal sac: Biochemical and histomorphometric investigations. Lab. Invest. *48*:428, 1983.
5. Wilson, G.P., and Hayes, H.M.: Castration for treatment of perianal gland neoplasms in the dog. J. Am. Vet. Med. Assoc. *174*:1301, 1979.

FATTY TUMORS

STAGING AND EXCISION

Definitions and Indications. Lipomas are encapsulated benign tumors of fat. Subcutaneous lipomas are usually soft and fluctuant, but lipomas arising within fascial planes or between muscle and fascia may be very fixed and firm. Usually lipomas are well circumscribed; however, a recently described variant, the infiltrative lipoma, maintains a benign histologic appearance and is encapsulated on several sides, but invades (or arises from) adjacent muscle and fascial structures on its deeper surface. Yet another variant characterized by mineralization and attachment to and/or invasion of bone is called a parosteal lipoma. Liposarcoma, the malignant fatty tumor, has been discussed with soft tissue sarcomas. Lipomas should be excised before they reach large proportions. They should be staged according to the procedure used for the skin and subcutaneous tissue, the TNM system (see Staging Cutaneous Neoplasms, this chapter).

Technique. Fine needle aspiration of lipomas usually reveals droplets of fat when the needle contents are expulsed onto a slide. The droplets do not dry, and attempting to fix the slide in alcohol dissolves the droplets. A stain for fat (Sudan III) must be used instead.

The skin is incised over the tumor and deepened until the glistening capsule is encountered. If the tumor is within fascial planes or muscle, the fibers are divided bluntly to expose the tumor and then the subcutaneous or fascial incision is enlarged to allow the tumor to be easily dissected. Encapsulated lipomas can usually be bluntly dissected digitally, separating at the interface of the tumor capsule and surrounding tissue (Fig. 10-16A).

Blunt digital dissection is possible for only a portion of the circumference of infiltrative lipomas (Fig. 10-16B). When this type of tumor is encountered, dissection is interrupted by adhesion of the tumor to the fascia and muscle adjacent in the deeper portions of the wound. When this adhesion is encountered, it is necessary to enlarge the incision to obtain adequate exposure. If the originating muscle belly is small or if the muscle is nearly replaced with infiltrating fat, it may be excised. More frequently, the affected muscle and a margin of normal muscle is excised (Fig. 10-16B). Vessels are ligated as they are encountered. Knowledge of the general topographical anatomy of a region is valuable when an infiltrative lipoma is encountered. Involvement is so extensive in some cases that amputation is required. Amputation is avoided until the limb becomes nonfunctional.

Usually it is unnecessary to place drains in the cavity that results from the excision of a lipoma. Excision of infiltrative lipomas, however, may result in partially excised muscles and significant capillary ooze. Drains may be helpful in this instance. The tissues are closed in layers and, when the wound location makes it practical, a light compression bandage is applied.

Aftercare. Bandages are changed as necessary to accommodate drainage. Drains, when used, are removed when they no longer serve for egress of fluid, and

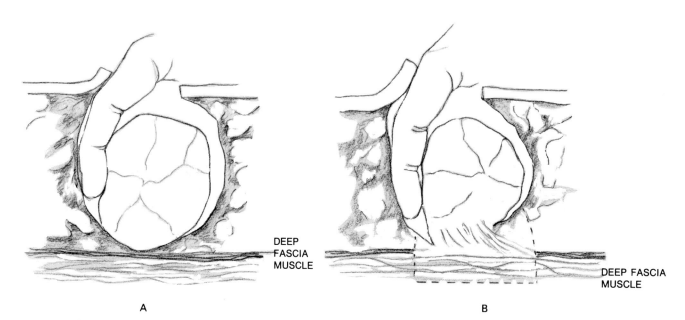

DEEP
FASCIA
MUSCLE

DEEP FASCIA
MUSCLE

A

B

FIG. 10-16. Surgical management of lipomas. A, Digital dissection of lipoma. B, Infiltration of deeper fascial plane by infiltrative lipoma requires fasciomyectomy (broken line).

bandages are removed 5 to 7 days postoperatively (see Drains and Wound Dressing Materials and Topical Medications, Chapter 3).

Advantages and Disadvantages. Cytology may be misleading when used in obese dogs or on fat-laden tissue. It is possible to obtain a mistaken diagnosis if fat is aspirated adjacent to a malignancy, missing malignant cells. For the same reason, when the "rubbery" to firm consistency of a tumor suggests malignancy, aspiration slides are stained using routine methods even when fat droplets are expulsed because malignant cells may be found.

Recurrence of lipomas is possible, but uncommon. Infiltrative lipomas are more likely to recur if inade-quately excised. The use of the above "shelling out" technique for lipomas is a serious error when the tumor is, in fact, a soft tissue sarcoma and is mistaken for a benign "fatty tumor" (see Surgical Excision of Soft Tissue Sarcoma, this chapter.)

REFERENCES AND SUGGESTED READING

1. Doige, C.E., Farrow, C.S., and Presnell, K.R.: Parosteal lipoma in a dog. J. Am. Anim. Hosp. Assoc. *16*:87, 1980.
2. McChesney, A.E., Stephens, L.C., Lebel, J. and Snyder, S., and Ferguson, H.R.: Infiltrative lipoma in dogs. Vet. Pathol. *17*:316, 1980.

INDEX

Page numbers in *italics* refer to illustrations; numbers followed by "t" refer to tables.